GUIDE TO

MECHANICAL VENTILATION
AND
INTENSIVE RESPIRATORY CARE

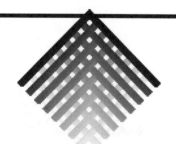

LYNELLE N.B. PIERCE, RN, MS, CCRN
The Washington Hospital Center
Washington, D.C.

W.B. SAUNDERS COMPANY
A *Harcourt Health Sciences* Company

Philadelphia   London   New York   St. Louis   Sydney   Toronto

W. B. SAUNDERS COMPANY
A *Harcourt Health Sciences Company*
The Curtis Center
Independence Square West
Philadelphia, PA 19106

Library of Congress Cataloging-in-Publication Data

Pierce, Lynelle N. B.
    Guide to mechanical ventilation and intensive respiratory care/
Lynelle N.B. Pierce. — 1st ed.
        p.   cm.
    ISBN 0-7216-6478-4
    1. Respiratory intensive care.   2. Respiratory therapy.
3. Artificial respiration.   4. Respirators.   I. Title.
    [DNLM: 1. Respiratory Therapy.   WB 342 1995]
RC735.R48P54   1995
615.8'36—dc20
DNLM/DLC   95-3948

GUIDE TO MECHANICAL VENTILATION   ISBN 0-7216-6478-4
AND INTENSIVE RESPIRATORY CARE

Printed in the United States of America

Last digit is the print number: 9   8   7   6   5

To my daughters—
Amanda Cheryl and *Natalie Naema*

They offer a fresh perspective on life
and their growing minds teach me something new every day.

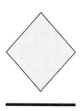

Reviewers

Linda Allen, RN, BSN, CEN, TNS
Trauma Service
Barnes Hospital
St. Louis, Missouri

Laura Crooks, RN, BSN
Allegheny General Hospital
Pittsburgh, Pennsylvania

Phillip Howard Cummings, RN, EdD
School of Nursing
University of North Carolina
Wilmington, North Carolina

Catherine A. Eddy, RN, MSN, CCRN
University of South Dakota
Rapid City, South Dakota

Hugh D. Fuller, MB, MSc, FRCPC
St. Joseph's Hospital and McMaster University
Hamilton, Ontario
Canada

Paul Joseph Mathews, Jr., MPA, EdS, RRT, RCP
Associate Professor
Respiratory Care and Physical Therapy Education
University of Kansas Medical Center
Kansas City, Kansas

Maureen McDonald, RN,C, MS, CNA, CS
Brockton Hospital School of Nursing
Brockton, Massachusetts

Peggy G. Pegg, RN, PhD
Respiratory Clinical Nurse Specialist
Associate Professor
California State University
Chico School of Nursing
Chico, California

Gary Persing, BS, RRT
Director of Clinical Education
Respiratory Therapy Program
Tulsa Junior College
Tulsa, Oklahoma

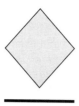

Preface

Guide to Mechanical Ventilation and Intensive Respiratory Care functions as both an educational manual and a clinical reference for those involved in monitoring, managing, and delivering care to patients requiring respiratory intervention or mechanical ventilatory support. Topics, ranging from the simple to complex, are addressed in an easy to read and understand manner. The range of coverage and practical approach make this guide valuable to both the beginning student and advanced practitioner. Individuals who will benefit from the manual are beginning and mid-level practitioners in critical care arenas including step-down and post-anesthesia care units; students in nursing, medicine, respiratory therapy, and nurse anesthesia; and acute care nurse practitioners and physician assistants.

The foundation for the book is in the opening chapters: anatomy basics and practical physiology. These chapters provide a scientific basis for patient care and for interpreting complex data. Clinical application begins in these opening chapters and continues throughout the text, which is full of pertinent facts relevant to patient management.

The chapters that follow progress to aspects of intensive and intermediate respiratory care. Airway maintenance, an essential facet of patient care, is covered in detail. The practitioner is provided with complete and easy to reference information on administration of oxygen, humidification and aerosol therapy, bronchial hygiene techniques, and lung expansion therapies.

The heart of the text, Chapters 6 to 11, details both fundamental and advanced, but practical, information about mechanical ventilation. These chapters evolved from lectures repeatedly delivered to diverse audiences and from teaching performed at the bedside. Every attempt has been made to answer the questions most commonly asked by the bedside practitioner. Mechanical ventilation is covered from the beginning decision-making process as to whom it should be applied and continues with ventilator performance of the respiratory cycle, choosing the appropriate settings, regulating ventilator settings based on objective patient-ventilator data, and adjusting alarm parameters. Chapters then proceed into essential information about complications of mechanical ventilation, a systematic approach to monitoring the patient-ventilator system, how to troubleshoot and respond to alarms, and in-depth information on how to intervene with patient and/or ventilator problems.

Traditional modes, nonconventional modes such as independent lung ventilation, and alternative methods such as noninvasive ventilation and permissive hypercapnia are described including their advantages, disadvantages, and unique facets of patient monitoring and intervention when a particular mode is applied. Respiratory muscle function and exercise physiology applied to the retraining of respiratory muscles are the groundwork within Chapter 10, Weaning from Mechanical Ventilation. Methods of weaning are then presented with a special emphasis on assessment of the patient and patient-machine interface.

The array of invasive and noninvasive techniques of patient monitoring used today as tools to gather real-time physiologic data and manage the patient's respiratory care are reviewed. Also covered are modifications of the traditional physical examination when assessing the mechanically ventilated patient and treatment of tissue oxygenation imbalances, because the ultimate goal of the respiratory system is to maintain adequate oxygenation to all of the tissues of the body.

Concepts are presented in a practical and logical format enabling the reader to relate the content directly to patient assessment data and interpretation of patient response to interventions. Throughout, there is extensive use of diagrams to illustrate key points and tables for summary and comparison. The book is organized in considerable detail making it easy for the reader to extract information. Appendixes provide reference to pulmonary symbols and abbreviations, drugs used in respiratory care, and chest drainage systems.

In the dramatically changing health care arena the critical care practitioner is challenged to become competent in an ever-broadening array of skills. Cross-training between and within the disciplines, a compelling new approach to providing patient-focused care efficiently, requires the acquisition of new and advanced knowledge. In various settings nurses and physician-extenders are training to manage aspects of the patient's respiratory care. The respiratory care professional retains a unique, expanding, and highly technological knowledge base of their own. However, other disciplines are being called upon to understand more fully, to intervene, and to communicate more effectively the patient's respiratory care needs. The intent of this manual is to assist, challenge, and inspire you to competence in caring for the critically ill patient requiring mechanical ventilatory support. These people entrust in your constant surveillance and in your wisdom as you put knowledge into practice.

Lynelle N. B. Pierce

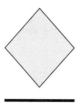

Acknowledgments

My deepest appreciation to my husband, Greg. Neither he nor I knew what was involved when he pledged his support of my desire to write this book. Two children and 3 years later we both feel a tremendous sense of accomplishment. He showed his greatest support through his dedication to our children. Either parenthood or authorship alone might have been enough for us over these years; simultaneously they turned life into an adventure.

I wish to express my gratitude to my family—my father who taught me about perseverance and commitment and my mother who taught me patience and tenderness. Also to my brother, Joe, and my sisters, Debbie and Cheryl, for their invariable love and support.

My gratitude to my colleague Pam Guillaume for her excellent contribution of Appendixes II and III. Working together was a pleasure. My heartfelt thanks to her for also donating her time to assist with the obtaining of permissions.

My sincere appreciation to the many colleagues and mentors who have both challenged and assisted me to grow as an educator and practitioner in critical care and the subspecialty of pulmonary care, particularly Sandra B. Marshall who has provided me with opportunities leading to tremendous professional growth. I am also grateful to the many students I have had the opportunity to teach. This material was refined through their questioning, enticing me to learn more.

I gratefully acknowledge others who have supported my writing of this book: Cindy Potts who nurtured my children during my working hours, Delois Meyer and Paul West for their consistent encouragement, and the many manufacturers of respiratory care products and others in the industry for their willing support of reference material, photos, and artwork. I am especially appreciative of the staff at W.B. Saunders for their characteristic quality editorial and production work.

Finally I wish to acknowledge the members of the health care team, especially the nurses who, with knowledge and compassion, care for the critically ill.

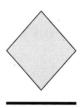

Contents

8 COMPLICATIONS OF MECHANICAL VENTILATION AND TROUBLESHOOTING THE PATIENT-VENTILATOR SYSTEM 206

9 NONINVASIVE RESPIRATORY MONITORING AND INVASIVE MONITORING OF DIRECT AND DERIVED TISSUE OXYGENATION VARIABLES 243

Pulmonary Anatomy

The respiratory system is both remarkable and complicated. Its overall function is to provide life-sustaining oxygen to all the cells of the body and to remove the byproduct of cellular metabolism, carbon dioxide. Therefore the efficient pulmonary system, along with the cardiovascular system, is intimately related to the body's metabolic processes. This becomes even more evident with an understanding of humoral control of ventilation. Knowledge of pulmonary anatomy provides a sound foundation for understanding the complex processes of respiration.

UPPER AIRWAY

The upper airway consists of the nasal passages, the sinuses, the pharynx, the epiglottis, and the larynx. Its functions are to conduct air to the lower airway, to protect the lower airway from foreign matter, and to warm, filter, and humidify the inspired air.

Nasal Passages

Beyond the olfactory function, the nose warms, filters, and moistens inspired air. The structure of the nose, with its two nasal cavities, turbinates, and rich vasculature, provides maximum contact between inspired air and the nasal mucosa (Fig. 1–1). Temperature adjustment and humidification begin as soon as air hits the anterior nasal cavity; thus, by the time inspired air reaches the alveoli, it is 100% saturated with water vapor. The nose clears debris from the inspired air in two ways. Strong hairs at the entry of the nostril trap the debris. Then nasal cilia, which are very fine microscopic hairlike projections, sway together in waves to move trapped particles posteriorly. When an artificial airway is in place, these functions of warming, filtering, and humidification of inspired air are bypassed and must be provided for the patient.

Sinuses

Sinuses are spaces that decrease the weight of the skull, provide mucus for the nasal cavity, and are important as resonance chambers of the voice. Named for the bone in which they lie, they are present in four of the cranial bones and one facial bone. The sinuses are divided into two groups: the paranasal (Fig. 1–2) and the mastoid sinuses. The paranasal sinuses are paired and include the frontal,

1

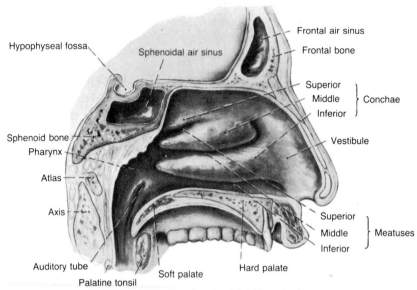

Figure 1-1 Lateral view of nasal cavity with nasal septum removed. Within the nasal cavity, convolutions of cartilaginous tissue known as turbinates provide an increased surface area for the warming, humidification, and filtering of inspired air. (From Jacob, S., et al.: *Structure and Function in Man*. 5th ed. Philadelphia: W.B. Saunders, 1982).

ethmoid, sphenoid, and maxillary sinuses. All are lined with ciliated mucus-producing cells and have small pathways that communicate with the nasal cavity, the pathway meatus lying underneath the nasal turbinates. Occlusion of the meatus causes fluid to accumulate in the sinuses, potentially leading to a sinus infection. Inflammation within the sinuses is called sinusitis. The mastoid sinus communicates with the middle ear. Lining the mastoid sinus is a mucus membrane that is continuous with the nasopharynx. Inflammation of this lining is called mastoiditis.

Pharynx

Air passes from the nasal cavity into the space behind the nasal cavity and the mouth called the pharynx. The pharynx extends to the point where the airway (larynx) and the digestive tube (esophagus) divide. There are three divisions of the pharynx: the nasopharynx, oropharynx, and laryngeal pharynx (or hypopharynx) (Fig. 1–3). The nasopharynx begins at the base of the nasal cavities and extends to the soft palate. It contains the eustachian tubes and the lymphoid mass known as the adenoids. The eustachian tubes form a connection to the middle ear. During swallowing, they open to equalize pressure across the middle ear. The oropharynx extends from the soft palate and uvula to the epiglottis and is visible with the mouth open and the tongue depressed. Two sets of tonsils are contained in the oropharynx, the palatine and the lingual. The laryngopharynx contains the larynx and is the critical dividing point of solids and liquids from air.

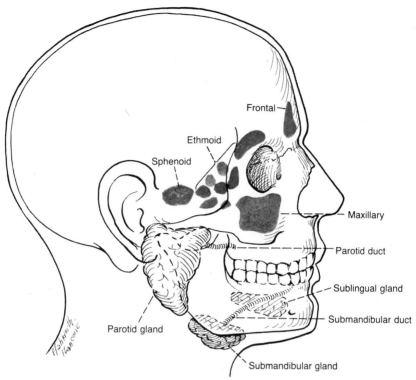

FIGURE 1–2   Lateral view of the head, showing the frontal, ethmoid, sphenoid, and maxillary sinuses. The mastoid sinus is not shown here. (From Jacob, S., et al.: *Structure and Function in Man*. 5th ed. Philadelphia: W.B. Saunders, 1982.)

Larynx

The larynx contains the vocal cords for phonation and is also an organ with sphincter functions that help prevent aspiration. The principal cartilages of the larynx are the thyroid, arytenoid, and cricoid (Fig. 1–4). The largest and most superior of the cartilages is the thyroid (meaning "shieldlike"), which is commonly referred to as the Adam's apple. The cricoid cartilage lies just below the thyroid and is attached to it by the cricothyroid membrane. It is this membrane that is incised to perform an emergency procedure, the cricothyroidotomy, for upper airway obstruction. The arytenoid cartilage serves as the attachment of the vocal cord ligaments. It swings in and out from a fixed point, thus opening and closing the space between the vocal cords, actions that are necessary to vary the pitch of sounds. Sound intensity is affected by the amount of air passing between the vocal cords. Thus, when an artificial airway is in place, the patient is unable to phonate.

The vocal cords are drawn apart during inspiration and relax toward midline during expiration. The glottis is the space between the vocal cords. The epiglottis is a leaf-shaped cartilaginous structure extending from the base of the tongue and attached to the thyroid cartilage by ligaments. It projects upward and poste-

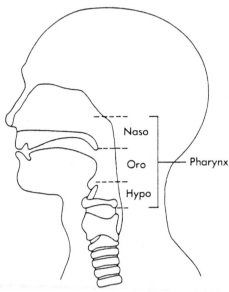

FIGURE 1-3 The three anatomic divisions of the pharynx are named for the respiratory structures that lie next to them. The hypopharynx is also known as the laryngeal pharynx. (From Spearman, C.B., and Sheldon, R.L.: *Egan's Fundamentals of Respiratory Therapy.* 4th ed. St. Louis: C.V. Mosby, 1982.)

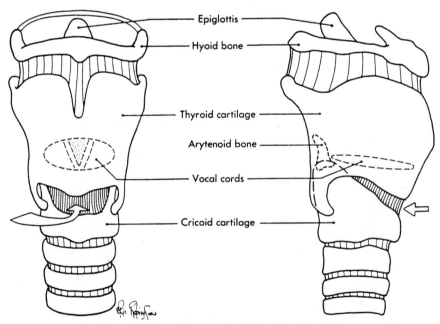

FIGURE 1-4 Cartilages of the larynx as seen from frontal and lateral views. Arrows point to the cricothyroid membrane. (From Spearman, C.B., and Sheldon, R.L.: *Egan's Fundamentals of Respiratory Therapy.* 4th ed. St. Louis: C.V. Mosby, 1982.)

riorly. During swallowing the epiglottis flaps down to direct swallowed material into the esophagus, thus guarding the opening of the larynx.

LOWER AIRWAY

The lower airway consists of a series of tubes that divide like the branches of a tree, becoming narrower, shorter, and more numerous as they penetrate deeper into the lung. Its functions are to conduct air, provide mucociliary defense, and, most important, perform external gas exchange.

Conducting Airways: Nonalveolate Region

Approximately the first 16 divisions of the tracheobronchial tree take no direct part in gas exchange and are thus designated the conducting zone (Fig. 1–5). The volume is approximately 150 ml and is known as the anatomic dead space.

The trachea, which is made of C-shaped rings of cartilage, extends from the cricoid cartilage in the larynx to the point where the right and left main-stem bronchi divide: the carina. The posterior portion of the trachea is made of

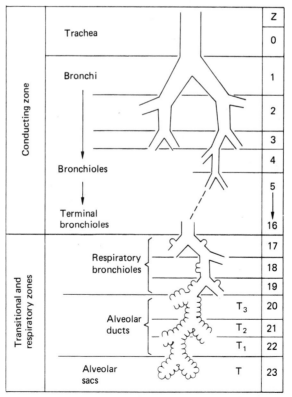

FIGURE 1–5   The twenty-three divisions of the tracheobronchial tree. Each time the airways branch, a new division, or generation, arises. (Reproduced with permission from Weibel, E.: Design and structure of the human lung. In Fishman, A. [Ed.]. *Assessment of Pulmonary Function*. New York: McGraw-Hill, 1980.)

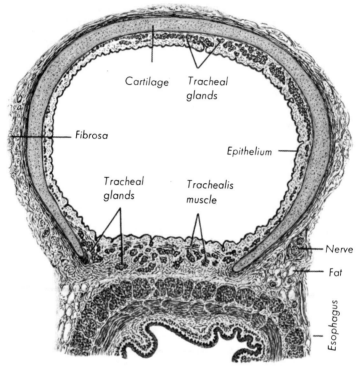

Figure 1–6 The trachea, which lies adjacent to the esophagus, is made of C-shaped rings of cartilage closed posteriorly by the trachealis muscularis muscle. (From Kelly, D.E., Wood, R.L., and Enders, A.C.: *Bailey's Textbook of Microscopic Anatomy.* 18th ed. Baltimore: Williams & Wilkins, 1984.)

smooth muscle and lies adjacent to the esophagus (Fig. 1–6). Excessive pressure on this smooth muscle by the cuff of an artificial airway can lead to erosion and tracheoesophageal fistula. The lining of the trachea consists of ciliated epithelium and mucus-producing goblet cells.

The main-stem bronchi consist of circumferential smooth muscle and plates of cartilage that irregularly encircle the airway. The smooth muscle constricts in response to certain stimuli. Lining the bronchi are ciliated epithelium and more mucus-producing goblet cells. Progressing distally in the airways there is a loss of cartilage, mucus-secreting cells, and cilia.

The trachea divides into the main-stem bronchi. The right main-stem bronchus lies almost vertical to the trachea. This position promotes both a greater incidence of aspiration into the right lung and accidental right main-stem intubation when an endotracheal tube is advanced too far into the airway. The left main-stem bronchus is shorter and narrower and lies more horizontal to the trachea. The point where the bronchi, nerves, lymphatic vessels, and blood supply leave the mediastinum and enter the lung is known as the hilum.

After penetrating the lung, the right main-stem bronchus divides into three lobar bronchi that supply the upper, middle, and lower right lung lobes. Two lobar divisions of the left main-stem bronchus supply the two lobes of the left lung: the upper and the lower. Lobar bronchi bifurcate and trifurcate into segmental bronchioles or terminal bronchioles that supply the lung segments on the left and right. The bronchioles lack cartilage and are made of connective tissue that contains elastic fibers and limited smooth muscle. Bronchioles are held open by radial traction from the elastic recoil forces of the lung tissue. With the lack of supporting cartilage, these airways are susceptible to bronchospasm.

Respiratory Zone: Alveolate Region

Alveolar buds begin to appear on the walls of the transitional airways, or respiratory bronchioles, which make up the seventeenth through nineteenth generations of airway branches. The terminal respiratory unit, or acinus, is that portion of the lung arising from a single terminal bronchiole. The acinus is the primary gas-exchanging unit of the lung, consisting of the respiratory bronchiole, alveolar ducts, alveolar sacs, and the alveoli (Fig. 1–7). The number of airway divisions, or generations, from the trachea to the alveolar sac is generally 23. The distance from the terminal bronchiole to the most distant alveolus is only about 5 mm, but the respiratory zone makes up most of the lung, its volume being about 3000 ml.

There are approximately 300 million alveolar-capillary units in the adult lung. The total surface area of the lung parenchyma is 50 to 100 m^2, about the size of a tennis court. The distance between the alveolus and the capillary is less than the diameter of a single red blood cell. The alveoli are surrounded by capillaries so dense that, when fully recruited, they form almost a complete sheet of blood. Small holes, known as pores of Kohn (Fig. 1–8), that are present in the walls of the alveoli provide for even gas distribution among the alveoli of an alveolar sac.

The cellular makeup of the alveolus makes it an efficient gas exchanger. Type I alveolar cells are squamous epithelium one cell layer thick that are structured to promote gas exchange and prevent fluid transudation into the alveolus. They are particularly sensitive to oxygen and inhaled agents. Type II cells differentiate into type I cells as needed and produce surfactant, a lipoprotein that reduces the surface tension within the alveolus. The alveolar macrophages, free-moving scavenger cells, phagocytize foreign materials that have evaded the cough reflex and the mucociliary clearance system.

Surfactant prevents the alveoli and bronchioles from collapsing, especially during expiration, by reducing surface tension. Surface tension is due to the liquid lining the alveoli. This liquid develops a cohesive force that tends to collapse the alveoli. The lung therefore consists of hundreds of millions of relatively unstable bubbles, each 0.3 mm in diameter. Surfactant makes it easier to expand the lung (increases compliance), thereby reducing the work associated with breathing. Surfactant and alveolar stability may be lost in some disease states; this loss leads to atelectasis, impaired gas exchange, and increased work of breathing. Surfactant-deficient states are now being treated in neonates with artificial or bovine surfactant.

Gas exchange occurs remarkably efficiently at the alveolar-capillary membrane. The pathway of a gas molecule beginning from inside the alveolus is illustrated in Figure 1–9. Blood passes through the capillaries in approximately $\frac{1}{2}$ second at rest. However, it is estimated that gas exchange is completed when

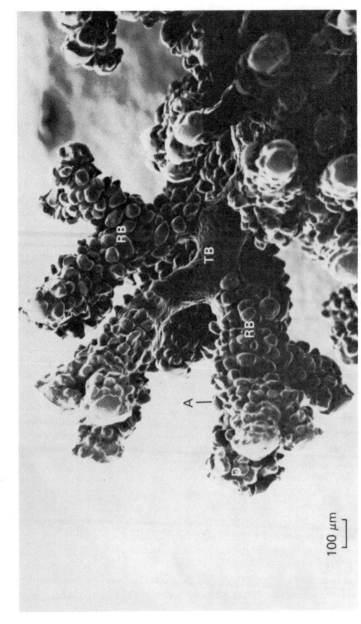

FIGURE 1–7 Scanning electron micrograph of a silicone-rubber cast of cat lung. Structure of the acinus, the site of external gas exchange in the lung, is made visible to the human eye. A, alveolus; D, alveolar duct; RB, respiratory bronchiole; TB, terminal bronchiole. (Reproduced with permission from Weibel, E.: Design and structure of the human lung. In Fishman, A. [Ed.]. *Assessment of Pulmonary Function*. New York: McGraw-Hill, 1980.)

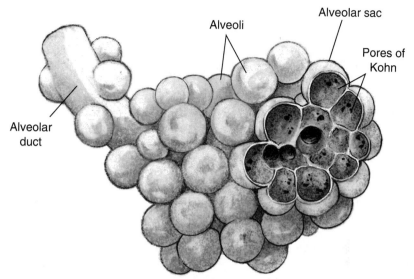

FIGURE 1-8 The pores of Kohn are small holes in the walls of the alveoli that provide for collateral airflow between the alveoli. Ventilation through these pores contributes to the synchronous ventilation of alveolar units that are receiving less gas because of airway obstruction or reduced compliance.

the blood has traversed only one fourth of the capillary distance. This efficiency provides for gas exchange reserve during disease and exercise states. Diffusion distance and time may be increased in alveolar congestion, interstitial or alveolar edema, or pulmonary fibrosis. Gas exchange at the alveolar-capillary membrane is known as *external respiration*, whereas the exchange of oxygen and carbon dioxide between the systemic capillaries and the cells of the various organ systems is known as *internal respiration*.

Airway Innervation

The tracheobronchial tree is innervated by both sympathetic and parasympathetic nerve fibers. Parasympathetic innervation is supplied by the vagus nerve. Stimulation of the vagus nerve by laryngeal irritation results in weak bronchoconstriction, primarily of the larger airways. Sympathetic receptors are primarily the beta-2 type. When these adrenergic receptors are stimulated by either of two catecholamines, epinephrine or norepinephrine, the result is bronchodilation. Patients with asthma or bronchial spasm may obtain relief by using drugs that induce bronchial dilation by either stimulating the beta-adrenergic receptors or blocking the effects of vagal nerve stimulation (see Appendix II: Drugs Used in Intensive Respiratory Care).

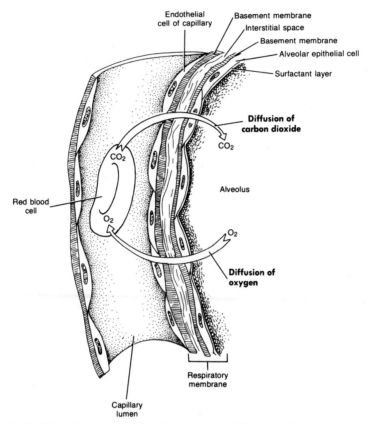

FIGURE 1-9 The pathway molecules of gas must travel for gas exchange to occur at the alveolar-capillary membrane. (From Sexton, D.L.: *Nursing Care of the Respiratory Patient.* Norwalk, Conn.: Appleton & Lange, 1990.)

VASCULAR SUPPLY

Bronchial Circulation

The lung has two different circulatory systems: the bronchial and the pulmonary. The bronchial circulation supplies the bronchi and bronchioles as far as the distal portion of the terminal bronchioles. As a division of the systemic circulation, the bronchial arteries arise from the aorta, traverse the bronchi, and drain into the pulmonary veins. This circulation receives only about 2% of the cardiac output.

Pulmonary Circulation

The pulmonary circulation begins in the main pulmonary artery, which receives unoxygenated blood from the right side of the heart. The main pulmonary artery then divides into right and left pulmonary arteries at the point where the main-stem bronchi divide in the hilum. The arteries then divide, running parallel to each division of the airways until they finally terminate in a capillary network so dense that, when fully recruited, the alveoli are nearly coated with blood

(Fig. 1–10). The walls of the pulmonary arteries are very thin. They contain smooth muscle but are much less muscular than the arteries of the systemic circulation. The oxygenated blood is collected by the pulmonary veins, which unite with other veins, eventually forming the four large pulmonary veins that drain into the left atrium. Unlike the systemic circulation, the pulmonary arteries carry venous blood and the pulmonary veins carry oxygenated blood.

Lymphatic System

The functions of the pulmonary lymphatic tissue are to maintain fluid homeostasis and to play a role in immunologic defense. The lymphatic system, made up of channels and lymph nodes, reabsorbs excess fluid in the lung interstitium and the peribronchial and pleural spaces and returns to the circulation the serum, escaped plasma protein, and products of cellular metabolism that cannot be absorbed by the capillaries. By reducing interstitial protein concentration, the lymphatic system decreases interstitial colloid oncotic pressure and assists in the prevention of pulmonary edema formation. The immunologic function of the lymphatic system is to filter out bacteria and other harmful substances that have escaped the mucociliary escalator. Filtering is performed in the lymph nodes before the lymphatic fluid is returned to the general circulation, thereby protecting the body from dissemination of foreign material.

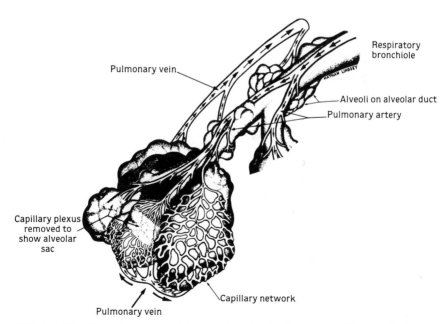

FIGURE 1–10   Alveoli are encased in a meshwork of pulmonary capillaries, which promotes extreme efficiency in gas exchange. (Adapted from Wilkins, R.L., Sheldon, R.L., and Krider, S.J.: *Clinical Assessment in Respiratory Care.* 2nd ed. St. Louis: C.V. Mosby, 1990.)

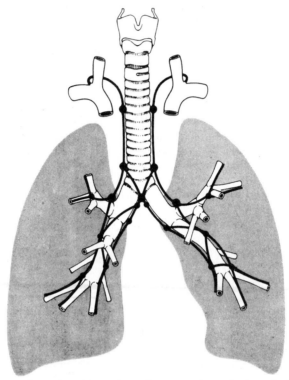

FIGURE 1–11 The main lymphatic channels course along the bronchial tree. Lymph nodes, which filter the lymph, are scattered along the channels. (Reproduced with permission from Weibel, E.: Design and structure of the human lung. In Fishman, A.P. [Ed.]. *Assessment of Pulmonary Function.* New York: McGraw-Hill, 1980.)

Lymphatic channels are present in the pleura and in the peribronchial and perivascular spaces, forming networks around the blood vessels that they accompany in the thoracic cavity. The channels contain valves that promote unidirectional lymph flow. Lymph is fluid that is formed by the normal processes of interstitial fluid development. Its flow is from the periphery toward the main lymphatic channels along the bronchial tree (Fig. 1–11), toward the lymph nodes clustered about each hilus, and from there onward to either the thoracic or the right lymphatic ducts, which drain into the right and left subclavian veins. Lymph nodes are scattered throughout the course of the lymphatic channels. These nodes are lymph-filtering stations; large particulate matter may therefore be deposited in them. The lymphatic vessels are not typically visualized on the chest x-ray film except in certain disease processes such as histoplasmosis, a fungal infection spread in the droppings of fowl, bats, and birds.

LUNGS: LOBES AND SEGMENTS

The lungs are conical in shape, their apices arising about 2 to 4 cm above the inner third of the clavicle and their bases resting on the upper diaphragm surfaces. The right lung, which accounts for about 55% of lung function, has three

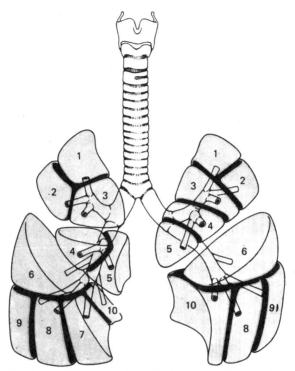

FIGURE 1-12 Divisions of the tracheobronchial tree and the bronchopulmonary segments. (Reproduced with permission from Weibel, E.: Design and structure of the human lung. In Fishman, A.P. [Ed.]. *Assessment of Pulmonary Function.* New York: McGraw-Hill, 1980.)

lobes: upper, middle, and lower. The left lung has two lobes: upper and lower. However, the left upper lobe has a superior and an inferior division. The inferior portion is known as the lingula and is thought of as being comparable to the right middle lobe.

The lobes of the lung are further divided into bronchopulmonary segments (Fig. 1–12). Each segment has its own airway and arterial and venous blood supply, which allows any diseased segment to be surgically removed. Understanding the location of the various pulmonary segments is useful in applying the pulmonary toilet techniques of postural drainage, percussion, and vibration and for anatomically defining and describing areas of abnormality.

PLEURA AND PLEURAL SPACE

The lungs and the thoracic cavity are lined with the pleura, a continuous sheet of elastic and collagenous fibers that is described in two portions: the visceral pleura and the parietal pleura (Fig. 1–13). The visceral pleura is a thin, delicate lining around the lungs, lung fissures, and hilar bronchi and vessels. The parietal pleura lines the inner surface of the thoracic cavity. The parietal pleura has nerve receptors for pain, but the visceral pleura does not. A mucous solution is produced by the cells of the pleura. This solution, which is probably less than

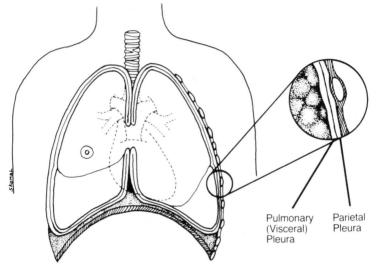

Pulmonary
(Visceral)
Pleura

Parietal
Pleura

FIGURE 1–13 Pleural linings of the lungs. (From Carroll, P. *Understanding Chest Drainage*. Fall River, Mass: Deknatel, Inc., 1992.)

10 ml, lubricates the pleural surfaces, allowing for smooth movement of the surfaces over one another. It also holds the two pleurae together by means of surface tension forces; thus the pleurae move in unison with the thoracic cage on inspiration. Surface tension is an attractive force between adjacent liquid molecules. This force preserves the integrity of the surface, preventing it from separating. It is the surface tension between the two pleurae, opposing the tendency of the lung to want to collapse because of its elastic recoil, that leads to the existence of a negative pressure of about −5 mm Hg within the intrapleural space.

The pleural space is essentially a potential space between the two pleural surfaces. If excessive fluid (pleural effusion) or air (pneumothorax) enters this space, lung expansion may be inhibited. If the decreased expansion is significant enough to compromise respiration, a chest tube may be needed (see Appendix III: Chest Drainage Systems). Because the right and left parietal and visceral pleurae are entirely separate, pleural space disease may exist in one hemithorax and be absent in the other.

THORACIC CAGE

The lungs are housed in the thoracic cage, which is bordered posteriorly by the vertebral column, anteriorly by the sternum, and laterally by the ribs. Its floor is formed by the dome-shaped diaphragm. The ribs, 24 in number, 12 on each side, attach posteriorly to the spinal column and then extend around and down, under the arms, where they turn upward again and extend, not as bone but as cartilage, to the sternum (Fig. 1–14). These resilient bars of cartilage, the costal cartilages, extend from all the ribs, except the last two pairs, toward the sternum. The first seven pairs of ribs, the true ribs, have cartilage that actually reaches the sternum. The last five pairs are the false ribs. Of the false ribs, numbers 8, 9, and

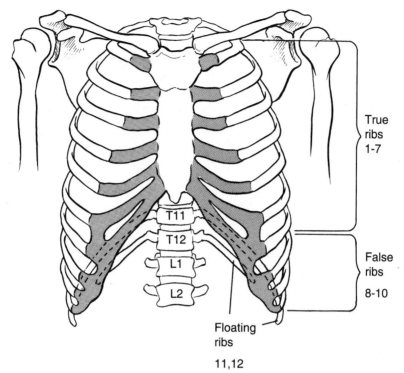

FIGURE 1-14   The bony thorax.

10 have costal cartilages that turn up and join the rib above. Ribs 11 and 12 are floating ribs in that they have no anterior attachment. The ribs provide not only protection of the lungs but also an attachment for the respiratory muscles.

The sternum has three parts: the handle (or manubrium) above, the body (or gladiolus) in the middle, and the xiphoid process below. The point where the manubrium and the body articulate, the sternal angle, is a prominent ridge that can be felt under the skin. At this point, the second rib articulates with the sternum and is a landmark for counting the ribs and the intercostal spaces (ICS). The ICSs are numbered according to the number of ribs above; therefore the space above the second rib is the first ICS.

RESPIRATORY MUSCLES

Inspiratory Muscles

The principal muscle of respiration is the *diaphragm*. The central portion is composed of fibrous tissue and is known as the central tendon. The muscular portion of the diaphragm attaches to the xiphoid process, the costal margins of the lower six ribs, and the vertebral column. The muscle fiber composition of the diaphragm makes it highly suited to the type of endurance work it must perform. When high-resistance workloads, which require strength, not endurance, are placed on the diaphragm, the muscle fibers may fatigue quickly

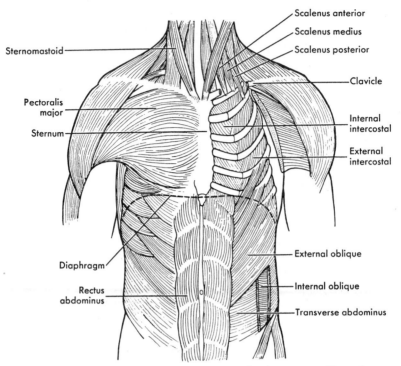

Scalenus anterior
Scalenus medius
Scalenus posterior
Sternomastoid
Clavicle
Pectoralis major
Internal intercostal
Sternum
External intercostal
External oblique
Diaphragm
Internal oblique
Rectus abdominus
Transverse abdominus

Figure 1-15 The muscles of ventilation. See text for description. (From Spearman, C.B., and Sheldon, R.L. *Egan's Fundamentals of Respiratory Therapy.* 5th ed. St. Louis: Mosby–Year Book, 1990.)

if energy demands exceed supply. (For further information on respiratory muscle composition, see Chapter 10: Weaning From Mechanical Ventilation.) The diaphragm can adapt with time to high-resistance workloads placed on it by some disease states.

In the resting position, the diaphragm is dome shaped. On inspiration the diaphragm contracts, flattening the dome. This action increases the superior-inferior dimension of the thoracic cavity, forces the abdominal contents downward, and elevates the lower ribs. The diaphragm normally accounts for approximately 70% of the tidal volume.

Playing a lesser role in inspiratory activities are the *external intercostal muscles*. These muscles arise from the lower border of the first 11 ribs and have fibers that extend downward and forward to the upper border of the rib below. On inspiration, the external intercostal muscles contract, elevating the ribs and increasing the anterior-posterior dimension of the thoracic cavity.

The accessory muscles of respiration are called into play with increased effort breathing. During inspiration the *scalene muscle*, which extends from the cervical vertebrae to the first two ribs, contracts to elevate the first two ribs. The *sternocleidomastoid muscle*, which extends from the jawline to the sternum, assists in elevating the sternum. Both muscles therefore attempt to increase the anterior-posterior diameter of the thorax. Figure 1–15 illustrates the ventilatory muscles.

Expiratory Muscles

Expiration during normal quiet ventilation is a passive activity that occurs because of relaxation of the inspiratory muscles and recoil of the lung parenchyma. During forceful expiration the *internal intercostal muscles* contract, decreasing the anterior-posterior diameter of the thorax by pulling the ribs downward and inward. These muscles lie under the external intercostals and have similar points of attachment but differ in that they have fibers that pass downward and backward.

The abdominal muscles used for increased effort expiration include the *internal and external oblique muscles*, the *rectus muscle*, and the *transverse abdominus muscle*. When contracted, these muscles force the diaphragm upward and depress the lower ribs, decreasing the superior-inferior diameter of the thorax.

Innervation of the Ventilatory Muscles

Knowledge regarding the nervous innervation of the muscles of respiration (Fig. 1–16; Table 1–1) provides a basis for understanding the respiratory effects of neuromuscular disease. This knowledge is particularly valuable when caring for patients with Guillain-Barré syndrome or spinal cord injury because one can

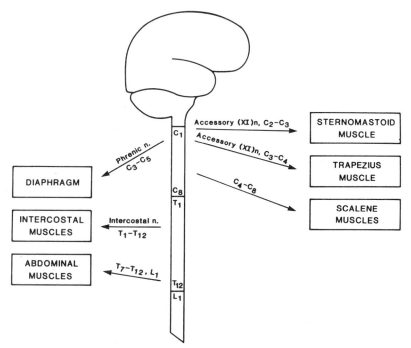

FIGURE 1–16 Motor innervation of ventilatory muscle groups. (From Tobin, M.J.: Respiratory muscles in disease. *Clin Chest Med* 9[2]:277, 1988.)

Table 1-1 Innervation of the Muscles of Ventilation

Muscles	Innervating Nerves
Diaphragm	Phrenic nerve. Arises from the cervical spinal cord, roots C3, C4, and C5. Susceptibility to injury increased during thoracic surgery or trauma because of course of nerve down the thoracic cavity. High cervical spinal cord injury may result in immediate loss of diaphragm function and death. Patients with high spinal cord lesions develop hypertrophy of sternocleidomastoid and trapezius muscles, which are spared because of innervation by cranial nerve XI.
External and internal intercostal muscles	Intercostal nerves. Arise from thoracic spinal nerves 1 to 12. Patient with thoracic spinal cord injury may learn to breathe without a ventilator by using diaphragm and neck muscles. Expiratory muscle paralysis results in reduced cough effectiveness and impaired secretion clearance.
Abdominal	Spinal nerves. Arise from T7 through L1. Reduced expiratory effort therefore results in less effective cough and secretion clearance.
Scalene	Spinal nerves C4 through C8. Function is lost in high-level spinal cord lesions.
Sternocleidomastoid	Cranial nerve XI, spinal accessory. Spared in cervical spinal cord injury.
Trapezius	Spinal nerves C3 and C4 and cranial nerve XI, spinal accessory. Partially spared in cervical spinal cord injury.

detect ventilatory failure early, determine what respiratory muscle function has been lost or spared, and develop a rehabilitation plan.

PROTECTIVE MECHANISMS

Cough

The coughing response represents an important protective mechanism for the body and utilizes forced expiration as the basic pattern for expelling foreign objects from the respiratory passages. The cougher inspires, closes the glottis and vigorously contracts the expiratory muscles in a Valsalva maneuver, and then suddenly opens the glottis. Because air is momentarily prevented from leaving the lungs, intrapleural and intrapulmonic pressures are built to maximum levels. On the sudden opening of the glottis, a blast of air is forced through the trachea, effectively ejecting the foreign object or mucous deposit from the airway. Mechanical, chemical, or physical stimuli initiate a cough, which is a cholinergic vagal reflex, the receptors for which are primarily located in the upper airway. When an endotracheal tube is in place, the mechanics of coughing are disrupted in that the glottis cannot close normally, potentially leading to a less efficient cough.

Sneeze

A sneeze is elicited by irritation of the mucous membranes of the nose by mechanical, physical, or chemical stimuli. It results when the sensory receptors of the trigeminal or olfactory nerves are stimulated. A deep inhalation is initiated, followed by a violent exhalation through the nose.

Mucociliary Clearance System

The mucociliary clearance system, consisting of mucus and ciliated cells, functions to trap and transport airborne particles not filtered in the nose and larger airways. Normal production of mucus in the lungs is about 100 ml/day. Mucus comes from two sources: the surface goblet cells and the submucosal glands, which produce a mixed serous and mucous secretion. The submucosal glands respond to vagal stimulation with increased output. Output is therefore decreased with vagal blocking agents (see Appendix II: Drugs Used in Intensive Respiratory Care) or pulmonary dennervation, as in pulmonary transplantation. Conversely, increased production of mucus, as in bronchitis or cystic fibrosis, can overwhelm the mucociliary system.

Ciliated epithelium is present from the upper airways down to the terminal bronchioles. Each cell contains about 200 to 275 cilia that beat upward in a co-ordinated, wavelike fashion projecting mucus upward at a velocity of 10 to 20 mm/min. Once the secretions reach the oropharynx, they are eliminated by ex-pectoration or swallowing. Many factors may affect the function of the mucocil-iary clearance system (Box 1–1).

Immunoglobulins and enzymes are also found in the mucous blanket of the lungs. IgA is the principal antibody found in normal mucous secretions. Im-munoglobulin deficiencies may lead to predisposition to respiratory infection. Enzymes play a role in the destruction of bacteria. Considering that the respira-tory tract is in constant contact with the environment, it is truly remarkable that the lower respiratory tract is almost sterile. Working together to achieve this feat are the mucociliary clearance system, enzymes, alveolar macrophages, the pul-monary lymphatic system, and immunoglobulins.

Box 1–1 Factors Adversely Affecting Mucociliary Function

Cigarette smoke
Hyperoxia and hypoxia
Hypercapnia
Lack of, or low, humidity in inspired air
Systemic dehydration
Artificial airways
Inhalation anesthetics
Narcotics
Sedatives
Alcohol
Acute respiratory tract infections
Cellular destruction caused by tracheal suctioning
Smoke inhalation
Dennervation as a result of lung transplantation
Increasing age
Sleep

CONTROL OF VENTILATION

Ventilation is controlled through an interplay of many complex processes to ensure that adequate oxygen is available for metabolism and that the by-product of cellular metabolism, carbon dioxide, is removed and acid-base homeostasis is maintained. Despite many years of study, our understanding of the control of ventilation is incomplete. Breathing is primarily controlled humorally, through the action of chemical stimuli on regulatory centers in the brain stem.

Voluntary Control: Cortical Centers

Though breathing continues rhythmically without our conscious effort, such as when sleeping or concentrating on work, conscious control of breathing is possible. Conscious regulation of breathing is mediated by the cerebral cortex, specifically in the motor cortex of the frontal lobe and the limbic area. An individual may voluntary hyperventilate, hold his breath, or alter his breathing pattern to sniff, sing, speak, hum, or perform isometric work such as straining at stool or lifting heavy objects. However, the ability of the cerebral cortex to override other central regulatory centers for breathing is limited. For example, holding one's breath to the point of unconsciousness is limited by carbon dioxide stimulation of spontaneous breathing.

Involuntary Control: Medullary, Pontine, and Peripheral Centers

Both peripheral and central centers take part in the involuntary control of breathing. Ventilatory centers are named according to their location within or outside the central nervous system (Fig. 1–17). Within the central nervous system there are at least three centers for the control of rhythmic breathing: one in the medulla oblongata and two in the pons. Input to these centers comes from proprioceptors and peripheral chemoreceptors via the glossopharyngeal and vagus nerves. Output (efferent) activity is via the phrenic nerve to the diaphragm and thoracic nerves 1 through 12 to the intercostal muscles.

The medullary center is the main coordinating center for all the sources of input from other centers involved in ventilatory control. Two subcenters, one for inspiration and one for expiration, lie within the medulla. It is by means of these subcenters that the medullary center sends efferent impulses, through the phrenic and thoracic nerves to the muscles of ventilation.

The two pontine centers are the apneustic and the pneumotaxic. The apneustic center acts on the medulla to promote deep and prolonged inspiration. Injury to the pons can lead to an abnormal breathing pattern known as apneustic breathing, which is a gasping type of ventilation with maximal inspiratory effort. Output from the apneustic center is limited by the pneumotaxic center, which acts to inhibit inspiration by sending impulses to the medullary inspiratory subcenter. The pneumotaxic center therefore encourages rhythmic ventilation by limiting inspiration. Peripheral receptors are located on the aortic arch and at the bifurcation of the internal and external carotid arteries. These tissues, being chemoreceptors, are sensitive to blood levels of oxygen, carbon dioxide, and hydrogen ion. Afferent impulses from the carotid bodies to the

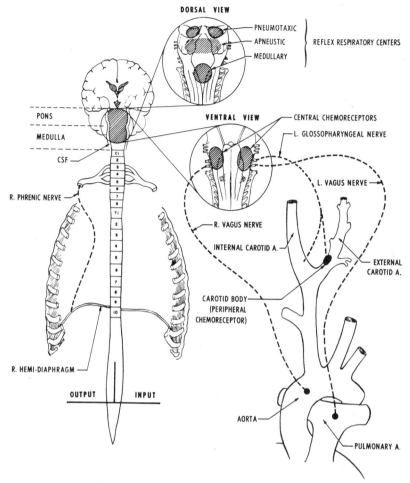

FIGURE 1–17 Central and peripheral centers responsible for the control of ventilation. (From Slonim, N.B., and Chapin, J.L.: *Respiratory Physiology*. St. Louis: C.V. Mosby, 1967.)

medulla are sent via the glossopharyngeal nerve (cranial nerve IX) and from the aortic bodies via the vagus nerve (cranial nerve X).

Humoral Control of Ventilation

Breathing is primarily controlled by a feedback mechanism that involves chemical stimuli acting on chemoreceptors in the brain stem and the periphery (Table 1–2). Afferent stimuli are received into the medulla and the aortic and carotid bodies via these chemoreceptors.

CENTRAL CHEMORECEPTORS

Chemoreceptors located in the medulla are primarily influenced by the hydrogen ion concentration (pH) of the cerebrospinal fluid (CSF). An increase in

TABLE 1-2   Location and Response of the Chemoreceptors Involved in the Control of Ventilation

Location	Category	Stimulus	Response
Medulla	Central	Increased hydrogen ion concentration of CSF (decreased pH)	Strong stimulus to increase the rate and depth of ventilation
Aortic arch and bifurcation of the carotid arteries	Peripheral	Decreased PaO_2	Increase in the rate and depth of ventilation
		Increased $PaCO_2$ or decreased pH	Mild increase in ventilation

$PaCO_2$ causes maximal increases in the hydrogen ion concentration of the CSF because it lacks the protein hydrogen buffers found in the blood. Central chemoreceptors, when stimulated by a decreasing pH because of increasing H^+ ion concentration, increase the depth and rate of respiration. A low concentration of CSF hydrogen ion, alkalosis, retards ventilation. Central chemoreceptors do not respond to a low PaO_2.

PERIPHERAL CHEMORECEPTORS
Peripheral chemoreceptors are extremely sensitive to decreases in both blood oxygen tension and content. Hypoxemia increases the activity of the peripheral receptors, leading to an increase in the rate and depth of ventilation. High oxygen tensions may result in mild hypoventilation; however, this response is generally overridden by the central respiratory center's response to a rising $PaCO_2$. The peripheral chemoreceptors also respond to increases in $PaCO_2$ and hydrogen ion concentration with an increase in ventilation, but do so less sensitively than the central receptors.

Mechanical Reflexes
STRETCH RECEPTORS
Stretch receptors are located in bronchial smooth muscle. When they are stimulated by lung hyperinflation, impulses are sent to the respiratory center, via the vagus nerve, to limit further inflation and increase expiratory time. This is known as the Hering-Breuer inflation reflex. The Hering-Breuer deflation reflex initiates inspiratory activity at very low lung volumes.

IRRITANT RECEPTORS
Activity of the irritant receptors, which lie between the epithelial cells of the airway, is mediated by the vagus nerve. When stimulated by inhaled particles such as cigarette smoke or cold air, the reflex response is bronchoconstriction and increased respiratory rate.

J-RECEPTORS
Receptors located in the alveolar walls near the capillary are appropriately named juxtacapillary receptors, or J-receptors. They are innervated by the vagus

nerve and, when stimulated, cause rapid, shallow breathing that may deteriorate to apnea with intense stimulation. Stimulants include fluid in the alveoli and distention of the pulmonary capillaries, conditions that are present in adult respiratory distress syndrome, left heart failure, and pulmonary edema.

OTHER RECEPTORS

Proprioreceptors in the joints are believed to be responsible for the increase in rate and depth of ventilation with increased movement of the joint, which occurs with exercise or even during passive range of motion. Gamma receptors in the intercostal muscles and the diaphragm muscle spindles may be responsible for the sensation of dyspnea when increased respiratory effort is required. An increase in body temperature or stimulation of pain receptors can lead to hyperventilation. In addition, stimulation of the carotid and aortic baroreceptors, by an increase in blood pressure, may cause reflex hypoventilation or apnea, whereas a decrease in blood pressure may result in hyperventilation.

RECOMMENDED READINGS

Kelly, D.E., Wood, R.L., and Enders, A.C. (1984). *Bailey's Textbook of Microscopic Anatomy*. Baltimore: Williams & Wilkins.

Selkurt, E.E. (1975). Respiratory gas exchange and its transport and Nervous and chemical control of respiration. In E.E. Selkurt (Ed.). *Basic Physiology for the Health Sciences* (pp. 419–438 and 439–454). Boston: Little, Brown.

Sexton, D.L. (1990). Anatomy and physiology. In D.L. Sexton (Ed.). *Nursing Care of the Respiratory Patient* (pp. 1–39). Norwalk, Conn.: Appleton & Lange.

Spearman, C.B., Sheldon, R.L., and Egan, D.F. (1982). *Egan's Fundamentals of Respiratory Therapy*. St. Louis: C.V. Mosby .

Tobin, M.J. (1988). Respiratory muscles in disease. *Clin Chest Med* 9(2), 263–286.

Weibel, E. (1980). Design and structure of the human lung. In A. Fishman (Ed.). *Assessment of Pulmonary Function* (pp. 18–68). New York: McGraw-Hill.

Williams, P.L., Warwick, R., Dyson, M., and Bannister, L.H. (Eds.) (1989). *Gray's Anatomy*. New York: Churchill Livingstone.

Practical Physiology of the Pulmonary System

Practice in many clinical arenas requires a strong understanding of physiologic processes. Physiology is utilized as the basis to interpret knowledgeably the large amounts of data gathered in patient care settings. It is from this physiologic vantage point that we interpret the cause of findings (i.e., high airway pressures, hypoxemia, hypercapnia) and therefore choose the appropriate therapy. We then evaluate the effects of therapies, using physiologic measures that provide quantifiable gauges of whether or not the patient is improving. For example, serial measures of oxygenation or ventilation, percent shunt, compliance, and resistance help us in reevaluating our therapies. Finally, physiology helps us understand the positive or adverse effects of therapies, such as the effects of changing the body position on ventilation/perfusion relationships and thus oxygenation, the effects of positive end-expiratory pressure (PEEP), and how to treat adverse PEEP effects. The foundation for caring for the patient supported by a mechanical ventilator begins with an understanding of how spontaneous ventilation is achieved.

VENTILATORY CONCEPTS

Mechanics of Spontaneous Ventilation

The purpose of ventilation is to supply fresh gas to the lungs, to be exchanged at the alveolar-capillary membrane. The basic principle underlying the movement of gas is that it travels from an area of greater concentration to a lower concentration, or from an area of higher to lower pressure. Physiologic pressures related to the flow of gases into and out of the lung are atmospheric pressure, intrapulmonic (or intraalveolar) pressure, intrapleural (or intrathoracic) pressure, and transpulmonary pressure (Table 2–1).

At rest, the pressure within the alveoli is atmospheric. When a spontaneous inspiration is initiated, muscular effort is exerted by the contraction of the diaphragm and the external intercostal muscles. Inspiration is thus an active process that requires the expenditure of energy. Contraction of the inspiratory muscles enlarges the thoracic cavity. The lungs expand because they are pulled outward, along with the movement of the thoracic wall. The lungs move with the chest wall because of surface tension created by the small amount of fluid be-

TABLE 2-1   Physiologic Pressure Related to Ventilation

Pressure/Definition	Inspiration	Expiration	End Expiration
Atmospheric: pressure exerted by the surrounding air on the earth's surface.	760 mm Hg or 0 cm H_2O	0 cm H_2O	0 cm H_2O
Intrapulmonic or intraalveolar (Palv): pressure within the bronchial tree and the alveoli.	-1 to -2 cm H_2O	$+1$ to $+2$ cm H_2O	0 cm H_2O
Intrapleural or intrathoracic: pressure within the pleural space; subatmospheric, or negative, because of the tendency of the lungs to want to collapse. Elastic recoil of the lungs continuously exerts a pull on the thoracic wall.	-8 to -9 cm H_2O	-4 cm H_2O	-5 cm H_2O
Transpulmonary or transmural: pressure difference across the lung; intraalveolar minus intrapleural pressure; created entirely by the elasticity of the lung; number is always positive. The gradient increases on inspiration, causing air to flow into the lungs.	$+7$ cm H_2O	$+5$ cm H_2O	$+5$ cm H_2O

tween the visceral and parietal pleurae. Negative pressure normally within the intrapleural space becomes even more negative on inspiration. Intraalveolar pressure also becomes negative, and then air at atmospheric pressure flows into the lung. Inspiration continues until intraalveolar pressure rises to equal atmospheric pressure (Fig. 2–1). Air does not have to be drawn, or sucked, into the lung. Air simply moves from an area of high pressure to one of low pressure.

Expiration is a passive process that occurs because of the elastic recoil of the lung. When contraction of the inspiratory muscles ceases, the thoracic cage and lungs recoil to their original size. Intrapleural pressure becomes less negative. Intraalveolar pressure becomes slightly positive on expiration, which ends when intraalveolar and atmospheric pressures equalize. In the spontaneously breathing individual, lung volume attained at end expiration is determined by the competing forces of elastic recoil and thoracic cage stiffness.

The increased negativity of the intrapleural pressure during inspiration is important for bringing air into the lungs and for promoting venous return to the right side of the heart (preload) by expanding the great veins. When an individual is placed on a positive-pressure ventilator, the normally low intrathoracic pressures are disrupted in that they become positive. Positive pressure within the thorax affects the distribution of gases and may also lead to hemodynamic embarrassment, primarily through a reduction in right heart preload (see Chapter 8).

Lung Volumes and Capacities: Spirometry

Air within the lung can be measured with an instrument called a spirometer. Total air is divided into subdivisions called *volumes*. When two or more volumes

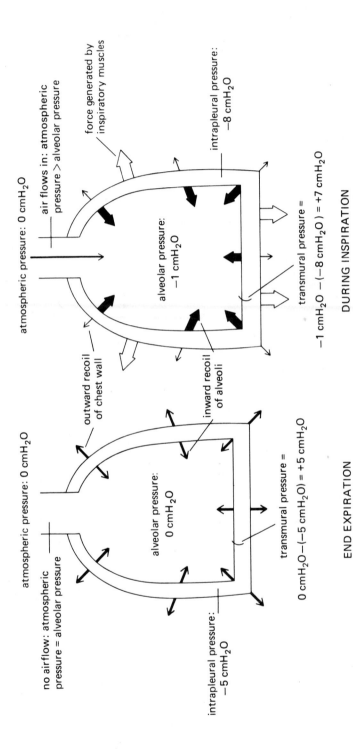

FIGURE 2-1 Pressure changes within the thoracic cavity during spontaneous ventilation. (*Left*) At end-expiration the muscles of respiration are relaxed. Lung volume is determined by the competing forces of elastic recoil of the lung and thorax. No airflow occurs because atmospheric and alveolar pressures are equal. (*Right*) Contraction of the respiratory muscles on inspiration enlarges the thoracic cavity. The lung is pulled outward with the chest wall and intrapleural pressure becomes more negative. Alveolar pressure drops below atmospheric pressure, and air, because of its tendency to move to an area of less pressure, flows into the lungs. (From Levitsky, M.G.: *Pulmonary Physiology.* 3rd ed. New York: McGraw-Hill, 1991.)

The figure labels read as follows:

atmospheric pressure: 0 cmH$_2$O

air flows in: atmospheric pressure > alveolar pressure

force generated by inspiratory muscles

intrapleural pressure: −8 cmH$_2$O

alveolar pressure: −1 cmH$_2$O

transmural pressure = −1 cmH$_2$O − (−8 cmH$_2$O) = +7 cmH$_2$O

DURING INSPIRATION

atmospheric pressure: 0 cmH$_2$O

outward recoil of chest wall

inward recoil of alveoli

no airflow: atmospheric pressure = alveolar pressure

alveolar pressure: 0 cmH$_2$O

transmural pressure = 0 cmH$_2$O − (−5 cmH$_2$O) = +5 cmH$_2$O

intrapleural pressure: −5 cmH$_2$O

END EXPIRATION

are added, they are called a lung *capacity* (Fig. 2–2). Measurement of lung volumes is useful because many pathophysiologic states alter lung volumes. The effect of therapies utilized specifically to enhance particular lung volumes can also be evaluated. The following definitions are relevant:

Tidal volume (VT). The volume of gas moved into or out of the lung in a single normal inspiration or expiration. It averages 500 ml, or 5 to 8 ml/kg. It represents the volume reaching the alveoli, about 350 ml, plus the volume in the conducting airways, known as the anatomic dead space, which is about 150 ml, or 2 ml/kg.

Inspiratory reserve volume (IRV). The volume of air that can be inspired at the end of a normal tidal inspiration. It is appropriately titled "reserve" volume. The IRV is called on when increased tidal breathing is necessary, as in exercise.

Expiratory reserve volume (ERV). The maximal volume of gas that can be exhaled after a normal exhalation.

Residual volume (RV). The volume of gas remaining in the lungs after a maximal expiration. This volume cannot be measured with spirometry. It is obtained indirectly by using the helium dilution test, nitrogen washout method, or body plethysmography to determine the functional residual capacity (FRC). The formula RV = FRC − ERV is then used to determine RV.

Inspiratory capacity (IC) = IRV + VT. The maximal volume of gas that can be inspired after a normal exhalation. Measurement of the IC as a determinant of maximal tidal volume capability is a more useful and accurate measurement than the IRV because when the IRV is measured, deciding when the tidal volume ends is extremely subjective.

Vital capacity (VC) = IRV + VT + ERV. The volume of gas that is exhaled after the deepest possible inspiration. This measurement can be obtained at the bedside with a handheld spirometer in a cooperative patient. It is clini-

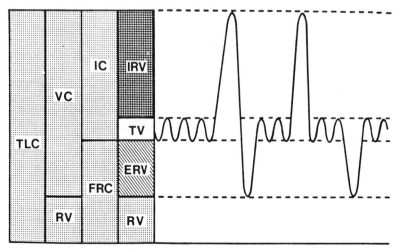

FIGURE 2–2 Measurement of lung volumes and capacities with a spirometer. (From Bonner, J.T., and Hall, J.R.: *Respiratory Intensive Care of the Adult Surgical Patient*. St. Louis: C.V. Mosby, 1985.)

cally useful in that it tells us the patient's maximal ventilatory capability. VC is often measured and trended as an indicator of the patient's ability to be weaned from mechanical ventilation.

Functional residual capacity (FRC) = ERV + RV. The volume of air remaining in the lungs at the end of a normal expiration. This is the volume where gas exchange is constantly taking place. The V_T can be thought of as the dilutional volume. Tidal breaths bring in fresh gas to mix with the volume already present in the lungs, the FRC, where steady-state gas exchange is occurring. In many pathologic conditions, such as atelectasis, secretion or fluid collection in the lungs, or pleural effusion, the FRC is reduced and thus gas exchange is affected. Direct measurement of the FRC cannot be performed with spirometry (see the definition of residual volume).

Total lung capacity (TLC) = IC + FRC. The maximal volume of air in the lungs after a maximal inspiration. TLC is the sum of all lung volumes (see also Table 2–2).

Closing Volume

The closing volume (CV) is that volume on expiration where small airways in the lung base begin to close. It is expressed as a percentage of the VC and is normally 10% but may increase with age and in disease processes that lead to a loss of lung elasticity. CV may actually exceed FRC in some diseases, and this leads to impaired gas exchange. CV cannot be measured with a spirometer.

The airways in the basilar portion of the lung close sooner than those above because the transpulmonary pressure gradient is less at the base. The reason is that intrapleural pressure is less negative at the lung bases because of the weight of the lungs hanging within the thorax. When lung elasticity or volume decreases, the intrapleural pressure at the base of the lungs may actually become positive, compressing the lung. Under these conditions, CV increases and alveolar ventilation decreases. These changes become evident in the patient's blood gases.

TABLE 2–2   Lung Volumes and Capacities

Measurement	Volume* (ml)
Tidal volume (V_T)	500
Inspiratory reserve volume (IRV)	3000
Expiratory reserve volume (ERV)	1200
Residual volume (RV)	1300
Inspiratory capacity (IC) = IRV + V_T	3500
Vital capacity (VC) = IRV + V_T + ERV	4700
Functional residual capacity (FRC) = ERV + RV	2500
Total lung capacity (TLC) = FRC + IC	6000

*Average volume in adult men. There is a range of normal values that vary by age, body size, build, and sex. Volumes are approximately 25% less in women.

FACTORS AFFECTING VENTILATION

Compliance

Compliance is a measurement of the distensibility of the respiratory tissue. The elasticity of the pulmonary tissues is primarily due to its interstitial makeup of elastin and collagen fibers. This interstitial network provides crucial support for airways, alveoli, and capillaries. In some disease states these fibers become less elastic, leading to "stiff" lungs.

Elastic recoil refers to the return of tissue to its resting position after being stretched. For example, pantyhose and rubberbands are both made of elastic fibers that should return to their resting state when an applied stretch is removed. Likewise, the lungs have very strong elastic recoil that makes them want to continually return to their resting state. Indeed, if the negative pressure in the intrapleural space (the pressure that opposes the lung's elastic recoil) is disrupted, the lungs collapse.

Distensibility refers to the stretchability of the lung, that is, the relative ease with which the lung can be stretched with a given force. Compliance is a measurement of the lung's distensibility. It is defined and measured as the volume change per unit of pressure change. The compliance of both the chest wall and the lung tissue is known as total lung compliance. The following is the physiologic formula for total lung compliance:

$$C_{TL} = \frac{\text{Change in volume}}{\text{Change in pressure}}$$

Various pathologic conditions such as adult respiratory distress syndrome (ARDS), pneumonia, pulmonary edema, pulmonary fibrosis, pneumothorax, and hemothorax lead to low compliance, or stiff lungs. Pathologic conditions that affect total compliance generally fall into three categories: disease of the lung interstitium, disease of the intrapleural space, and disease of the chest wall.

A decrease in compliance affects ventilation. As an example, if the patient is not able to increase the *work* required to generate greater muscular effort to expand the thorax and overcome the stiffer elastic recoil of the lung, a decrease in V_T will result. The distribution of ventilation is also affected in that it will be uneven. Ventilation will be preferentially distributed to the areas of best compliance.

In the clinical setting, treatments that improve compliance can be implemented. Measures of compliance are then used to evaluate the effectiveness of the chosen therapy and to decide whether the patient is progressing. These serial measures actually quantify whether a treatment is decreasing the abnormality and improving the compliance.

Begin by gathering assessment data and determine whether they are suggestive of disease processes that adversely affect compliance (i.e., congestive heart failure [crackles, rales], pneumothorax, atelectasis, infiltrates, pleural effusion, lobar collapse). If a consolidative or infiltrative disease process is present, then the patient will need therapies designed to mobilize secretions, such as chest physiotherapy (CPT), suctioning, and turning, coughing, and deep breathing. The diuresing of edema, however, may also be a choice. If the patient has pleural space disease, therapies should be directed toward evacuating the pleural effusion, pneumothorax, hemothorax, or empyema and then maintaining the chest tube drainage system. If the reduction in compliance is due to a decrease in chest wall movement, then the therapies may include pain control, sedating the patient to promote synchrony with the ventilator, or, in the case of a circumferential chest burn, an escharotomy.

Two forms of compliance—static and dynamic—can be measured. In settings that use the new microprocessor ventilators, they can be obtained very easily because the ventilator performs measurements of respiratory mechanics after the operator inputs only a few simple commands. Static compliance is the truest measure of the compliance of the *lung* tissue. It is measured while there are no gases flowing into or out of the lungs. The following is the physiologic formula for static compliance:

$$C_{ST} = \frac{\text{Exhaled tidal volume}}{\text{Plateau pressure } - \text{ PEEP}}$$

During care of a patient who requires a ventilator, the measurements of exhaled tidal volume, plateau pressure, and PEEP are easily obtained. The exhaled tidal volume is the most accurate measure of the volume actually in the lungs at the time the pressure measurement was taken; therefore it should be utilized as the volume measurement (see the discussion in Chapter 6 of exhaled tidal volume). The plateau pressure is obtained by instituting a 2-second inspiratory pause at the peak of inspiration. This pause creates the condition of no gases flowing into the lungs. At the point where no gases are flowing, and with the glottis open, the pressure within the alveoli is obtainable in the form of the plateau pressure. The reading taken during the inspiratory pause, the plateau pressure, reflects pressure, due to the elastic recoil forces of the lung tissue alone, on the volume of gas in the lungs. No pressure resulting from the flow of gases is measured. When the calculation is performed, any artificial pressure placed in the airway, such as PEEP, must be subtracted from the plateau pressure. When a patient does not have an endotracheal tube in place, measurement of static compliance is still possible. This is achieved by measuring pleural pressure, which reflects alveolar pressure, with an esophageal balloon.

A normal value for static compliance is 70 to 100 ml/cm H_2O. This means that for every 1 cm H_2O pressure change in the lungs, there is a change in volume of 70 to 100 ml of gas. A decrease in static compliance implies abnormalities of the lung parenchyma, pleural space, or chest wall. An increase in compliance from normal, though it may sound good, is a significant problem. Increased compliance occurs in disease processes that destroy the lung's elastic tissues, such as emphysema. Deteriorating elasticity leads to a decrease in the transpulmonary pressure, the force that holds small airways open. Small airways decrease in size and may even collapse, airway resistance increases, and expiratory flow decreases. The inspiratory work of breathing also increases when the transpulmonary pressure decreases because a greater force is required to achieve a change in pressure that will promote sufficient inspiratory flow.

Dynamic compliance is a measurement taken while gases are moving in the lungs; therefore it measures not only compliance of the lung tissue but resistance to gas flow. It may be used as a measurement of compliance because it is somewhat easier to obtain than static compliance, the reason being that it does not require the use of the inspiratory hold maneuver. However, one must remember that dynamic compliance is not a pure measurement of lung compliance. The following is the physiologic formula for dynamic compliance:

$$\text{C}_{\text{DYN}} = \frac{\text{Exhaled tidal volume}}{\text{Peak inspiratory pressure} - \text{PEEP}}$$

Again, the exhaled tidal volume should be used as the numerator because it is the most accurate measurement of the volume actually in the lungs at the time the pressure measurement was taken. The exhaled tidal volume is then divided by the pressure in the airway at the peak of inspiration. At this point, gases are still flowing in the lungs, and some pressure measured will be due to the movement of the gas particles (resistance). Any artificial pressure, such as PEEP, must be subtracted from the pressure measurement when the calculation is performed.

The normal value for dynamic compliance is 50 to 80 ml/cm H_2O. Dynamic compliance measures are always smaller than static compliance because peak airway pressure is always greater than plateau. A decrease in dynamic compliance may indicate a decrease in lung compliance or an increase in airway resistance.

No single value of compliance is as useful as a trend of the variable with time. Measures are used to quantify the extent of the compliance problem and monitor patient progress after therapy is instituted.

Resistance

Resistance is a measurement of the opposition to the flow of gases through the airways. There are two types of resistance: tissue and airway. Tissue resistance, which is caused by tissue friction during inspiration and expiration, normally makes up about 20% of total resistance. Airway resistance (Raw) is the opposition to the flow of gases caused by friction between the walls of the airway and the gas molecules, as well as viscous friction between the gas molecules themselves. Resistance to gas flow is measured in the clinical setting with the following physiologic formula:

$$\text{Raw} = \frac{\text{Peak pressure} - \text{Plateau pressure}}{\text{Flow}}$$

Airway resistance is driving pressure divided by flow rate. Driving pressure is the difference in the pressure between the beginning of the circuit, the mouth (peak pressure), and the end of the circuit, the alveoli (plateau pressure). Flow rate is the speed at which a gas travels, or to look at it another way, the volume of gas delivered in a given amount of time. Its unit of measure is liters per minute. The normal value for airway resistance is 0.5 to 3.0 cm H_2O/L per second, measured at a standard flow rate of 0.5 L/sec.

Factors that affect airway resistance include *airway length, radius,* and *flow rate*. If the length of the airway is increased, resistance to flow will increase. This is one of the reasons that ventilator tubing length is standardized. Moreover, a lengthy endotracheal tube will create higher resistance than a tracheostomy tube of the same diameter. Airway radius affects resistance in that, if the size of an airway is doubled, resistance decreases 16-fold. Likewise, if the airway radius is decreased, the resistance to gas flow is increased. Therefore the flow of gas into the lungs is decreased. The airway radius can be variable in clinical situations. This is an important concept to remember when an artificial airway is chosen or in the management of a disease that decreases the diameter of the airways, such as asthma. Airway radius may also be affected by such factors as a mucous plug or fluid in the ventilator tubing.

Flow rate and the pattern of flow also affect resistance. If the flow rate is increased, pressure in the airway increases and therefore resistance also increases. This becomes easier to understand if the analogy of a garden hose is used. Begin with a garden hose of a given radius and length. You turn on the water at the spigot at a certain flow rate, and a degree of pressure (which you can think of as resistance) is created in the hose. Now turn up the flow rate of water running through the hose. What is going to happen? The pressure (and thus resistance to flow) within the hose increases. The same is true for the flow of gases through the airways. At higher flow rates, airway pressures rise and resistance increases. This occurs during rapid breathing and in the mechanically ventilated patient when high flow rates are required (see the discussion of flow rates in Chapter 6).

Pressure in the airway rises with increasing flow rates primarily because of the patterns of flow created (Fig. 2–3). Laminar flow is characterized by parallel lines of gas traveling together; it is streamlined and low pressure. Turbulent flow is disorganized; there are eddies and whorls that create friction between the molecules of gas. Turbulent flow, which occurs more often when the flow rate is high, causes higher airway resistance. Transitional flow is a mixture of laminar and turbulent flow.

When a patient is being mechanically ventilated, the number used to roughly assess resistance is the peak inspiratory pressure. This can be read on the airway pressure gauge manometer. For a more thorough discussion of interpreting airway pressures in terms of compliance and resistance, see Chapter 8.

High airway resistance may be caused either by patient factors or by the factors related to ventilator circuitry. Examples of patient-related factors include bronchoconstriction, secretions in the airway, or bronchial mucosal edema, as in thermal injury. Examples of ventilator circuit factors are as follows: "biting" or kinking of the endotracheal tube, kinking of the vent tubing between the bed rail and the mattress, and water in the ventilator tubing. In all these conditions that cause increased resistance, gas flow into the lungs is decreased if the pressure getting the air into the lungs is not increased. Increased airway resistance therefore decreases the patient's tidal volume and alveolar ventilation. It also increases the amount of pressure required to get air into the lungs. Finally, the distribution of ventilation is affected in that it becomes uneven. The areas of the lung that have the least resistance are ventilated better than high-resistance areas.

Time Constants for Lung Elasticity

It should now be clear that uneven distribution of ventilation in the lung may be due to regional differences in compliance or resistance. These regional differences may be expressed as a time constant, the formula for which is as follows:

$$\text{Time constant (seconds)} = \text{Resistance} \times \text{Compliance}$$

Different time constants may exist for different regions of the lung. Areas of the lung that have either increased resistance or decreased compliance will have

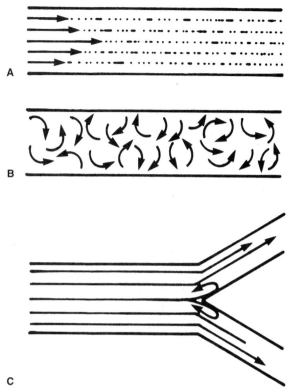

FIGURE 2–3 Patterns of airflow within the respiratory tract. A represents laminar flow, which creates an olive-shaped velocity head. This smooth, rounded velocity head eases into even the smallest airways while creating minimal pressure. B represents turbulent flow, which creates higher pressure and greater shearing forces on the walls of the airways. C represents a transitional pattern that is created when orderly flow is disrupted at points where the airways bifurcate. (From Kelley, M.A. The pulmonary system. In Carlson, R.W., and Geheb, M.A.: *Principles and Practice of Medical Intensive Care*. Philadelphia: W.B. Saunders, 1993.)

a longer time constant. Lung units with longer time constants require a longer inspiratory time to inflate (Fig. 2–4). If the respiratory rate is high, then only lung units with short time constants will inflate fully. The overall results are regional maldistribution of gases and decreased alveolar ventilation. An understanding of time constants is useful in the application of forms of mechanical ventilation using inverse inspiratory to expiratory (I:E) ratios. Inverse I:E ratios are designed to improve the distribution of gases within the lung, and thus alveolar ventilation, by improving ventilation to lung units with longer time constants (see Chapter 6).

Work of Breathing

Breathing requires mechanical work, which is performed by the respiratory muscles, and metabolic work, which is the expenditure of energy. Mechanical

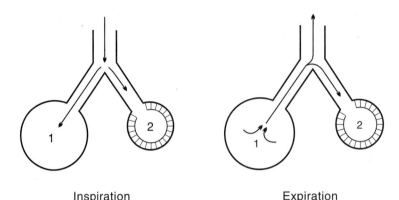

Inspiration   Expiration

FIGURE 2-4 Effect of uneven time constants on the distribution of ventilation. Compartment 2 has a long time constant because of poor compliance or increased resistance. During inspiration, gas is slow to enter compartment 2, and therefore it does not fill as well as the lung unit with a normal time constant (compartment 1). At expiration the abnormal units may still be inhaling though the lung units with normal time constants have begun to exhale.

work is defined as force times distance, meaning that work is performed whenever an applied force causes displacement. In the lung, mechanical work equals pressure (force) times volume (distance factor). The work that the respiratory muscles must perform is that which will overcome elastic and nonelastic forces: compliance and resistance, respectively. When compliance decreases or resistance increases, a greater force is required to move volume in the lung—that is, the work of breathing (WOB) increases.

The WOB, though measurable for research purposes, is generally not calculated with a physiologic formula or trended numerically in the clinical setting. Methods by which this can be done have been described (Dupuis, 1992; Marini, 1990). The WOB is an important factor to take into account when one is considering initiating mechanical ventilation, choosing an appropriate mode of ventilation, altering ventilator settings, weaning a patient from a ventilator, or advancing a patient's activity level. That is, one must ask, Does the patient have sufficient muscle strength to maintain the WOB, given the compliance and resistance of the pulmonary tissue, the work imposed by the ventilator circuitry, and the ventilatory demands?

Physical assessment of the patient may provide some of the most useful clues as to patient tolerance of imposed ventilatory demands. If the WOB is manageable, the respiratory examination will reveal a normal respiratory rate, absence of the use of accessory muscles of respiration, and no abdominal paradox. Moreover, the patient will demonstrate no increase in blood pressure or heart rate from baseline, barring any concurrent processes that could account for such changes.

Clinically meaningful is the WOB expressed in metabolic terms, commonly called the oxygen cost of breathing. Normal quiet breathing requires only about 5% of the total resting oxygen consumption. In disease processes in which compliance or resistance is affected, the oxygen cost of breathing can increase markedly, to as much as 25% of total oxygen consumption. A considerable portion of the total body energy expenditure may be required to maintain respiratory efforts, carbon dioxide production may exceed alveolar ventilation, and respiratory acidosis may ensue.

PERFUSION
Distribution of Perfusion in the Lung

It is commonly believed that the distribution of perfusion is even throughout the lung; however, this is not true. There are two significant factors that lead to the natural, uneven distribution of perfusion within the lung. These factors are the interplay of arterial, venous, and alveolar pressures within the pulmonary system and gravitational forces.

When a human being is standing upright, blood flow increases linearly down the lung, in such a way that it is greatest in the bases. This changes with alterations in body position; thus, when one is lying supine, blood flow is greatest in the posterior lung zones, and when one is lying on one's side, blood flow is greatest in the dependent lung (Fig. 2–5). Blood flow is therefore gravity

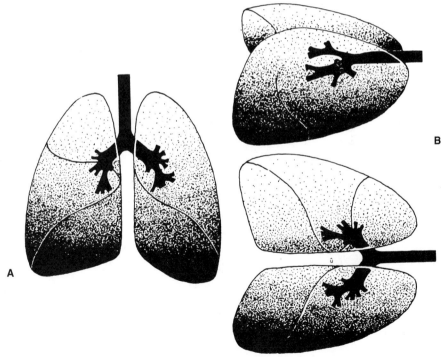

FIGURE 2–5 Blood flow in the lung is gravity dependent in nature. The greatest percentage of blood is in the most dependent lung regions. This is true regardless of body position, as shown in the erect (A), supine (B), and lateral decubitus (C) positions. (From Shapiro, B.A., et al.: *Clinical Application of Blood Gases*. 4th ed. Chicago: Year Book Medical Publishers, 1989.)

dependent in nature, and the hydrostatic pressure differences within the blood vessels explain the regional differences in perfusion distribution. Understanding these pressure differences and their effect on perfusion distribution is explained in a model of three lung zones described by West (Fig. 2–6).

An underlying principle of West's model is that alveolar pressure remains relatively constant down the lung, whereas there is a vertical gradient to pulmonary arterial and venous pressures. Pressure within the alveoli easily influences the adjacent pulmonary capillaries because they have such thin walls. Indeed, the capillaries may actually become compressed during mechanical ventilation when alveolar pressure is high, as when tidal volumes are too large or maldistributed or inflating pressures are high.

The apices of the lungs represent zone I, a region above the heart and therefore not well perfused because alveolar pressure may exceed arterial pressure. If alveolar pressure rises, as may occur with positive-pressure ventilation, or if arterial pressure falls, as in hemorrhage or other causes of decreased perfusion pressure, then no flow will occur in zone I. The absence of flow in areas where ventilation is intact is known as alveolar dead space, or wasted ventilation.

Zone II is the middle portion of the lung. Perfusion through zone II lung areas is dependent on the pressure difference between the pulmonary arteries and the alveolar pressure. Because perfusion is now occurring at the level of the heart, arterial pressures are higher and the lung is better perfused.

In zone III, venous pressure exceeds alveolar pressure; perfusion is therefore determined by the usual mechanism of the arterial-venous pressure differ-

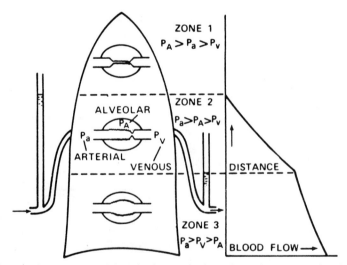

FIGURE 2–6 Three-zone model of the lung, which explains the uneven distribution of blood flow in the lung. The basis of this model is that alveolar and pulmonary venous pressures both affect capillary perfusion pressure. In the patient who is lying supine, the three lung zones, obeying gravitational laws, occur at right angles to that shown above. See text for explanation. (From West J.B.: *Respiratory Physiology: The Essentials*. 3rd ed. Baltimore: Williams & Wilkins, 1985.)

ence. Perfusion is greatest in zone III because of gravitational, or hydrostatic, forces.

Overall lung perfusion increases during exercise or other causes of increased cardiac output. The distribution of perfusion is also influenced by several therapies used in critically ill patients, such as positive end-expiratory pressure, vasodilators, and inotropic agents.

Pulmonary Vascular Resistance

The pulmonary circulation is a high-volume, low-pressure system. The entire cardiac output is received into the pulmonary circulation from the right side of the heart at a systolic pressure of 25 mm Hg and a diastolic pressure of 8 mm Hg. The result is a mean perfusion pressure of 15 mm Hg, compared with a mean systemic pressure of 100 mm Hg. The resistance in the pulmonary circuit is only one tenth that of the systemic circuit. As a result of this low-pressure system, the work of the right side of the heart is kept small and the entire cardiac output is perfused with minimal pressure over the vast vascular surface area of the pulmonary circulation.

Pulmonary vascular resistance (PVR) can be calculated if the patient has a pulmonary artery catheter in place. Resistance in the pulmonary vasculature is determined by measuring the pressure at the beginning of the circuit (mean pulmonary artery pressure) minus the pressure at the end of the circuit (pulmonary capillary wedge pressure) and dividing by flow rate (cardiac output).

$$\text{Pulmonary vascular resistance (PVR)} = \frac{\text{PA} - \text{PCWP}}{\text{CO}} \times 80$$

$$\text{Normal} = <250 \text{ dyn} \cdot \sec \cdot \text{cm}^{-5}$$

where PA is the mean pulmonary artery pressure, PCWP is the pulmonary capillary wedge pressure, 80 is the factor used to convert units of measure from millimeters of mercury per liter per minute, to dynes per second per centimeter^{-5}, and CO is cardiac output.

Regulation of the PVR occurs even though the pulmonary capillaries do not contain a significant amount of muscle. Recall that in a resting state all the pulmonary capillaries are not perfused. Alteration in the number of vessels perfused (capillary recruitment) and alteration in the amount of perfusion that any given vessel receives (capillary distention) are two main mechanisms of maintaining a low pressure in the pulmonary vascular system (Fig. 2–7).

Hypoxic Vasoconstriction

A second unique characteristic of the pulmonary circulation is its response to changing respiratory gas tensions. The effects of changing PO_2 and PCO_2 are opposite to the effects in the systemic circulation. Pulmonary blood vessels dilate in response to increased PO_2. Conversely, the response to alveolar hypoxia is potent pulmonary vasoconstriction, known as hypoxic pulmonary vasoconstriction. This response increases pulmonary vascular resistance and can significantly increase the work of the right side of the heart—that is, the right heart afterload

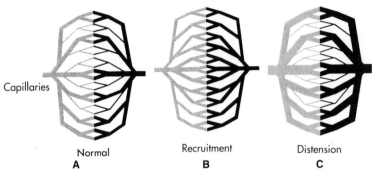

Capillaries

| Normal | Recruitment | Distension |
| A | B | C |

FIGURE 2–7   Physiologic mechanisms that assist in maintaining a low pulmonary vascular resistance (PVR). (A) In the normal lung, some capillaries are minimally perfused. (B) The mechanism of *recruitment* calls in more capillaries to conduct blood when the pulmonary artery pressure rises. This is the main mechanism for decreasing PVR. (C) Capillary *distention* occurs with increasing pressure or cardiac output. A distended capillary offers less resistance to blood flow. (From Dettenmeir, P.A.: *Pulmonary Nursing Care.* St. Louis: Mosby–Year Book, 1992.)

is increased. However, this mechanism is important in maintaining homeostasis in gas exchange. Vasoconstriction, in areas of low alveolar PO_2, diverts blood flow toward alveoli with more optimal oxygen tensions, thereby better matching perfusion to the well-ventilated areas. The overall result is improved gas exchange. For example, if a patient has a left lower lobe (LLL) pneumonia, ventilation to this area of the lung will be decreased and alveolar oxygen tension in the LLL will therefore be decreased. Hypoxic vasoconstriction will occur in this lung region, diverting blood flow to areas of adequate alveolar ventilation and thus improving overall gas exchange. Other humoral factors that may affect pulmonary vascular tone are outlined in Box 2–1.

Box 2–1   Factors Affecting Pulmonary Vascular Resistance

Increase (Pulmonary Constrictors)	*Decrease (Pulmonary Dilators)*
Low alveolar oxygen tension	Oxygen
Hypercapnia	Hypocapnia
Acidosis	Alkalosis
Hypothermia	Beta-adrenergic agonists
Sympathetic stimulation	Isoproterenol
Alpha-adrenergic agonists	Dobutamine
Norepinephrine	Sodium nitroprusside
Increased pulmonary blood flow	Nitroglycerin
Increased airway pressure	Prostaglandin E_1
Pulmonary embolism	Theophylline
Angiotensin II	

DIFFUSION

Once the gas reaches the alveoli, the next process of external respiration, diffusion, begins. Diffusion is the movement of gas molecules from an area of relatively high partial pressure to one of low partial pressure. The driving force for the molecules is the pressure gradient of the gases across the alveolar-capillary (A-C) membrane. The normal pathway that gas molecules must travel at the A-C membrane is illustrated in Chapter 1 (Fig. 1–9). Factors affecting diffusion include the total surface area of the A-C membrane, the thickness of the tissue through which the gases must diffuse, the diffusion coefficient of the gas (how readily the gas diffuses relative to the other gases in the solution), and the difference in partial pressure of the gases between the two sides of the membrane.

Factors that decrease surface area, such as significant pulmonary vascular disease or lobectomy, may decrease the diffusion of gases. However, the lung has a tremendous surface area for gas exchange, approximately 70 square meters. Disease processes that increase the thickness of the A-C membrane and thus increase the diffusion distance for gases include pulmonary edema and chronic lung conditions that cause fibrotic changes.

Both oxygen and carbon dioxide diffuse readily across the A-C membrane. Carbon dioxide diffuses 20 times more readily than oxygen; factors that adversely affect diffusion are therefore less likely to affect the diffusion of carbon dioxide than that of oxygen. Despite the many factors that may affect diffusion, gas exchange is completed by the time the red blood cell is only one third of the way along the capillary: about 0.3 to 0.4 second. Because the red blood cell is in the pulmonary capillary almost a full second at rest, there is an enormous reserve time for gas exchange to take place. Only when accompanied by other factors that adversely affect diffusion, such as illness or exercise, would very high cardiac output states adversely affect diffusion.

The final factor that affects diffusion, the partial pressure of gases across the A-C membrane, warrants further discussion. To understand diffusion gradients, one must become familiar with the normal partial pressures of gas in the inspired air, the alveolus, and the pulmonary capillary (Fig. 2–8).

Inspired air at sea level has a total pressure of 760 mm Hg. Each gas in inspired air—oxygen (O_2), carbon dioxide (CO_2), and nitrogen (N_2)—exerts a partial pressure, which is determined by the percentage of that gas in relation to the total gases. For example, oxygen, which is 21% of inspired air, exerts a partial pressure of 159 mm Hg. Once the air is inspired, it is warmed and humidified by the upper airway and the partial pressure of the water vapor becomes 47 mm Hg. Since the total partial pressure can still be only 760 mm Hg, the partial pressure of all the other gases must change by the time they become alveolar gases. Furthermore, the partial pressure of alveolar gases (P_A) is affected by the fact that inspired air is mixed with gases already in the alveoli, because exhalation does not result in complete emptying of the alveolus.

Respiratory gases in the pulmonary blood exert partial pressures as well. Venous blood returning from the tissue beds of the body normally has partial pressures of gases that reflect tissue use of oxygen and excretion of carbon dioxide: Pv_{O_2} = 40 mm Hg, Pv_{CO_2} = 46 mm Hg, pH = 7.36, and Sa_{O_2} = 75%.

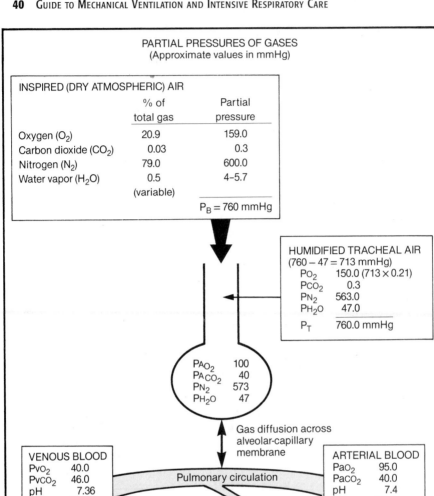

Figure 2-8 Partial pressures of dry inspired and humidified tracheal and alveolar gases. Alveolar pressures are in millimeters of mercury at sea level under BTPS conditions (body temperature of 37° C, ambient pressure, and saturated with water vapor). Also shown are the partial pressures of gases in the venous and arterial blood. (From Kersten, L.D.: *Comprehensive Respiratory Nursing*. Philadelphia: W.B. Saunders, 1989.)

This review of the partial pressures of gases in the alveolus and the pulmonary capillary shows that a pressure gradient exists for the movement of oxygen from the alveolus into the pulmonary capillary and for the movement of carbon dioxide from the capillary into the alveolus. Under normal conditions, complete equilibration of gases occurs at the A-C membrane; the partial pressures of alveolar and arterial gases are therefore assumed to be the same.

The blood, after traversing the pulmonary capillaries, travels to the left atrium. There the venous blood from the bronchial circulation, which is not oxygenated, is mixed with the arterialized blood, which is in equilibrium with the alveolar gas. This has the effect of decreasing the partial pressure of oxygen in arterial blood relative to that in the alveolus. This alveolar-arterial gradient (A-a gradient), called the anatomic shunt, is normally 10 mm Hg in healthy individuals.

Though many factors can affect the diffusion of gases at the A-C membrane, the lung has significant diffusion reserve, which promotes remarkable function even in disease. Factors other than diffusion defects, such as ventilation/perfusion inequalities, are the major contributors to abnormal gas exchange in the lung.

VENTILATION/PERFUSION RELATIONSHIPS

Distribution of Ventilation and Perfusion in the Lung

The ratio of alveolar ventilation ($\dot{V}$) to pulmonary blood flow ($\dot{Q}$) determines the composition of the gas leaving the lung. Ideally, each alveolus would be matched to well-perfused capillaries, leading to a $\dot{V}/\dot{Q}$ ratio of 1.0; however, ventilation and perfusion are not equally distributed throughout the lung. Recall that perfusion is greater at the base than at the apex of the lung. This is due to gravitational forces; therefore, if the patient changes body position, blood flow will always be greatest in the most dependent lung regions.

Ventilation also increases linearly down the lung in the spontaneously breathing individual. This is due to regional differences in lung compliance that result from regional differences in intrapleural pressure. The lung hangs in the thoracic cavity in such a way that the weight of the lung is greatest at its base. The result is an intrapleural pressure of about -10 cm H_2O at the apex of the lung and about -2 cm H_2O at the base (Fig. 2–9). The alveoli at the apex are far more expanded and have a larger resting volume, so that with inspiration there is relatively less change in volume in these apical alveoli. At the base of the lung, the alveoli have a smaller resting volume and, on inspiration, the transpulmonary pressure change is greater; therefore more volume is distributed to the base of the lung.

Regional differences in ventilation and perfusion result in relatively greater ventilation than perfusion at the apex of the lung, making the $\dot{V}/\dot{Q}$ ratio high (3.0). Perfusion, however, is relatively greater than ventilation at the bases, making the $\dot{V}/\dot{Q}$ ratio low (0.6).

Normal $\dot{V}/\dot{Q}$ Ratio

The *overall* $\dot{V}/\dot{Q}$ ratio represents an average of all the ratios throughout the lung. Normally, alveolar ventilation is 4 L/min, whereas cardiac output is 5 L/min. The $\dot{V}/\dot{Q}$ ratio for the whole lung, then, averages 4/5, or 0.8, despite regional differences. Normal pulmonary gas exchange is dependent on this ratio of ventilation to perfusion in the lung. Disturbances in this $\dot{V}/\dot{Q}$ ratio, which include shunt and dead space units, account for the abnormal arterial blood gas values in most respiratory disorders (Fig. 2–10).

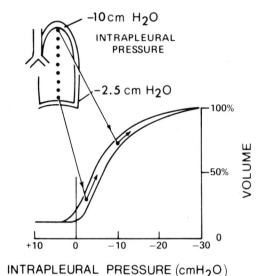

FIGURE 2-9 Ventilation down the lung and the reason it varies regionally. The weight of the lung hanging in the thorax creates greater negative pressure at the apex than at the base. At the apex there is less change in transpulmonary pressure on inspiration, relative to the base, and consequently less change in volume. Therefore, in spontaneously breathing man, ventilation is preferentially distributed to the base of the lung. This is true regardless of body position. (From West J.B.: *Ventilation/Blood Flow and Gas Exchange.* 3rd ed. Baltimore: Williams & Wilkins, 1977.)

$\dot{V}/\dot{Q}$ INEQUALITIES

Low $\dot{V}/\dot{Q}$: Shunt ($\dot{Q}s/\dot{Q}T$)

One type of $\dot{V}/\dot{Q}$ inequality is known as shunt. Shunt occurs when blood enters the arterial system without perfusing ventilated areas of the lung. There are two types of shunt: anatomic and physiologic. Anatomic shunt has been discussed previously. It is the 2% to 5% of the cardiac output that normally bypasses the pulmonary arterial system. This blood is part of the bronchial, pleural, and coronary circulations. *Physiologic shunt* occurs when pulmonary blood flow is adequate but the alveolus is not well ventilated. In effect, perfusion is wasted.

Shunt is the most common cause of hypoxemia in the critical care setting. This hypoxemia results in increased myocardial and ventilatory work. Blood passes through the lungs; however, in some lung regions it never interfaces with well-ventilated alveoli and therefore is not oxygenated. It is for this reason that in pure shunt the administration of supplemental oxygen will not result in an increase in PaO_2. Increasing the PO_2 to those alveoli that are well ventilated does not help either, because the hemoglobin molecules traversing these alveoli are already carrying their maximum capacity of oxygen. Causes of shunt include atelectasis, consolidative-infiltrative disease processes, bronchospasm, and the use of vasodilators, which overcomes hypoxic vasoconstriction when this compensatory mechanism is in place.

It is possible to quantify the percentage of shunt in the clinical setting. Calculation of this percentage can be useful as a baseline measure. Then, after the

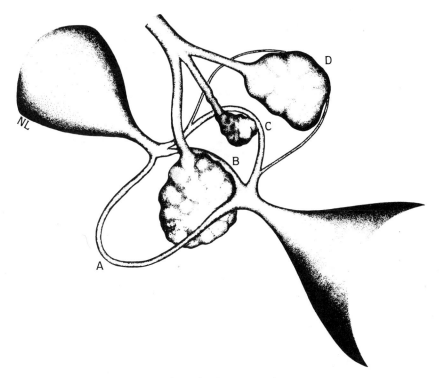

Figure 2-10 Spectrum of ventilation/perfusion matching in the lung. A, Anatomic shunt: blood flow through nonventilated areas. B, Normal matching of ventilation and perfusion. C, Shunt: perfusion in excess of ventilation. D, Dead space: ventilation in excess of perfusion. (Modified from Wilkins, R.L., Sheldon, R.L., and Krider, S.J.: *Clinical Assessment in Respiratory Care*. 2nd ed. St. Louis: C.V. Mosby, 1990.)

abnormality causing the shunt has been determined and treatment initiated, additional measures can facilitate evaluation of the effects of therapy, and plotting the trend of measures can help guide the therapeutic plan and its revision, if necessary.

The form of shunt that is due to $\dot{V}/\dot{Q}$ mismatching caused by disease, and the one we want to measure, is physiologic shunt. There are several methods of measuring shunt. The shunt equation, however, is the gold standard, the truest measure of physiologic shunt (Fig. 2–11). It requires a pulmonary artery (PA) catheter to determine oxygen content of mixed venous blood. The use of a PA catheter is not indicated in all patients, and therefore the estimated shunt equation (see below) was developed as an alternative method of trending the changes in the physiologic shunt. In this equation the arterial-venous oxygen content difference (a-vDo$_2$) is assumed to be 3.5 vol%. This value is representative of the a-vDo$_2$ of the critically ill patient with an adequate cardiovascular reserve.

$$\dot{Q}s/\dot{Q}T = \frac{(Cc_{O_2} - Ca_{O_2})}{3.5 + Cc_{O_2} - Ca_{O_2}}$$

This equation is useful when the patient does not have a PA catheter in place. The equation assumes cardiovascular stability. The estimated shunt has a

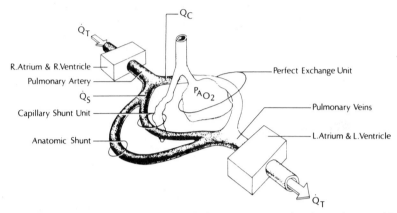

FIGURE 2–11 Calculation of intrapulmonary shunt using arterial and mixed venous blood samples:

$$\dot{Q}_S/\dot{Q}_T = \frac{(Cc_{O_2} - Ca_{O_2})}{(Cc_{O_2} - C\bar{v}_{O_2})}$$

Where: Cc_{O_2} = oxygen content of pulmonary capillary blood, which mathematically represents the portion of the cardiac output that exchanges perfectly with alveolar air

Ca_{O_2} = oxygen content of arterial blood

$C\bar{v}_{O_2}$ = oxygen content of mixed venous blood.

Shunted blood ($\dot{Q}_S$) is expressed as a ratio of the total blood flow ($\dot{Q}_T$). Normal value = 2% to 5%. A percent shunt of 28%, for example, would indicate that 28% of the cardiac output traveled through the lungs without the occurrence of oxygenation. (From Shapiro, B.A., et al.: *Clinical Application of Blood Gases*. 4th ed. Chicago: Year Book Medical Publishers, 1989.)

stronger correlation to the measured shunt than other shunt indices primarily because the calculation utilizes oxygen content rather than tension.

In an effort to try to find an equation that can be used when the patient does not have a PA catheter, gas exchange indices that use oxygen tension rather than oxygen content measures have been developed. Shunt calculations using oxygen tension variables have all been shown only to estimate the shunt and may be unreliable with changes in FIO_2. If this fact is kept in mind, then the use of these equations has their place in the clinical setting. The use of oxygen tension (Pa_{O_2}) in calculating shunt is based on comparing what the Pa_{O_2} should be, on a particular FIO_2, with its actual value. Box 2–2 provides examples of these equations.

In some settings, as part of the assessment of the adequacy of oxygenation, the alveolar-arterial gradient (PA-a_{O_2}) is calculated. The normal value, 10 mm Hg when a patient is breathing room air and 100 mm Hg when breathing 100% oxygen, is due to normal $\dot{V}/\dot{Q}$ differences down the lung and the normal small physiologic shunt. The normal value increases with age because of airway closure at the bases in older individuals, caused by loss of elastic recoil, and can be calculated by the following equation: $2.5 + (0.43 \times age)$. An increase in the A-a gradient is strictly an indication that there is a defect in oxygenation ability. It is not a specific measure of shunt. In fact, of the estimated shunt equations, the

Box 2-2 Gas Exchange Indices Used to Estimate Physiologic Shunt

1. *Arterial/Alveolar Ratio (a/A Ratio):*

$$\frac{PaO_2}{PAO_2}$$

PAO_2 is calculated by the alveolar air equation:

$$PAO_2 = FIO_2 (PB - PH_2O) - PaCO_2/0.8$$

Where: PB =   Barometric pressure
         PH_2O =   Vapor pressure of water at 37° C (the value of
                      which is 47 mm Hg)
           0.8 =   Assumed respiratory quotient (ratio of CO_2 pro-
                      duction to oxygen consumption)

Normal value for the a/A ratio is 0.8, meaning that 80% of the alveolar oxygen is reaching the arterial system.

Moderate shunt = 0.50 − 0.80
Significant shunt = 0.25 − 0.50
Critical shunt = <0.25

The a/A ratio remains relatively stable with changes in the FIO_2. Calculation can be used to predict the FIO_2 required for a desired PaO_2.

2. *PaO_2/FIO_2 Ratio:*

Normal ratio is 550 (a person breathing FIO_2 of 1.0 at sea level should have a PaO_2 of 550 to 600 mm Hg). The obtained value is subtracted from the normal value (550), and for every difference of 100 the shunt is 5%.
Example:

PaO_2 of 68 on FIO_2 of 0.4,
68 mm Hg/0.4 FIO_2 = 1.7, then
1.7 × 100 = 170 (estimation of PaO_2 on 100% oxygen)
550 − 170 = 380, then
380/100 = 3.8, then
3.8 × 5 = 19% shunt

The percent shunt can also be roughly estimated from the PaO_2/FIO_2 ratio as follows:

500 ≈ 5% shunt
300 ≈ 15% shunt
200 ≈ 20% shunt

3. *A-a Gradient (on 100% O_2):*

$$PAO_2 - PaO_2$$

Where: PAO_2 is calculated by the alveolar air equation previously presented. The patient must receive 100% oxygen for at least 15 minutes to eliminate all other causes of A-a gradient other than shunt. Ideally, the PAO_2 would be near 670, with the PaO_2 close to 550.
Every 20 mm Hg difference is equal to a 1% shunt.

A-a gradient is the weakest predictor. The gradient also changes unpredictably with changes in FIO_2.

If the A-a gradient is normal in the presence of hypoxemia, the cause is hypoventilation. If hypoxemia is accompanied by an increase in the gradient, the cause may be anatomic right-to-left shunt, diffusion limitation, or $\dot{V}/\dot{Q}$ inequality. Therefore an increase in the A-a gradient alerts one to a problem in oxygenation; however, the cause of the problem may fall within any of the previously mentioned categories. If the problem is shunt and the FIO_2 is increased, there will be no change in the PaO_2, whereas the PaO_2 should increase in a diffusion defect.

One clinical use of the A-a gradient is to determine whether the cause of hypoxemia accompanied by hypercapnia is simply due to hypoventilation alone, or to hypoventilation complicated by another disease process affecting pulmonary function. In the patient with both hypoxemia and hypercapnia, if the A-a gradient is normal, the cause is hypoventilation alone. If the A-a gradient is increased, a complicating process such as pneumonia, pulmonary edema, or atelectasis is present.

High $\dot{V}/\dot{Q}$: Dead Space (V_D/V_T)

In the second type of $\dot{V}/\dot{Q}$ inequality, ventilation is present but the alveoli are poorly perfused; in effect, ventilation is wasted. This is known as dead space ventilation. There are two types of dead space: anatomic and physiologic. Anatomic dead space, as discussed previously, is the amount of air in the conducting airways. It is normally about 2 ml/kg, or approximately 150 ml. Though the anatomic dead space in any one individual is a fixed volume, in shallow breathing a greater percentage of the inspired volume will be ventilation to the anatomic dead space. Physiologic dead space occurs when ventilation is normal but perfusion to some alveoli is reduced or absent. Either there is not enough blood, or the blood is blocked from reaching the alveoli. Causes of physiologic dead space include pulmonary embolus; decreased pulmonary perfusion, as in low cardiac output or acute pulmonary hypertension; mechanical ventilation with large tidal volumes or pressures that overdistend the alveoli to such a degree that alveolar pressure exceeds capillary pressure; and diseases in which extensive capillary damage and intravascular coagulation occur, such as sepsis, burns, or adult respiratory distress syndrome. Dead space increases the $PaCO_2$ because the blood carrying the CO_2 back from the tissues does not interface with the alveolus. Increased dead space demands an increased minute ventilation and therefore an increase in the work of breathing if a normal $PaCO_2$ is to be maintained.

Measurements of dead space ventilation that can be performed in the clinical setting are illustrated in Box 2–3. Measurement of end-tidal CO_2, required in equation 1 (Box 2–3), is further explained in Chapter 9.

EFFECT OF BODY POSITION ON $\dot{V}/\dot{Q}$ MATCHING

Body position may affect gas exchange by altering the matching of ventilation to perfusion in the lung. Postural variations in gas exchange may be clinically significant, particularly in patients with unilateral or asymmetric lung disease. Improved oxygenation has been demonstrated in patients with predominantly unilateral lung disease from various causes by positioning the patient in the lateral

---

Box 2–3   Measurements of Dead Space Ventilation

---

1. *Arterial/Alveolar* P_{CO_2} *Gradient (a-A P_{CO_2}):*

$$\text{Arterial } P_{CO_2} - \text{Alveolar } P_{CO_2}$$

Where: Alveolar P_{CO_2} is measured by means of end-tidal P_{CO_2}. Normal gradient is an alveolar P_{CO_2} 2 mm Hg less than arterial. Acute increase reflects increase in physiologic dead space.

2. *Minute Ventilation ($\dot{V}_E$) — Pa_{CO_2} Disparity:*

When an increase in the $\dot{V}_E$ is not associated with the expected decrease in Pa_{CO_2}, dead space ventilation should be suspected. An increase in the metabolic rate (and thus production of CO_2) must be ruled out. This is useful clinically because it does not require measurement of exhaled CO_2.

3. *Dead Space/Tidal Volume Ratio:*

$$V_D/V_T = \frac{Pa_{CO_2} - P_{E_{CO_2}}}{Pa_{CO_2}}$$

Where: Pa_{CO_2} = partial pressure of CO_2 in arterial blood
$P_{E_{CO_2}}$ = partial pressure of CO_2 in expired air

Normal value = 0.25–0.40 (25%–40%).
The total exhaled gases must be collected into a large balloon for a 5-minute period. The patient must have a constant respiratory pattern; therefore, this measurement is most accurately taken when controlled modes of ventilation are used. The metabolic rate must be in a steady state. If the V_D/V_T ratio is 0.6 or greater, an attempt to wean the patient from the ventilator will usually be unsuccessful because ventilatory reserve will generally be exceeded by the necessary increase in $\dot{V}_E$.

---

decubitus position, where the more healthy lung is dependent (good lung down). Improved oxygenation is attributed to positionally induced enhancement of the matching of ventilation to perfusion. This conclusion has been supported by investigators who have demonstrated a decrease in the percentage of shunt when the patient is positioned with the good lung down. Therefore an awareness of the effect of changes in position on pulmonary ventilation and perfusion may permit therapeutic application of patient positioning.

Perfusion, being gravity dependent in nature, is greatest to the less diseased lung when that lung is placed in the dependent position. Ventilation, because it is preferentially distributed to areas of best compliance and least resistance, will also be best in the dependent lung. The duration of the immediate effect of body position on gas exchange is unpredictable. A patient with unilateral disease who initially shows enhanced oxygenation with the good lung down may demonstrate a gradual fall in oxygenation during a period in which the position is maintained. The mechanism responsible for this deterioration is atelectasis and airway closure by secretions that gradually migrate from the upper lung into the more dependent, and previously relatively less diseased, lung; this leads to a fall in PaO_2. In the mechanically ventilated patient, hypoventilation related to three factors may also contribute to a decreasing oxygenation status when the patient is placed in the lateral decubitus position. These three factors are decreased dependent lung motion from mediastinal weight, dependent diaphragm elevation as a result of the weight of the abdominal contents, and relative immobility of the dependent chest wall. Therefore the use of body position to achieve optimal oxygenation requires careful evaluation of individual patient response over time.

There are several clinical implications for the use of therapeutic positioning to enhance oxygenation in patients with predominantly unilateral lung disease. First, having the patient lie in a position with the good lung down will allow ventilation with lower levels of FiO_2 and PEEP. Second, recognition of the phenomenon should help to prevent the diagnostic error of overall worsening respiratory status when, in fact, the arterial blood gas may have been obtained when the patient was positioned in the less favorable lateral position. Third, changing body position without considering its possible ill effects may be life threatening in patients with severe respiratory insufficiency and unilateral involvement.

The efficacy of position changes is widely recognized. In the critical care setting, position changes are often difficult to accomplish effectively because of various tubes, catheters, and other technologic apparatuses that are impediments to movement. Additionally, patients are often required to remain in the supine position for extended periods so that data gathering and treatments may be employed. Nonetheless, even though turning a patient may be cumbersome, if done properly it has far fewer detrimental effects on the patient than relative immobility. In the patient with predominantly unilateral lung disease, the incorporation of chest x-ray interpretation data into the decision to perform the routine patient care intervention of turning the patient ascribes an additional patient benefit to the maneuver: enhancement of oxygenation. Therefore, in selected cases in the intensive care setting, the physiologic basis for turning patients may be related to the distribution of ventilation and perfusion in the lung.

OXYGEN TRANSPORT IN THE BLOOD

Oxygen is transported in the blood in two ways: dissolved in the serum and in combination with hemoglobin. The oxygen dissolved in the serum is measured as the PaO_2. The PaO_2 constitutes only 2% to 3% of the total O_2 transported in the body. There is 0.0031 ml of O_2 dissolved in each 100 ml blood for each 1 mm Hg partial pressure of O_2. Thus, at a PaO_2 of 100 mm Hg, only 0.3 ml of O_2 would be carried per 100 ml of plasma. This is only a very small part of the total oxygen content of the blood. If this were the only method of carrying O_2 in the blood, then the cardiac output would have to be almost 160 L/min to deliver enough oxygen to the tissues to meet resting metabolic needs!

Most oxygen in the body (97% to 98%) is transported to the cells in combination with hemoglobin and is measured as the percentage of O_2 saturation (SaO_2). The percentage of saturation of blood is that portion of the total hemoglobin saturated with O_2. It is a relationship between the amount of O_2 that is carried and the amount that can be carried. Each gram of hemoglobin can transport 1.34 ml of O_2 per 100 ml of blood.

Oxygen binds loosely and reversibly with the heme portion of the hemoglobin molecule. When the PO_2 is high, as at the alveolar-capillary membrane, O_2 readily binds to hemoglobin, forming oxyhemoglobin. At the capillary level, where tissue partial pressures of oxygen are low, hemoglobin readily releases O_2. The relationship between the PaO_2 and the SaO_2 is expressed in an S-shaped curve of great physiologic significance, the oxyhemoglobin dissociation curve (Fig. 2–12).

The affinity, or strength of the bond, between hemoglobin and oxygen is affected by various physiologic states that cause the curve to shift to the right or left. The clinical significance is in one's awareness of how these factors affect the patient's ability to unload oxygen at the tissue level. The affinity of hemoglobin is expressed as the PaO_2 value at which 50% of the hemoglobin is saturated (P_{50}). Under standard conditions on the normal curve, the PaO_2 is 27 mm Hg at P_{50}.

Factors that cause a shift of the curve to the left (increase O_2 affinity to hemoglobin) include a decreased H^+ ion concentration, alkalemia, decreased body temperature, and decreased 2,3-diphosphoglycerate (2,3-DPG), which is an intermediate metabolite of glucose that facilitates dissociation of O_2 from hemoglobin at the tissues. A shift to the left results in a lower P_{50}, that is, less oxygen tension is required to saturate 50% of the hemoglobin. Thus, for any given SaO_2, the PaO_2 is lower than it would be on the normal curve. Hemoglobin is not giving up oxygen readily at the tissues.

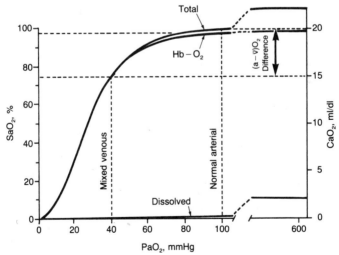

FIGURE 2–12 Oxyhemoglobin dissociation curve, relating the partial pressure of O_2 in arterial blood (PaO_2) to the percentage of hemoglobin saturated with O_2 in the arterial blood (SaO_2). The upper, flat part of the curve is the arterial portion, whereas the steeper part is the venous dissociation portion. The lower line represents O_2 dissolved in the blood. Note that dissolved O_2 contributes very little to total oxygen content (CaO_2). The middle line depicts O_2 bound to hemoglobin at that PaO_2, and the upper line shows a combination of O_2 bound to hemoglobin and dissolved in the blood. (From Luce, J.M., Pierson, D.J., and Tyler, M.L.: *Intensive Respiratory Care*. Philadelphia, W.B. Saunders, 1993.)

Factors that cause a shift of the curve to the right (decrease O_2 affinity to hemoglobin) include an increased H^+ ion concentration, acidemia, increased body temperature, and increased 2,3-DPG. A shift to the right results in a higher P_{50} value, meaning that it takes a higher PaO_2 to saturate 50% of the hemoglobin. When the curve has a right shift, for any given SaO_2 the PaO_2 is higher than it would be on the normal curve because hemoglobin is readily giving up oxygen to the tissues. Under the conditions listed above, especially increased body temperature and acidemia, the ready release of O_2 by hemoglobin is favorable because, under these conditions, oxygen demand at the tissues is higher than normal.

RESPIRATORY CHEMISTRY: ACID-BASE REGULATION

The respiratory and renal systems work constantly to keep the body within a normal acid-base balance that provides a milieu for the optimal function of metabolic processes. Acid-base balance is a reflection of H^+ ion concentration in the body, which is represented by the pH. The pH is the negative logarithm of the concentration of H^+ ions; therefore, as the H^+ ion concentration increases, the pH will decrease and vice versa.

The normal pH (7.35 to 7.45) is maintained by a balance of acid to base in the body. An acid is a substance that liberates H^+ ions when it dissociates in solution. A base is a substance that can bind or accept H^+ ions. Normally the body has 20 acid ions for every base ion. This relationship can be calculated with the Henderson-Hasselbach equation:

$$pH = pK + \log \frac{[HCO_3^-]}{PaCO_2}, \text{ or } \frac{\text{Kidneys}}{\text{Lungs}}, \text{ or } \frac{20}{1}$$

where pK $=$ a constant of 6.1. The Henderson-Hasselbach equation defines the relation between pH, PCO_2, and bicarbonate (HCO_3^-). Bicarbonate is regulated mainly by the kidney, and CO_2 is regulated by the lung. The ratio of bases to acids must remain at 20:1 to maintain a normal pH. When this ratio becomes imbalanced, resulting in an increase in H^+ ions, the pH decreases (becomes <7.35) and the patient is said to have acidemia. The *process* of becoming acidemic is called acidosis (e.g., diabetic ketoacidosis). Conversely, if the ratio of acids to bases in the body is imbalanced in that there is an excess of bases, the pH increases (becomes >7.45) and the patient is said to have alkalemia. The process of becoming alkalemic is correctly termed alkalosis.

Hydrogen ions are added to body fluids as a by-product of metabolic processes. These acids must be eliminated or neutralized by the body so that the patient does not develop acidemia. The hydrogen ion or acid produced is either fixed or volatile. Carbon dioxide is a volatile acid that is eliminated through the respiratory system by means of adequate alveolar ventilation. Fixed acids, such as hydrochloric acid and carbonic acid, must be excreted by the kidney. Therefore the lungs and the kidneys are primary organs in maintaining acid-base regulation.

To some extent, both volatile and fixed acids are neutralized in the body through combination with a base. Conversely, strong bases may be neutralized through combination with weak acids. These processes are called chemical buffering. Chemical buffers, therefore, are substances that minimize changes in pH when either acids or bases are added. Buffer systems occupy various locations in the body. Proteins and phosphates are buffers in the cells, hemoglobin is a buffer in the red blood cells, and bicarbonate, and proteins again, are buffers in the extracellular fluid. The combination of all the buffer systems is called the total buffer base. By far the most important buffer system is the bicarbonate buffer system (Fig. 2–13), because it accounts for more than half of total buffering.

The respiratory system controls the carbon dioxide tension of the blood by regulating alveolar ventilation, a process that may very quickly correct an acid-base disturbance. Alveolar ventilation (V_A) is the volume of gas within the respiratory bronchioles and alveolar ducts (i.e., the respiratory zone of the lung). The V_A does not reflect the volume of gas moved into and out of the mouth. The volume of gas moved into and out of the mouth per minute, the minute ventilation ($\dot{V}_E$), consists of the alveolar ventilation plus the dead-space ventilation. Therefore, $V_A = \dot{V}_E - V_D$. V_A strives to maintain the Pa_{CO_2} at 35 to 45 mm Hg (eucapnia).

Hypoventilation, or decreased alveolar ventilation, results in excessive acid. When the Pa_{CO_2} is >45 mm Hg, hypercapnia is present. If the pH is <7.35 and the Pa_{CO_2} is >45 mm Hg, the patient is said to have *respiratory acidosis*. Hyperventilation, or increased alveolar ventilation, causes acids to be blown off. When the Pa_{CO_2} is <35 mm Hg, hypocapnia is present, a condition known as *respiratory alkalosis* when the pH is >7.45. It is important to note that hyperventilation is not synonymous with a rapid respiratory rate. For example, the patient may be breathing 40 times per minute and still have a Pa_{CO_2} of 50 mm Hg.

The kidneys defend blood pH by controlling bicarbonate concentration. This is accomplished by excretion of hydrogen ions in the urine when the blood is too acidic, and excretion of bicarbonate in the urine when the blood is too alkaline. It may take hours to days for the kidney to affect pH.

If there is an abnormal rise in HCO_3^- concentration in the serum or a significant loss of hydrogen ions, accompanied by a pH of >7.45, the patient is said to have *metabolic alkalosis*. Conversely, if there is a loss of bicarbonate or a rise in hydrogen ions or both, accompanied by a pH of <7.35, the patient has *metabolic acidosis*. Causes, symptoms, and treatment of respiratory and metabolic acidosis and alkalosis are shown in Table 2–3.

Compensation refers to a return of the blood pH back to normal by the lungs or the kidneys. The system, respiratory or renal, opposite the primary disorder will attempt the compensation. For example, in respiratory alkalosis the body will first attempt to compensate by decreasing alveolar ventilation. However, hypoventilation cannot occur to a significant degree because hypoxemia will eventually stimulate the drive to breathe. The renal system will then attempt to com-

$$\text{Lungs} \qquad\qquad\qquad\qquad\qquad\qquad\qquad \text{Kidneys}$$
$$\nwarrow \qquad\qquad\qquad \text{CA} \qquad\qquad\qquad\qquad \nearrow$$
$$CO_2 + H_2O \rightleftharpoons H_2CO_3 \rightleftharpoons H^+ + HCO_3^-$$

FIGURE 2–13 Bicarbonate buffer system. Carbonic acid (H_2CO_3) is formed by the combination of carbon dioxide (CO_2) to water (H_2O) in the presence of the enzyme carbonic anhydrase (CA). Carbonic acid then quickly dissociates into hydrogen and bicarbonate (HCO_3^-). The bicarbonate buffering system then operates by using the lungs to regulate CO_2 and the kidneys to regulate HCO_3^-.

pensate for the respiratory acid-base imbalance by excreting HCO_3^-. If the compensation is *complete*, the pH will be returned to normal. If the compensation is *partial*, then the pH will be working its way toward normal. The body does not overcompensate.

TABLE 2–3   Causes, Symptoms, and Treatment of Acid-Base Disturbances

Disturbance	Causes	Symptoms	Treatment
Respiratory acidosis	Hypoventilation, acute process aggravating chronic lung disease, severe obesity, respiratory center depression (e.g., stroke, head trauma, drug overdose), respiratory neuromuscular disease, airway obstruction	Acute CO_2 retention: confusion, lethargy, stupor, coma	Decrease hypoventilation: treat underlying cause; cough and deep breathing, IPPB, incentive spirometry, bronchodilators, intubation, and mechanical ventilation
Respiratory alkalosis	Hyperventilation, hypoxemia, anxiety reaction, CNS irritation (e.g., central hyperventilation), metabolic acidosis, excessive artificial ventilation	Complaints of shortness of breath, anxiety, muscle cramps, tetany, perioral tingling, seizures	Decrease alveolar ventilation: sedation, improve oxygenation, rebreather bag, change ventilator settings (decrease RR or tidal volume)
Metabolic acidosis	Excessive acids: diabetic ketoacidosis, renal failure, lactic acidosis, starvation, salicylate overdose, ethylene glycol	Kussmaul respirations (deep, rapid), disorientation, restlessness, coma	Treat underlying abnormality
	Bicarbonate loss: diarrhea, pancreatic, biliary, or small bowel fluid loss; renal disease		Replace HCO_3^-
Metabolic alkalosis	Loss of acids: emesis, nasogastric suction (chloride will be lost as well)	Apathy, mental confusion, shallow breathing, tetany, spastic muscles	Control emesis or GI losses; if unable to control, replace chloride with Ringer's lactate solution or sodium chloride. Chloride replacement allows HCO_3^- to exit the cell to be excreted. Reduce use of alkaline antacids; monitor diuretic use, administer acetazolamide to increase renal HCO_3^- excretion, correct potassium depletion
	Excessive base: overuse of antacids, milk of magnesia, or $NaHCO_3^-$; citrate in blood transfusions, lactate in hyperalimentation		
	Diuretic therapy resulting in K^+, Na^+, and Cl^- losses; H^+ moves into cell, HCO_3^- concentration increases		

IPPB = Intermittent positive-pressure breathing; CNS = central nervous system; RR = respiratory rate; GI = gastrointestinal.

INTERPRETATION OF ARTERIAL BLOOD GASES

Using the information about respiratory chemistry presented above, and given an arterial blood gas (ABG) measurement, you should be able to determine whether the primary disturbance of acid-base imbalance is respiratory or metabolic. An ABG measurement provides more information than just the acid-base balance. It also enables one to assess the adequacy of oxygenation and ventilation. Before one can proceed to determination of abnormalities, it is essential to know the normal values of the variables obtained with an ABG measurement.

Oxygenation is assessed with the PaO_2, the normal value of which is 80 to 100 mm Hg in adults. Hypoxemia is a state in which the PaO_2 is <60 mm Hg, whereas hypoxia is a state in which there is inadequate oxygen at the tissue level. Factors affecting PaO_2 that must be considered in an interpretation of the value include age and altitude, both of which decrease the PaO_2, and the administration of supplemental oxygen. Oxygenation may be further assessed with the SaO_2, the normal value of which is 92% to 100%. At 92% saturation, the PaO_2 is approximately 60 mm Hg; a lower value indicates hypoxemia (see oxyhemoglobin dissociation curve, Fig. 2–12).

Ventilation is assessed with the $PaCO_2$. Normal values have been discussed previously and are reiterated below. Acid-base status is assessed with the pH, $PaCO_2$, HCO_3^-, and the base excess. The base excess (BE) reflects an increase or decrease in the total buffer base. It is an indicator of the metabolic makeup of acid-base disturbances. A decrease in the BE indicates loss of base and metabolic acidosis, whereas an increase in BE indicates metabolic alkalosis. Normal values for the ABG variables are as follows:

	Acidemia	Alkalemia	Hypoxemia
pH: 7.35-7.45	↓	↑	
PaO_2: 80-100 mm Hg			Mild: <80 mm Hg
			Moderate: <70 mm Hg
			Severe: <60 mm Hg
$PaCO_2$: 35-45 mm Hg	↑	↓	
HCO_3^-: 22-26 mEq/L	↓	↑	
BE: −2 to +2 mEq/L	↓	↑	
SaO_2: 92% to 100%			<92%

Systematic analysis of ABG values involves five steps:

1. Begin by looking at each number individually and labeling it. Decide whether the value is high, low, or normal and label the finding; for example, a pH of 7.50 would be high and labeled as alkalemia.
2. Describe the adequacy of oxygenation by assessing the PaO_2 and the SaO_2.
3. Determine acid-base status by assessing the pH.
4. Decide whether the acid-base disorder is respiratory or metabolic. Check the $PaCO_2$ (respiratory) and the HCO_3^- (metabolic) to see which one is altering in the same manner as the pH. Use the base excess to confirm your interpretation, especially when the disorder is mixed. In a mixed disturbance, there is an acid-base imbalance in both systems.

5. Determine the extent of compensation.
   a. Look at the system (respiratory or metabolic) that does not match the pH to determine whether it is moving out of its normal range in an effort to correct the acid-base disturbance.
   b. *Absent:* The value of the opposite system is normal, indicating that no compensation is occurring. The pH is assumed to be abnormal.
   c. *Partial:* If the value that does not match the pH status is above or below the normal range and the pH is still outside the normal range, then partial compensation has occurred.
   d. *Complete:* The value that does not match the pH is above or below normal and the pH is normal.

Examples of Arterial Blood Gases

EXAMPLE 1

pH	7.34	(acidemia)
Pao$_2$	129	(adequate oxygenation)
Paco$_2$	48	(acidemia)
HCO$_3^-$	26	(normal)
BE	+1	(normal)
Sao$_2$	99%	(normal)

Interpretation: Respiratory acidosis with no compensation, adequate oxygenation.

EXAMPLE 2

Patient with chronic bronchitis, emphysema, and cor pulmonale, treated with digitalis and diuretics.

pH	7.40	(normal pH)
Pao$_2$	57	(hypoxemia)
Paco$_2$	58	(acidemia)
HCO$_3^-$	35	(alkalemia)
BE	+9	(alkalemia; use to determine whether the primary disorder is respiratory or metabolic)
Sao$_2$	89%	(hypoxemia)

Interpretation: Metabolic alkalosis with complete respiratory compensation, hypoxemia.

EXAMPLE 3

Sixty-two year old man with history of cancer; status-post abdominal surgery for drainage of abscess.

pH	7.29	(acidemia)
Pao$_2$	192	(normal)
Paco$_2$	40	(normal)
HCO$_3^-$	19	(acidemia)
BE	−5.6	(acidemia)
Sao$_2$	97.5%	(normal)

Interpretation: Metabolic acidosis with no compensation, adequate oxygenation.

EXAMPLE 4

Thirty-four year old man; status-post 85% total body surface area burn in a house fire. Initially presented with a pH of 7.18. Resuscitated with 40 L lactated Ringer's solution and 6 ampules of $NaHCO_3^-$. The patient is sedated, medically paralyzed, and being mechanically ventilated with a $\dot{V}E$ of 17 L/min.

pH	7.37	(normal)
Pao_2	126	(normal)
$Paco_2$	40	(normal)
HCO_3^-	20	(acidemia)
BE	−3.1	(acidemia)
Sao_2	98%	(normal)

Interpretation: Fully compensated metabolic acidosis, adequate oxygenation.

Interpreting ABGs in Terms of $\dot{V}/\dot{Q}$ Mismatches

Abnormalities in $\dot{V}/\dot{Q}$ matching are evident in the patient's ABG values. Low $\dot{V}/\dot{Q}$ units, shunt, cause hypoxemia, whereas high $\dot{V}/\dot{Q}$ units, dead space, result in a rising $Paco_2$. The patient's clinical presentation also provides significant information regarding the possible presence of a $\dot{V}/\dot{Q}$ mismatch.

The patient who initially has an increasing $\dot{V}E$ and a rising $Paco_2$ may have a hypermetabolic or other state resulting in CO_2 production that exceeds the patient's ventilatory capabilities, or they may have increasing dead space. Possible causes of increased dead space have been delineated previously. When dead space increases, the ventilatory demand increases. Of concern to the clinician is what is causing the increased VD/VT and whether the patient has sufficient ventilatory reserve to meet the increased demand. In the following example, both patients have an increased $\dot{V}E$ as a result of increased VD/VT.

	Compensated Patient	Uncompensated Patient
$\dot{V}E$ minute ventil	18	16
$Paco_2$	40	55
pH	7.40	7.33

Only one patient is able to maintain acid-base balance. Both patients are at risk of developing fatigue and ventilatory failure because of the high demands placed on their systems and need to be monitored carefully. However, the uncompensated patient is at higher risk of developing ventilatory failure and likely needs intubation and mechanical ventilation. The underlying mechanism resulting in increased VD/VT (e.g., pulmonary embolus, decreased cardiac output) needs to be determined and appropriate therapy implemented. Treatments of pulmonary emboli include (but are not limited to) low-dose heparin therapy, inferior vena cava interruption of emboli with an umbrella or a bird's nest, and thrombolytic therapy. If the decreased pulmonary perfusion is due to low cardiac output, therapies need to be implemented that will achieve an optimal hemodynamic state. Alveolar overdistention caused by overzealous mechanical ventilation is managed by adjustment of the ventilator settings. Changes may include decreasing the V_T, or changing the flow pattern or ventilatory mode in an effort to decrease the inspiratory pressures.

The patient who has hypoxemia despite supplemental oxygen likely has increasing shunt. Recall that shunt is the most common cause of hypoxemia in the intensive care unit. Many therapies may be implemented in an effort to decrease shunt. Pulmonary hygiene interventions range from cough and deep breathing to therapeutic bronchoscopy; pulmonary edema may be managed partly with diuresis, and bronchospasm with a bronchodilator. If mechanical ventilation is used, PEEP may be used to reexpand the alveoli and decrease physiologic shunt. It must always be remembered, however, that the ventilator serves as a mechanism to support oxygenation and ventilation, not as a primary treatment for ventilation/perfusion abnormalities. Returning the patient to health requires identification and management of the underlying pathology, application of physiologic measures to monitor patient progress, and dynamic revision of the plan of care.

RECOMMENDED READINGS

Ahrens, T. (1989). Blood gas assessment of intrapulmonary shunting and dead space. *Crit Care Nurs Clin North Am* 1(4), 641–648.

Baba, L.N. (1986). *The effect of body position on oxygenation in mechanically ventilated patients with unilateral lung disease.* Unpublished master's thesis, University of Maryland at Baltimore.

Demling, R.H., and Knox, J.B. (1993). Basic concepts of lung function and dysfunction: Oxygenation, ventilation, and mechanics. *New Horizons* 1(3), 362–370.

Dettenmeier, P.A. (1992). *Pulmonary nursing care.* St. Louis: Mosby–Year Book.

Dupuis, Y.G. (1992). Work of breathing. In Y.G. Dupuis (Ed.). *Ventilators: Theory and Clinical Application* (pp. 209–216). 2nd ed. St. Louis: Mosby–Year Book.

Gottlieb, J.E. (1988). Breathing and gas exchange. In M.R. Kinney, D.R. Packa, and S.B. Dunbar (Eds.). *AACN's Clinical Reference for Critical Care Nursing,* (pp. 160–192). 2nd ed. New York: McGraw-Hill.

Kinasewitz, G.T., and Gray, B.A. (1993). Physiology of gas exchange. In R.W. Carlson and M.A. Geheb (Eds.). *Principles and Practice of Medical Intensive Care* (pp. 732–748). Philadelphia: W.B. Saunders.

Luce, J.M., Pierson, D.J., and Tyler, M.L. (1993). *Intensive Respiratory Care.* 2nd ed. Philadelphia: W.B. Saunders.

Marini, J.J. (1990). Strategies to minimize breathing effort during mechanical ventilation. *Crit Care Clin* 6(3), 635–661.

Shapiro, B.A., Harrison, R.A., Cane, R.D., and Kozlowski-Templin, R. (1989). *Clinical Application of Blood Gases.* 4th ed. Chicago: Year Book Medical Publishers.

Tobin, M.J. (1988). State of the art: Respiratory monitoring in the intensive care unit. *Am Rev Respir Dis* 138, 1625–1642.

West, J.B. (1985). *Respiratory Physiology: The Essentials.* 3rd ed. Baltimore: Williams & Wilkins.

Airway Maintenance

The purpose of airway maintenance is to ensure adequate ventilation. Artificial airways may be used to establish patency and control of the airway. Vigilant airway monitoring and possible use of an airway adjunct are indicated in the following circumstances:

- Partial or complete upper airway obstruction
- Prevention of aspiration when upper airway protective reflexes are inadequate
- Facilitation of secretion removal
- Provision of a closed system for the initiation of mechanical ventilation

Assess the patient for adequacy of ventilation. The patient may be making respiratory efforts but not moving sufficient air through the upper airway. There are many causes of upper airway complete or partial obstruction, such as the presence of food, vomitus, secretions, blood, expanding hematoma, and edema. In the patient with a depressed level of consciousness, muscle tone of the upper airway itself may be lost, resulting in an anatomic obstruction.

In partial airway obstruction the patient may present with increased respiratory effort and changes in voice tone. Signs and symptoms may progress to hoarseness and to complaints of difficulty in obtaining enough air. Complete obstruction is an emergency. Patients may grab at their throats and be extremely agitated, or they may have a depressed level of consciousness. The work of breathing is dramatically increased and suprasternal and intercostal retractions may be noted. A classic sign of severe upper airway obstruction is stridor, a shrill, crowing sound made on inspiration.

Many airways are available for airway maintenance. The appropriateness of one over another depends on the specific indications and individual patient considerations. The limitations and complications of each airway must also be considered.

HEAD-TILT TECHNIQUE, WITH CHIN-LIFT OR JAW-THRUST MANEUVER

Indication

When loss of tone in the natural airway is the cause of loss of patency, the head-tilt technique, with the chin-lift or jaw-thrust maneuver, is indicated. When the mandibular muscles lose tone, the tongue falls back, obstructing the

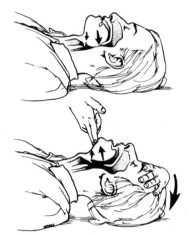

FIGURE 3-1 Opening the airway. (*Top*) When patients are unconscious, upper airway muscle tone is decreased, which leads to obstruction of the airway by the tongue and epiglottis. (*Bottom*) Relief of obstruction by the head-tilt technique with the chin-lift maneuver. (Reproduced with permission. From *Textbook of Advanced Cardiac Life Support*, 1987, 1990. Copyright American Heart Association.)

pharynx, while the epiglottis may occlude the airway at the level of the pharynx. Positioning of the head and jaw reinstates a patent airway.

Technique

The basic technique is to extend the patient's neck, or tilt the head backward into the "sniffing" position. This position is achieved by firmly placing the palm of one hand on the forehead and tilting the head backward. The chin is then brought forward either by lifting it with two fingers or by thrusting the jaw forward with the fingers placed behind the mandible (Fig. 3–1). When pulling the chin forward, ensure that the fingers are not jutted into the soft tissue under the chin, causing the tongue to be pushed farther back into the airway.

NOTE: The head-tilt position is contraindicated in trauma patients for whom the stability of the cervical spine has not been determined. In these patients, use the chin-lift or jaw-thrust maneuver only. If a patent airway is still not established, then use an airway adjunct.

OROPHARYNGEAL AIRWAY

The oropharyngeal airway, which can be made of rubber, metal, or, most commonly, plastic, when it is properly placed, holds the tongue away from the posterior portion of the pharynx. When the device is in position, it curves over the tongue, with its tip in the posterior pharynx (Fig. 3–2).

Indications

The use of the oropharyngeal airway is indicated when the patient has a depressed level of consciousness resulting in loss of muscle tone and airway obstruction. The device is also used to prevent biting, and thus occlusion, of an en-

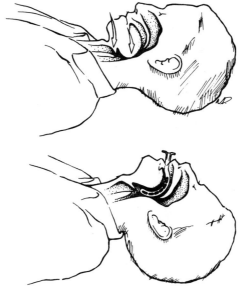

Figure 3-2 When correctly placed, the oropharyngeal airway holds the tongue away from the posterior portion of the pharynx, relieving airway obstruction. *(Top)* Obstructed airway, with incorrect head position. *(Bottom)* Correct head-tilt position and placement of oropharyngeal airway. (Reproduced with permission. From *Textbook of Advanced Cardiac Life Support*, 1987, 1990. Copyright American Heart Association.)

dotracheal tube. It is contraindicated in an awake and alert patient because it may stimulate the gag reflex, creating patient discomfort with possible emesis and aspiration.

Technique

The proper size oropharyngeal airway is chosen by measuring the airway on the patient. When the tip of the oropharyngeal airway is placed at the edge of the patient's mouth, it should extend to the bottom of the ear. An airway that is too short will force the patient's tongue back into the pharynx. An airway that is too long will stimulate the gag reflex.

There are two methods of insertion. The airway may be inserted "upside down," with its tip against the hard palate. The airway is slid into the mouth until the soft palate is reached, at which point it is rotated so that its curvature matches that of the tongue. The tip is advanced to the back of the mouth to ensure its position in the posterior portion of the pharynx. The end of the airway should rest between the teeth but not compress the lips against the teeth, which leads to mucosal trauma. The second method of insertion utilizes a tongue blade to depress the patient's tongue while inserting the airway, matching its curvature with that of the natural curvature of the tongue.

Management Principles

After insertion of the airway, the adequacy of ventilation must be assessed by observation and auscultation of the breath sounds. The chin-lift maneuver should accompany the use of the oropharyngeal airway, if its use is not contraindicated, to provide optimal airway control.

NASOPHARYNGEAL AIRWAY

The nasopharyngeal airway is a soft tube made of rubber or latex that is placed in the nose and extends to the posterior portion of the pharynx. It is sometimes called a nasal trumpet (Fig. 3–3).

Indications

The use of a nasopharyngeal airway is indicated when the patient has a depressed level of consciousness resulting in loss of muscle tone and airway obstruction and when an oropharyngeal airway would be contraindicated or technically difficult to place. Examples include distortion of the oral cavity because of trauma, tight closure of the jaw during a seizure, or closure of the jaw with wire for stabilization post injury. The nasopharyngeal airway is also used to facilitate the passage of a suction catheter, thus reducing nasal trauma when nasopharyngeal suctioning is indicated. This airway may be contraindicated in the presence of coagulopathy because severe epistaxis may result.

Technique

The proper length of the nasopharyngeal tube is chosen by measuring from the nare to the tip of the ear. The internal diameter of the tube will vary with tube length. A tube that is too long may enter into the esophagus and cause gastric distention. If a tube is too short to enter into the posterior portion of the pharynx, a patent airway cannot be established.

To insert the airway, lubricate it with a water-soluble lubricant or water. The correct nare is chosen by positioning the beveled tip to the patient's midline. Insert the airway along the floor of the nose for minimal trauma to the turbinates and minimal discomfort to the patient. Gentle, steady pressure should be used. If

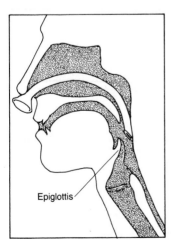

Epiglottis

FIGURE 3–3 The nasopharyngeal airway is used to relieve upper airway obstruction and to facilitate passage of a suction catheter. (From Luce, JM, Pierson, DJ, and Tyler, ML: *Intensive Respiratory Care*. Philadelphia: WB Saunders, 1993.)

resistance is met, then the use of the other nare or a smaller tube should be attempted. When the airway is properly positioned, the flanged portion of the airway will rest against the nare.

Management Principles

Assess the condition of the nares and prevent skin breakdown by pressure necrosis. Immediately after insertion, assess the adequacy of ventilation. Suction the airway if necessary to remove from the lumen any secretions or blood. If adequate ventilation has not been established, recheck head and jaw positions. Use a pocket face mask or manual resuscitation bag and mask to deliver positive-pressure ventilation if necessary.

POCKET FACE MASK

The pocket face mask provides a method of ventilating a patient's lungs that is more aesthetic than mouth-to-mouth ventilation. It does not establish a patent airway and may need to be used with the oropharyngeal or nasopharyngeal airway and/or the head-tilt and chin-lift maneuvers. The pocket face mask is made of a soft plastic material that allows the mask to be compressed into a flat position for storage. When needed, the mask is popped up into its expanded position (Fig. 3–4). Its use eliminates the need for direct contact with the patient's mouth and nose. It provides effective ventilation, placement and technique are easy to teach to individuals of variable skill levels, and some models allow for the supplemental administration of oxygen. For these reasons, placement of a pocket face mask in strategic locations in patient care areas is strongly recommended.

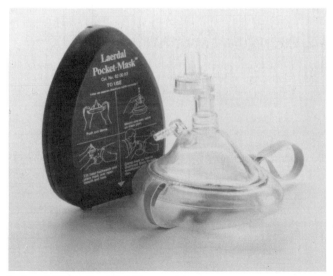

FIGURE 3–4 Laerdal™ Pocket Mask™ in its fully expanded position with filter in place. (Courtesy of Laerdal Medical Corporation, Armonk, N.Y.)

Technique

Pop the mask up into its fully expanded position. Connect the one-way valve and filter to the mask to prevent exposure to exhaled gases. The ideal position from which to approach the patient is from the top of the patient's head. Use the head-tilt maneuver and place the mask over the patient's mouth and nose. Grasp the jaw with your fingers and apply upward pressure while using the thumb side of your palms to press downward and hold the mask in place. Finally, blow into the opening of the mask.

Management Principles

Observe the rise and fall of the patient's chest to determine the adequacy of ventilation. Limitations to adequate ventilation include a small rescuer vital capacity, loss of volume because of an inadequate seal around the patient's mouth and nose, and inability to ventilate because of an obstruction of the airway by mucus, emesis, blood, or a foreign object.

ENDOTRACHEAL INTUBATION

Endotracheal intubation is accomplished by placing a tube, either nasally or orally (Table 3–1), through the larynx and into the trachea.

TABLE 3–1 Nasal Versus Oral Endotracheal Intubation

	Nasal	Oral
Indications	Nonemergent, elective intubation Suspected or known cervical spine injury	Emergency airway Technically difficult with suspected cervical spine injury
Advantages	Situations where oral access is difficult or impossible, such as oral trauma, maxillomandibular wiring More comfortable for patient Easier to stabilize and maintain good oral hygiene Less gagging Communication by mouthing of words possibly enhanced	Allows passage of larger tube: less airway resistance to gas flow, improved secretion removal Less kinking Easier to insert
Disadvantages	More difficult to place Requires use of smaller-lumen tube: greater airway resistance to gas flow, more difficult secretion removal Kinks more easily Epistaxis possible during insertion May contribute to development of sinusitis, otitis media	Less comfortable for patient: may cause gagging and stimulate oral secretion production More difficult to stabilize Patient may bite down on airway, reducing gas flow More difficult to maintain good oral hygiene and to communicate by mouthing words

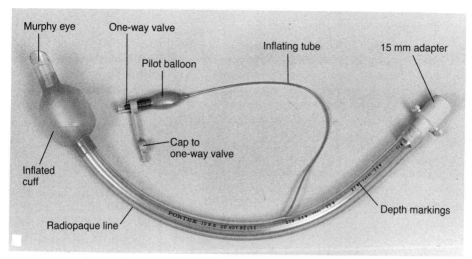

FIGURE 3-5 Basic design features of the endotracheal tube. (Modified from Kersten, LD: *Comprehensive Respiratory Nursing*. Philadelphia: WB Saunders, 1989.)

Indications

The following are indications for the use of endotracheal intubation: (1) airway obstruction that persists despite the use of previously discussed methods (i.e., airway edema), (2) secretion management, because an endotracheal tube provides a conduit for suctioning, (3) airway protection from regurgitation or aspiration in patients with a depressed level of consciousness or ineffective upper airway reflexes, and (4) the need for high concentrations of oxygen, mechanical ventilation, or general anesthesia.

Tube Design

The basic design of the endotracheal tube (ETT) is standardized (Fig. 3–5). The *connector* fits into the tube at the proximal end. It has a standard 15 mm outside diameter that permits connection to mechanical ventilator circuitry, a bag-valve-mask device, or anesthesia devices. The *tube body* has a standard curvature, centimeter markings that allow for the determination of depth of insertion, and radiopaque markings either running the length of the tube or at the distal end, so that the tube can be located on a chest x-ray film. The *distal tip* of the ETT has a beveled edge, which allows for easier passage of the tube through the glottic slit. A Magill type of ETT has an opening only at the distal end of the tube, whereas a Murphy type of tube also has a small hole opening opposite the beveled edge. This hole allows for ventilation in the event that the bevel becomes lodged against the tracheal wall. Adult ETTs are equipped with a *cuff*, which when inflated seals the trachea allowing for the application of positive-pressure ventilation and minimizing aspiration (see the section Monitoring and Managing Cuffs, below). Finally, the *inflating system* is a small-bore tube fused within the wall of the ETT, which allows for inflation of the cuff. At the proximal end of this small lumen is a spring-loaded valve that is activated by inserting a syringe. Air can then be inserted into the cuff. The valve closes when the syringe is removed, thus preventing the escape of air from the cuff. Adjacent to this valve is the *pilot balloon*, a small balloon that, when felt for air pressure, indicates the general inflation state of the cuff.

Endotracheal tubes come in different sizes. The tube size is determined by the internal diameter (ID) of the lumen and is measured in millimeters. The ID is marked on the outside of the tube. Tube size increases in increments of 0.5 mm. The risk of glottic injury is reduced by using a tube that approximates the patient's glottic dimensions. Glottic size is related to sex, not height, weight, or body surface area. The usual size of a tube needed for an adult woman is 7.0 or 7.5 and for an adult man 8.0 or 8.5. In an emergency situation an 8.0 mm ID tube serves as a good standard-sized tube.

Technique

INTUBATION EQUIPMENT

Intubation must be performed only by persons trained in this difficult skill. Endotracheal intubation is most often facilitated by direct laryngoscopy. Laryn-

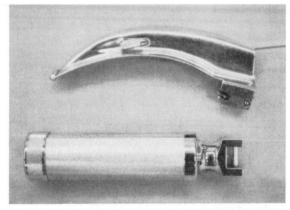

A

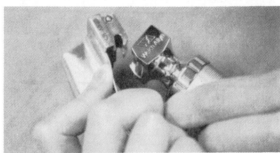

B

FIGURE 3-6 Laryngoscope, used during endotracheal intubation for direct visualization of the vocal cords. (A) The two basic parts of the laryngoscope, the handle and the blade. (B) The U-shaped indentation on the base of the blade hooks over the bar on the laryngoscope handle. The blade is then snapped upward into place. When the blade forms a 90-degree angle with the handle, it is correctly placed. (From Levitsky, MG, Cairo, JM, and Hall SM: *Introduction to Respiratory Care*. Philadelphia, WB Saunders, 1990.)

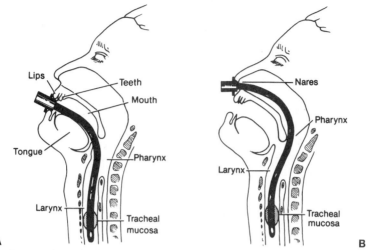

Lips
Teeth
Mouth
Tongue
Pharynx
Larynx
Tracheal mucosa

Nares
Pharynx
Larynx
Tracheal mucosa

A

B

FIGURE 3–7 Endotracheal intubation may be performed (A) orally or (B) nasally. (Reproduced by permission from GA Traver [Ed.]: *Respiratory Nursing: The Science and the Art.* New York: John Wiley & Sons, 1982. Copyright © 1982 John Wiley & Sons.)

goscopy, which is the direct visualization of the vocal cords or glottic slit, is performed with the use of a laryngoscope. The laryngoscope consists of two basic parts: the handle and the blade (Fig. 3–6). The handle, which is textured to allow for a good grip, houses batteries to supply power to the built-in light source on the blade. The indentation of the blade fits into the bar on the handle, and the light is illuminated when it is properly snapped into its right-angle position. Laryngoscope blades may be either curved (MacIntosh) or straight (Miller) and come in a variety of sizes to allow for variation in patient size. The laryngoscope handles and blades should be checked periodically and batteries and lights changed as necessary to keep the equipment in a ready state.

Equipment necessary for endotracheal intubation includes the following:
- The ETT
- Suction equipment in good working order, along with a rigid-tip suction catheter (Yankauer) and a suction catheter
- Oxygen source, connecting tube, and a manual resuscitation bag and mask
- Water-soluble lubricant
- A 10 ml syringe for cuff inflation
- Tape for stabilization of the tube
- Magill forceps for directing the tube into the larynx or removing foreign material
- A plastic-coated, malleable stylet that can be inserted into the tube to make it more rigid, thus facilitating insertion

The individual who assists with an intubation, especially in an emergent situation, should ensure that all equipment is ready, anticipate the needs of the intubationist, and assist in patient positioning, teaching, and medication administration as necessary. A good assistant is always appreciated and will help to achieve the common goal: the establishment of either an oral or a nasal patent airway (Fig. 3–7).

Oral Endotracheal Intubation

Assemble all equipment and check the tube cuff for patency and symmetry by inflating it with air. Lubricate the tube. Explain the procedure to the patient and provide sedation as necessary. Position the patient supine, with a rolled towel placed vertically between the shoulder blades (to facilitate viewing of the glottis). Preoxygenate the patient with 100% oxygen. Hyperextend the patient's head if this maneuver is not contraindicated. Holding the laryngoscope with the left hand, insert the blade into the mouth. The tip of the curved blade is inserted into the vallecula, which is the space between the base of the tongue and the epiglottis. The tip of the straight blade is inserted under the epiglottis. Upward traction is then exerted to expose the glottic opening. (Care must be taken to avoid using the upper teeth as a fulcrum.) The tube is then inserted with the right hand through the vocal cords and slightly beyond (5 to 6 cm), into the trachea. The laryngoscope is removed, the stylet is removed, and the cuff is inflated. Breath sounds are immediately auscultated, while the patient's lungs are ventilated with a manual resuscitation bag to determine whether the procedure has been successful. The tube should then be stabilized immediately, and a chest x-ray film should be obtained to confirm placement. If an attempt at intubation is prolonged (>30 seconds) or if the O_2 saturation drops significantly, the heart rate or rhythm changes, or cyanosis develops, then the procedure should be interrupted and the patient oxygenated with 100% oxygen with a manual resuscitation bag and mask device.

Nasal Endotracheal Intubation

Assemble all equipment and check the tube cuff for patency and symmetry by inflating it with air. Lubricate the tube. Explain the procedure to the patient and provide sedation as necessary. Position the patient according to the intubationist's preference: semi-Fowler's, high Fowler's, or supine. Nasal intubation is usually performed blindly; that is, no laryngoscope is used to visualize the vocal cords, no hyperextension is utilized, and the head remains in the midline position. The tube is inserted into the nostril that appears to have the greatest patency, after a topical anesthetic has been liberally applied. While the tube is gently advanced along the floor of the nostril, breath sounds are listened for at the proximal tube end. At the time of inspiration, the intubationist advances the tube through the open vocal cords. If the tube has been placed correctly, a vapor column (cloudiness) will be visible in the endotracheal tube. In nasal endotracheal intubation in which a laryngoscope blade is used, Magill forceps may also be used to assist in advancing the tube through the glottic slit once it has been visualized. Once the tube is in place, the cuff is inflated, and while the patient is undergoing ventilation with a manual resuscitation bag, breath sounds are immediately auscultated to ascertain the presence of bilaterally equal breath sounds. The tube is then stabilized to the upper lip, with caution exercised to prevent upward pressure on the nare. A chest x-ray film should be obtained immediately to confirm placement.

Complications

Endotracheal intubation is a highly technical skill that is not without complications (Box 3–1). Vigilant monitoring and care of the patient will lead to the prevention of many complications.

Box 3-1   Complications Associated With Endotracheal Intubation

During the Intubation Procedure

Vomiting with possible aspiration
Trauma: laryngeal, pharyngeal, tracheal, dental
Bradycardia caused by vagal stimulation
Hypoxemia caused by delay in procedure
Cardiac arrhythmias
Right main-stem intubation
Esophageal intubation

While the Tube Is in Place

Tube malposition: too high, too low
Right main-stem intubation
Laryngeal or tracheal erosion, necrosis
Pharyngeal edema
Mouth, lip, or nare pressure-sore development
Inadequate ventilation or oxygenation as a result of tube obstruction or
    kinking
Loss of cuff integrity
Unplanned (self) extubation
Aspiration
Sinusitis/otitis media

After Extubation

Laryngeal spasm or edema potentially leading to airway obstruction
Tracheal dilation, stenosis, or tracheomalacia
Laryngeal or tracheal granuloma
Laryngeal stenosis: glottic or subglottic
Vocal cord paresis or paralysis potentially causing aspiration

---

Tube Stabilization Techniques

Each time the patient is assessed, the security of the airway should be viewed as the highest of priorities. Endotracheal tubes may be secured with either tape or harnesses specially designed for this purpose (Fig. 3–8). Whenever an ETT securing device is removed, two persons must be present, one to hold the airway to prevent dislodgment if the patient coughs or gags and the other to perform oral and nare care and stabilize the tube. Inflation of the cuff should never be viewed as a method of tube stabilization.

There are several techniques for taping an ETT. General principles common to each technique include the following:

- Secure the tape completely around the patient's head to provide stabilization superior to that of tape placed only across the cheeks.
- Prevent the patient's hair from sticking to the tape by placing a second piece of tape, 6 to 8 inches long (sticky sides together), along that portion of the tape that will be at the patient's occiput.

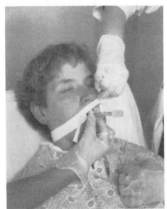

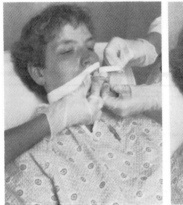

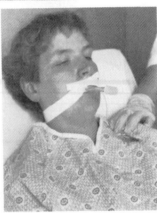

A

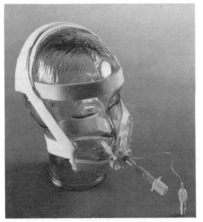

B

Figure 3-8 Two methods of securing the endotracheal tube: (A) tape and (B) harness device. Harness device shown is the SecureEasy Endotracheal Tube Holder. Its nonelastic headgear reduces the risk of self-extubation without putting excessive pressure on the patient's face. A soft bite-block comfortably prevents tube occlusion. (A from Perry, A, and Potter, P: *Clinical Nursing Skills and Techniques*. 3rd ed. St. Louis: Mosby–Year Book, 1994. B, Courtesy of IPI Medical Products, Chicago, Ill.)

- Tape an oral endotracheal tube to the upper lip, not to the mandible, which moves with talking.
- Tape a nasal endotracheal tube to the upper lip, not to the bridge of the nose, so as to reduce traction on the nares.
- Apply tincture of benzoin to the skin to promote adhesiveness of the tape.
- Fold the end of the tape to create a pull tab and thus promote easier removal for tape changes.
- Reposition oral endotracheal tubes once every 24 hours to prevent pressure necrosis.
- Avoid securing multiple tubes together (e.g., an endotracheal tube and a nasogastric tube) because if the patient pulls on one, both tubes will be dislodged.

The quest for an optimal method of stabilizing endotracheal tubes has led to the production of harness devices that are particularly useful when tape cannot be used, such as in patients with tape allergies or facial burns. The device must be removed at least once every 8 hours for oral care and assessment of the mouth for pressure areas. At least one harness model also has a built-in bite block. A combination headgear and faceplate holds the tube securely and reduces tube movement, thus easing frictional trauma to the mouth and trachea. Such devices are more costly than cloth tape; however, they can be washed and reused. Though these devices cannot eradicate unplanned extubation, in patients who tongue at their tubes in an attempt to dislodge them, the harness holds the tube more securely than does tape.

TRACHEOSTOMY TUBES

Tracheostomy tubes provide an airway directly into the anterior portion of the neck, usually at the level of the second or fourth tracheal rings. The tracheotomy procedure is performed by a surgeon, preferably in the controlled setting of the operating room.

Indications

Tracheostomy tubes are indicated (1) for long-term secretion management, (2) to reduce dead-space ventilation and airway resistance (in comparison with endotracheal tubes) and therefore to reduce the work of breathing, (3) for protection of the airway from aspiration, (4) when upper airway obstruction prevents placement of an endotracheal tube, (5) and when prolonged mechanical ventilation is necessary. Tracheostomy tubes are better tolerated and create less airflow resistance than oral or nasal endotracheal tubes, allow for oral intake and better oral hygiene, and, in the case of some tube designs, even allow for talking. They prevent further laryngeal injury by the translaryngeal tube, are more securely fixed and thus decrease the incidence of accidental extubation, and often facilitate the transfer of the patient from the intensive care unit. There are no existing clear-cut data that delineate the ideal timing of tracheostomy in patients with an endotracheal tube in place for long-term mechanical ventilation. Each case must be reviewed individually, and the potential risks and benefits weighed carefully. Whether a tracheostomy should be performed is ultimately decided on the basis of the team's projections regarding the length of time that mechanical ventilation or an artificial airway will be required. In general, after 7 days of intubation, the case review should be performed. If 7 or more additional days of intubation will be required, then tracheostomy should be considered.

Tracheostomy Tube Designs

Tracheostomy tubes are available in a variety of sizes, styles, and materials. Primarily they are made of either plastic or metal. General design features (Fig. 3–9) include the *neck flange,* which should lie flush against the patient's neck. The flange has holes on either end in which tracheostomy ties are inserted for securing of the airway. Some tracheostomy tubes have flanges that are adjustable so that the extratracheal portion of the tube can be made shorter or longer, a useful feature when there is soft tissue swelling or when the patient is obese. The flange should lie securely against the patient's skin so that movement of the tube into and out of the stoma, and thus airway trauma, are minimized. The *tube body* has both extratracheal and intratracheal portions, being divided by the neck flange. A radiopaque marker is located on the body. Near the end of the body is the *cuff* (uncuffed tubes are also available). When inflated, the cuff seals the trachea, allowing for the application of positive-pressure ventilation and minimizing aspiration. Finally, the *inflating system,* a small-bore tube fused within the wall of the tracheostomy tube, allows for the inflation of the cuff. At the proximal end of this small lumen is a spring-loaded valve that can be opened by inserting a syringe to allow air to be inserted into the cuff. The valve closes when the syringe is removed, thus preventing the escape of air from the cuff. Adjacent

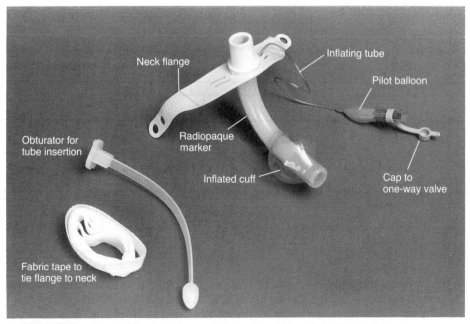

FIGURE 3–9 General design features of the tracheostomy tube. (Modified from Kersten, LD: *Comprehensive Respiratory Nursing.* Philadelphia: WB Saunders, 1989.)

to this valve is the *pilot balloon*, a small balloon that, when felt for air pressure, indicates the general inflation state of the cuff. The *obturator* is inserted into the lumen of the tracheostomy tube, its rounded end extending slightly farther than the body. The obturator creates a smooth tube tip, which will prevent injury to the tracheal wall when the tube is initially inserted. It must always be removed after the tube is inserted to allow for the passage of air and should be kept in a visible place at the patient's bedside should emergency reinsertion of a misplaced tube be necessary.

CUFFED VERSUS UNCUFFED TUBES

The choice of a cuffed tube over an uncuffed tube is made if the patient will require mechanical ventilation or if aspiration may be a problem. Cuffed tubes are most often used in the acute care setting. Uncuffed tubes are useful in long-term care settings when the patient has competent glottic function and aspiration is therefore not a problem. Uncuffed tubes are also used in the pediatric population.

SINGLE VERSUS DOUBLE CANNULAS

Tracheostomy tubes may be single or double cannula. The cannulas of the double-cannula tube are referred to as the inner cannula and the outer cannula. The inner cannula is removable to facilitate cleaning of the inner tracheal lumen, a useful feature because tracheal tubes tend to be left in place for prolonged periods and accumulation of secretions may become a problem. When the inner cannula is not in place, the ventilator cannot be connected to the tracheostomy because the outer lumen is not the same size as a standard-size connector. Therefore, if the patient cannot tolerate being off the ventilator, a spare inner cannula must be available for use when tracheostomy care is being performed.

The inner cannula is secured to the outer cannula by various mechanisms. Some cannulas twist to lock into place, others snap-lock into place, and still others have a hinge on the outer cannula that swings to lock over and thus secure the inner cannula. Caregivers must ensure that they know how to secure and remove the inner cannula.

Inner cannulas may be reusable or disposable. Reusable cannulas are washed and replaced, whereas disposable ones are used only once and then discarded. Disposable inner cannulas (DICs) reduce the time required for performing tracheostomy care and reduce the possibility of caregiver contamination by splashing, which can occur when an inner cannula is cleaned. Whether DICs are more or less cost-effective than reusable inner cannulas is unknown (Fig. 3–10).

METAL TUBES

Metal tubes are indicated for long-term use in chronic care populations because of the durability of the metal. Another material used for long-term tracheostomy tubes is nylon. Metal tubes are also used for weaning patients from their tracheostomy in preparation for decannulation (see section on decannulation, below).

The most commonly used metal tube is the Jackson tube. Made of sterling silver or, more commonly, stainless steel, it is an uncuffed tube with an inner cannula and a metal obturator (Fig. 3–11). Dr. Chevalier Jackson originally developed the tracheostomy tube sizing system. This method (e.g., sizes 00, 0, 1, 2) serves as a sizing reference in the industry. However, within the industry there is no standard for tracheostomy tube sizing. This means that tubes of the same

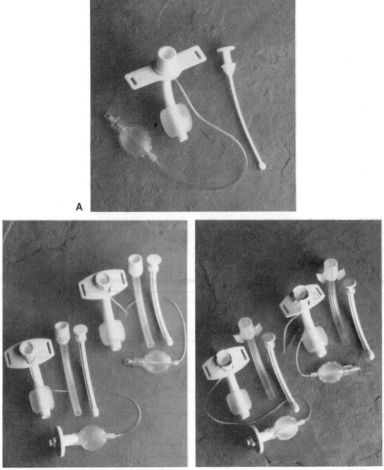

Figure 3-10 Tracheostomy tubes. (A) Single cannula (B) Double cannula. Shown are both reusable (*left*) and disposable (*right*) inner cannulas. (Courtesy of Mallinckrodt Medical Tracheostomy Products Inc., Irvine, Calif.)

numeric size from different companies may not have the same internal or external diameters. Table 3–2 is presented to assist the clinician in comparing sizes between the Jackson tube and those of other manufacturers. When a change is made from a plastic to a metal tube, the most important number to consider is the external diameter, because this is sized to the patient's tracheal stoma.

A second important principle in the management of the patient with a metal tracheostomy tube concerns ensuring adequate manual ventilation when necessary. The standard 15 mm connector on a manual resuscitation bag (MRB) does not fit onto a metal tracheostomy tube. An adapter, which is standard in size at one end, must be attached to the MRB. The opposite end of this adapter narrows to a smaller lumen that fits into the inner lumen of the metal tube, allowing for a closed system for manual ventilation. The adapter must be the appropriate size

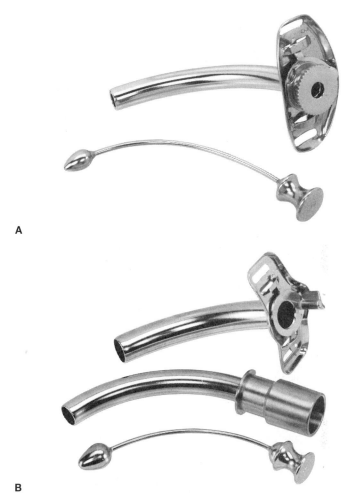

A

B

FIGURE 3-11 (*A*) Metal tracheostomy tube, which is uncuffed, comes with an obturator and a reusable inner cannula. Fitting a manual resuscitation bag (MRB) to this tube requires a special adapter. The end of the adapter, which fits to the MRB, has a standard 15 mm connector; the other end, which fits into the inner cannula of the tracheostomy tube, is much smaller and varies by tube size. (*B*) Metal tracheostomy tube with 15 mm adapter incorporated into the inner cannula. (Courtesy of Pilling Weck, Research Triangle Park, N.C.)

for the size of the metal tube. In the clinical setting, one must always ensure that an adapter of the appropriate size is readily available at the bedside. Alternatively, metal tracheostomy tubes may be fit with an inner cannula with a 15 mm connector.

SPEAKING TRACHEOSTOMY TUBES

A tracheostomy tube that allows for speech is indicated to provide the patient with a mechanism for voice communication, thereby reducing frustration,

TABLE 3–2 Conversion Chart for Comparing Sizes of Jackson Metal Trach Tubes With Various Other Tracheostomy Tubes

Jackson Size	Outside Diameter (mm)	Inside Diameter (mm)
00	4.5	2.4
0	5.0	2.8
1	5.5	3.0
2	6.0	3.4
3	7.0	4.3
4	8.0	5.3
5	9.0	6.2
6	10.0	7.2
7	11.0	8.3
8	12.0	9.2
9	13.0	9.9
10	14.0	10.6
11	15.3	12.3
12	16.3	12.7

Data from Tracheostomy and laryngectomy tubes. In *Pilling Endoscopic Instruments*. Catalog No. 99–1001. Research Triangle, N.C.: Pilling Weck, Inc., 1987.

improving patient and caregiver understanding, cultivating adaptation to illness, and promoting increased independence and self-esteem.

Communication mechanisms include either specially made tracheostomy tubes or a valve attached to the patient's tracheostomy tube. The special "talking" tracheostomy tubes have a channel through which air flows, exiting above the cuff and allowing for speech when the cuff is inflated (Fig. 3–12). This extra channel is attached to a standard air or oxygen flowmeter by a supply tube. A thumb valve on the air line controls the flow of gas. The practitioner needs to assist the patient in learning how to use the thumb valve to control the flow of gas. The flowmeter should be adjusted to provide the degree of flow needed for comfortable, audible speech (usually 4 to 6 L/min). For prevention of drying of the upper airway, the air source should be disconnected when not in use. Talking tracheostomy tubes that work by this mechanism can be used without interrupting mechanical ventilation.

The Passy-Muir Tracheostomy Speaking Valve (Fig. 3–13) is a one-way valve that attaches to a standard tracheostomy tube. At the end of inspiration the valve closes so that, on exhalation, air is forced up through the vocal cords. An added advantage is that secretions are also forced into the oral cavity for expectoration. The patient must be carefully assessed for tolerance, because the work of breathing is increased with the use of the valve. Valves are available for use both when a patient is using a ventilator and when he or she is not. When the valve is attached, the cuff must be deflated.

Before the Passy-Muir valve is used, a thorough assessment of several issues must be performed. Successful use of the valve requires the patient to be able to exhale efficiently around the tracheostomy tube and through the mouth and nose. Glottal patency assessment may be performed by deflating the cuff and instructing the patient to attempt vocalization on expiration. The patient should also be assessed for hemodynamic stability, sufficient pulmonary compliance to

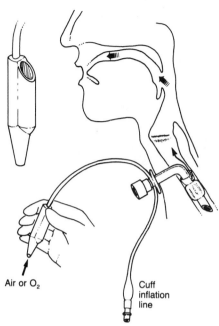

Air or O₂

Cuff
inflation
line

FIGURE 3-12 "Talking" tracheostomy tube. Air or oxygen, which is instilled through a special channel, exits from holes above the cuff, allowing for phonation. (From Luce, JM, Pierson, DJ, and Tyler, ML: *Intensive Respiratory Care*. Philadelphia: WB Saunders, 1993.)

maintain an effective functional residual capacity, intact cognitive function, and ability to handle secretions. Assessment for the presence of contraindications should also be performed. Contraindications include use of a foam-cuffed tube, presence of an artificial airway that is too large to allow for adequate air passage around its perimeter, and delayed or absent swallow reflex because of the increased potential for aspiration when the cuff is deflated.

When the Passy-Muir valve is used on mechanically ventilated patients, adjustment of the ventilator settings is necessary to compensate for air leak around the deflated tracheostomy cuff. Tidal volume will need to be increased by approximately 200 cc, by increasing either the set tidal volume or, when pressure support ventilation is used, the inspiratory pressure. The inspiratory flow rate may also have to be increased if a larger tidal volume is used or if a longer expiratory vocalization period is needed. The set positive end-expiratory pressure (PEEP) should be reduced because the valve creates auto-PEEP. Ventilator alarms that will need to be turned off are the exhaled tidal volume and minute ventilation alarms, because the tidal volume will no longer be returning to the ventilator.

While the valve is in place, the patient should be carefully monitored for respiratory stability and tolerance. Monitoring should include O₂ saturation, skin color, heart rate, respiratory rate, blood pressure, patient perception of the experience, anxiety, work of breathing, and secretion management. The amount of time that the valve is in place should be gradually increased. Eventually some patients may even learn to place the valve themselves, increasing their

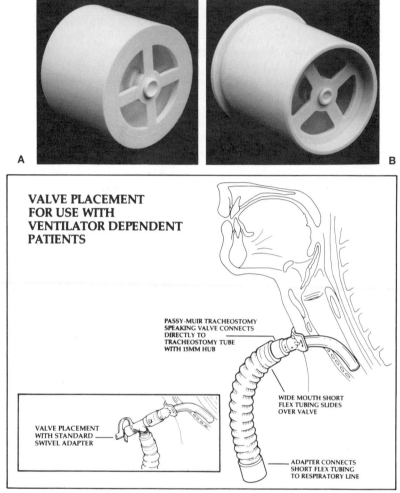

A

B

VALVE PLACEMENT FOR USE WITH VENTILATOR DEPENDENT PATIENTS

PASSY-MUIR TRACHEOSTOMY SPEAKING VALVE CONNECTS DIRECTLY TO TRACHEOSTOMY TUBE WITH 15MM HUB

WIDE MOUTH SHORT FLEX TUBING SLIDES OVER VALVE

VALVE PLACEMENT WITH STANDARD SWIVEL ADAPTER

ADAPTER CONNECTS SHORT FLEX TUBING TO RESPIRATORY LINE

C

FIGURE 3-13 Two examples of the Passy-Muir Tracheostomy Speaking Valve. Valve designs are for (A) patients who are not undergoing mechanical ventilation and (B) those who are being mechanically ventilated. (C) Options for valve placement within the ventilator circuitry. (Courtesy of Passy-Muir Inc., Irvine, Calif.)

independence. The valve should be removed while the patient is sleeping and during respiratory therapy treatments.

In the absence of a specially designed tube or valve, the patient may still be able to speak. The patient will need to be taught to use a finger to occlude the tracheostomy lumen on exhalation so that air can be redirected up through the vocal cords. This technique is particularly easy to use with uncuffed tubes because if the tube has a cuff, it must be let down. Problems with finger occlusion include contamination from the patient and the environment, difficulty with hand control, patient embarrassment because finger occlusion is conspicuous, and limited duration of vocalizations. With finger occlusion the patient generally can speak only in phrases, whereas with a device such as the Passy-Muir valve the patient can communicate in complete sentences.

FENESTRATED TUBES

The fenestrated tube has one or more pea-sized holes (fenestrae) in the upper one-third, posterior portion of the outer cannula. When the inner cannula is removed, air flows out of this hole and up through the vocal cords so that phonation can occur (Fig. 3–14). Increasing the airflow through the upper airway also possibly helps to reduce the patient's psychologic dependence on the tube before weaning. The inner cannula is removed to facilitate talking, and then the patient is instructed to hold a finger over the tracheal lumen on expiration to promote flow of air through the fenestration and vocal cords. Another method is to let the cuff down, remove the inner cannula, and place a plug over the tracheal opening. The patient will then be ventilating both through the fenestration and around the tracheostomy. With the use of either method, a fair amount of resistance to ventilation is created; however, this may be tolerated long enough to allow the patient the opportunity to speak. When the inner cannula is replaced, mechanical ventilation and pulmonary treatments may be readily applied. Table 3–3 provides guidelines for the state of the cuff and the inner cannula during suctioning, talking, and eating.

TRACHEOSTOMY BUTTONS

Tracheostomy buttons are small cannulas that extend only from the skin to the anterior surface of the trachea. They are generally made of plastic.

Indications. Buttons are used to prevent stoma closure and ensure easy access to the airway in the event that it becomes necessary to institute mechanical ventilation, suction the airway, or provide an airway on an occasional basis.

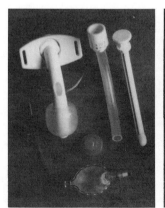 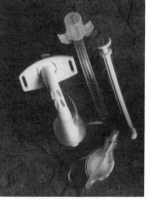

A   B

FIGURE 3–14 Fenestrated tracheostomy tubes. *(A)* Reusable inner cannula. *(B)* Disposable inner cannula. Removal of the inner cannula allows for phonation. Removal of the inner cannula with the cuff down and the decannulation plug in place facilitates air movement not only around but through the tube, preparing the patient for breathing through the natural airway. (Courtesy of Mallinckrodt Medical Tracheostomy Products Inc., Irvine, Calif.)

Table 3-3   **Guidelines for the State of the Cuff and Nonfenestrated Inner Cannula on a Fenestrated Tracheostomy Tube**

	Cuff Inflated	Cuff Deflated	Inner Cannula
Suctioning	X		In
Talking		X	Out
Eating	X		In

Examples of patients that may need an intermittent airway are those with ob-structive sleep apnea or burn and trauma patients requiring repeated trips to the operating room. Use of the tracheostomy button may also be the final step in weaning a patient from a tracheostomy to the natural airway. The button, if sized and inserted properly, creates very little resistance to gas flow through the trachea.

Management Principles. Ensure that the button is not protruding into the trachea. The distal end should be snug against the anterior surface of the trachea. Spacers, which look like washers, may be applied between the patient's neck and the proximal end of the button to ensure proper fit. If the button is too short, its distal end will lie in the anterior cervical tissue. This will lead to premature stoma closure or accidental dislodgment by the patient during coughing.

The Kistner button comes in a fixed length with a white spacer that is used to customize patient fit (Fig. 3–15). The proximal end may be either covered with a one-way valve attachment or plugged. The one-way valve allows air to flow in during inspiration but closes during expiration. If the valve becomes moist, it may stick and should be replaced. If the proximal end is fitted with a plug, the patient breathes completely through the natural airway.

The Olympic button (Fig. 3–16), which may have both outer and inner can-nulas, comes in a variety of sizes and lengths. The appropriate size needed for a particular patient is determined with the use of a measuring probe. At the distal end, the outer cannula has flanges that should lie snug against the anterior tra-cheal wall to help secure the button in place. Spacer rings may be placed exter-nally to prevent the button from extending too far into the trachea. Insertion of the inner cannula creates a standard-size external adapter for the institution of breathing treatments or for the use of a manual resuscitation bag. Alternatively, a closure plug may be inserted into the outer cannula, which allows the patient to breathe entirely by using the natural airway.

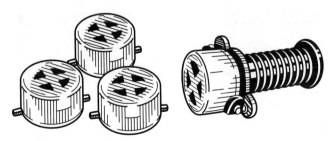

Figure 3-15   Kistner tracheostomy tube, also commonly referred to as a tracheostomy button. (Courtesy of Pilling Weck, Research Triangle Park, N.C.)

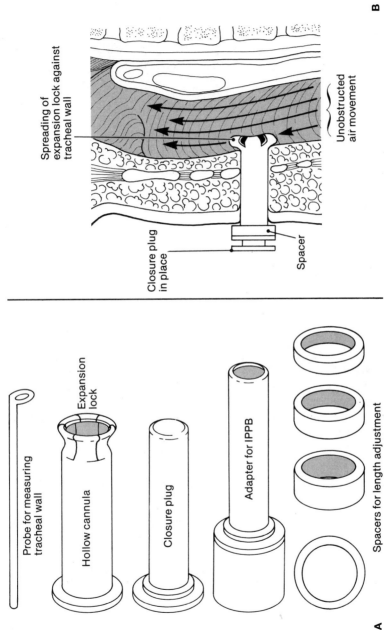

FIGURE 3-16 Olympic tracheostomy button. (A) Individual parts. (B) Breathing with the closure plug in place. Insertion of the closure plug, or intermittent positive-pressure breathing (IPPB) adapter spreads the flanged tip of the button. The flanged tip is known as the expansion lock. (From Kersten, LD: *Comprehensive Respiratory Nursing.* Philadelphia: WB Saunders, 1989.)

Probe for measuring tracheal wall

Expansion lock

Hollow cannula

Closure plug

Adapter for IPPB

Spacers for length adjustment

A

Spreading of expansion lock against tracheal wall

Closure plug in place

Unobstructed air movement

Spacer

B

Routine Tracheostomy Care

Routine tracheostomy care involves cleaning the stoma, the external portion of the tracheostomy tube, and the inner cannula. If dressings are being used, they also should be changed. The purpose of this procedure is to keep the tube free of mucus and other secretions that may be a source of infection or of encrustations that may impede airway patency. Tracheostomy ties must also be changed once a day, or more often if soiled.

Many facilities carry tracheostomy care kits (Fig. 3–17) that include all necessary supplies. These kits are particularly useful for cleaning the inner cannula because they contain sterile pipe cleaners or brushes. In general, the following supplies are needed: gloves, hydrogen peroxide, sterile saline solution, sterile cotton-tipped applicators, pipe cleaners, or a brush, and a tracheal dressing. If the ties are to be changed, scissors and twill tape are also needed.

Immediately after a surgical procedure, the tracheostomy site should be assessed frequently. Some venous oozing is normal and may require dressing changes as often as every 2 hours to prevent collection of blood with possible aspiration. If bleeding is excessive, the surgeon may choose to pack the site. Many surgeons suture the tracheostomy tube in place and prefer that these sutures not be disrupted for the first 48 hours. Even in these cases, it is still necessary to perform meticulous, sterile stoma care, as gently as possible, under the neck flange.

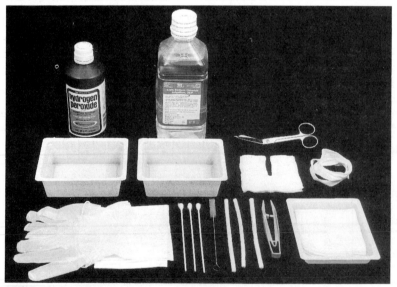

Figure 3–17 Equipment for tracheostomy care. Supplies may come prepackaged in a kit or be individually assembled. *Top row:* hydrogen peroxide (H_2O_2); normal saline (NS); scissors. *Center row:* containers for H_2O_2 and NS; sterile precut tracheostomy dressing (sterile 4 x 4 gauze without cotton filler is also acceptable); clean tracheostomy tape. *Bottom row:* sterile gloves; cotton swabs (Q tips), brush or pipe cleaners; sterile 4 x 4s. (From Kersten, LD: *Comprehensive Respiratory Nursing.* Philadelphia: WB Saunders, 1989.)

Tracheostomy care should be performed a minimum of once every 8 hours. Care of the single-cannula tracheostomy tube involves cleaning around the stoma and the external portion of the tube, changing the dressing, and changing the ties as necessary. When a double-cannula tube is used, care includes, in addition to the steps described above, the cleaning of the inner cannula. When the inner cannula is disposable, care involves removal of the inner cannula, replacement with a new cannula, and disposal of the old one. No attempt should be made to clean a disposable inner cannula, especially with the use of hydrogen peroxide, which disrupts the integrity of the structural material. Because hydrogen peroxide will also cause pitting of a metal inner cannula, only sterile saline solution should be used for cleaning a metal tracheostomy tube. Reusable inner cannulas made of plastic may be cleaned with hydrogen peroxide, followed by rinsing with normal saline solution before reinsertion. Cleansing of the inner cannula is assisted with the use of a sterile pipe cleaner or brush.

When care of an inner cannula used by a patient who cannot tolerate disruption of mechanical ventilation must be performed, it is necessary to have two inner cannulas of identical size and type available. When the inner cannula that needs to be cleaned is removed, the spare is inserted. After the inner cannula is cleaned, it is stored in a sterile container in readiness for the next care procedure.

Changing of tracheostomy ties is always a two-person procedure. One individual changes the tie, and the other holds the tracheostomy tube securely in place in case the patient coughs, gags, or simply makes a sudden movement during the procedure. Basic principles are, first, that the tie must be fastened with a knot, not a bow (which may be attractive but is impractical because it is not secure). Second, it should be tied firmly; that is, only one finger should be able to be inserted between the neck and the tie. A tie that is too loose will allow tracheostomy tube movement, which could lead to erosion and possible dislodgment.

There are no hard-and-fast rules regarding the use of dressings. Generally they are recommended for the first 2 postoperative weeks, while the stoma is maturing and peritracheal secretions are more prevalent. The dressing will help prevent irritation to the healing stoma and absorb some of the drainage. However, as an essential infection control measure, the dressing must be changed as often as necessary to prevent prolonged local contact of wet secretions with the stoma. Sources of peritracheal secretions are the sinuses and the oral cavity, pulmonary secretions coughed up and around the tracheostomy tube cuff, or exudate from a stoma infection. If the stoma is infected, then treatment may be necessary with either an antibiotic ointment or local cleansing with a 25% acetic acid solution every 6 to 8 hours, followed by frequent dressing changes.

MONITORING AND MANAGING CUFFS

The purpose of cuffs on airways is twofold: to allow for the application of positive-pressure ventilation without a loss of tidal volume and to prevent aspiration of oral and gastric secretions. For the cuff to perform these two functions, it must exert some pressure against the tracheal wall. The pressure between the cuff and the tracheal wall is appropriately termed the cuff–to–tracheal wall (C/T) pressure. The C/T pressure should be as low as possible so that the cuff may perform its functions while the complications of excessive pressure are prevented. The cuff may be inflated with one of two techniques: the minimal leak technique

(MLT) or the minimal occlusive volume (MOV) technique, also known as the minimal occlusive pressure or no-leak technique (Table 3–4). With either of these techniques the C/T pressure should be no higher than necessary to prevent excessive loss of volume, aspiration, and tracheal damage. Regardless of which technique is used to inflate the cuff, serial measurement of cuff pressure or volume is advised as a means of cuff monitoring (see Measuring Cuff Pressure and Measuring Cuff Volume, below).

Overinflation of a cuff creates excessive pressure on the tracheal wall. This constant pressure can lead to weakening of the tracheal muscles and softening of cartilage. The area of contact dilates, and volume must be added to the cuff to achieve an effective seal. The trachea may then further dilate, requiring more volume in the cuff, and a dangerous repetitive cycle has been set up. This process is referred to as the "chasing" of the trachea by the cuff.

All cuffs made today are of low-pressure design; that is, they are made of softer materials than in the past (low-volume, high-pressure cuffs). When even high volumes are inserted into these low-pressure, compliant cuffs, less *pressure* is created than in a cuff made of a more rigid material. The softer materials of the low-pressure, high-volume cuffs are also malleable. They more easily conform to the varying (C, D, O, oval) shapes of the trachea and therefore keep the formation of cuff folds to a minimum. Cuff folds serve as potential sites for aspiration of se-

TABLE 3–4 Comparison of the Minimal Occlusive Volume (MOV) and Minimal Leak Techniques (MLT) of Cuff Inflation

Minimal Occlusive Volume	Minimal Leak Techniques
Definition	
Sufficient air in cuff to abolish air leak on inspiration	Sufficient air in cuff to allow small leak on inspiration
Procedure	
During auscultation over trachea, inject air into cuff until no leak is heard.	During auscultation over trachea, inject air into cuff until no leak is heard.
Remove air until small leak is heard, usually 0.5 cc.	Remove air in 0.1 ml increments until small leak is heard.
Reinstill air until no leak is auscultated on inspiration.	
Advantages	
Less potential for aspiration because trachea is sealed	Avoidance of pooling of secretions above cuff because they either will be forced up by air passing around cuff or will drain into lungs to be coughed out
No loss of tidal volume	Potentially less injury to trachea because cuff to tracheal wall pressure will be less than in MOV
Disadvantages	
Greater potential for injury to tracheal wall than with MLT	Aspiration caused by secretions filtering around cuff into lungs
	Loss of tidal volume

cretions that pool above the inflated cuff. The practitioner should not be lulled into a false belief that tracheal damage will not occur just because improved material is used in today's cuffs. The C/T pressure may still become excessive if the tube is too small for the trachea or if the cuff is overinflated. In the past in some clinical settings, it was recommended that the cuff be let down for 5 minutes every 4 to 8 hours. This practice stemmed from the use of the high-pressure, low-volume cuffs and is no longer necessary with the newer cuffs.

Complications Associated With Cuffs

If pressure in a cuff is higher than capillary arterial perfusion pressure, which is generally estimated to be 30 to 32 cm H_2O in a normotensive patient, erosion and ischemic damage may occur to the tracheal tissues. Because venous and lymphatic flow occurs at even lower perfusing pressures, and critically ill patients may have episodes of hypotension, ideally the cuff pressure should remain as low as possible (25 cm H_2O or less) while still meeting the goals of cuff use. Complications of the use of cuffs range from mild inflammation and tracheitis to complete erosion of the trachea.

Ischemic injury may progress from areas of ulceration to hemorrhage and necrosis formation. The trachea may become dilated, as evidenced by the need for larger cuff volumes to seal the trachea. A tracheoesophageal fistula may form or tracheomalacia may develop if tracheal cartilages are affected. Granuloma and scar formation occurs when areas of injury heal. These areas may then become areas of stenosis or obstruction after extubation or decannulation.

Vascular injury may present as profuse bleeding if innominate artery erosion has occurred. If the bleeding is not rapidly controlled, exsanguination or suffocation caused by blood aspiration may occur. In the patient with a tracheotomy a gloved finger should be inserted into the stoma and an attempt made to compress the bleeding artery against the posterior portion of the sternum. Definitive therapy involves surgical ligation of the artery.

Measuring Cuff Pressure

Intracuff pressure provides an approximation of C/T pressure. The measurement of cuff pressure is therefore one mechanism advocated to prevent complications related to excessive C/T pressure. The maintenance of cuff pressures within the "normal" range, however, do not ensure the prevention of tracheal damage. Ongoing evaluation of the pressure may nevertheless alert the clinician to a problematic situation and prompt troubleshooting.

As stated previously, the cuff should first be inflated by either the MLT or the MOV technique. The cuff pressure is then maintained at 25 cm H_2O (18.5 mm Hg) or less, which is below tracheal capillary perfusion pressure in the normotensive patient. The pressure should be monitored every 4 to 8 hours while an attempt is made to control factors that can alter the parameter—primarily, patient position and state of wakefulness. Wakefulness, and thus tracheal muscle tone, are altered by anesthetic agents, paralytic agents, sedatives, and so on. Pressure may be measured with a standard sphygmomanometer (Fig. 3–18) or with an aneroid cuff-pressure manometer. The method for using a sphygmomanometer is described in Box 3–2. This method is useful when one of the newer devices

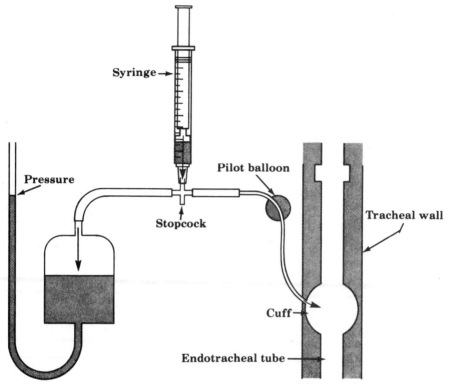

Figure 3–18 Setup for measuring cuff pressures with a standard sphygmomanometer (see Box 3–2 for procedure). (From Pilbeam, SP: *Mechanical Ventilation: Physiological and Clinical Applications.* 2nd ed. St. Louis: Mosby–Year Book, 1992.)

is unavailable. A Cufflator or similar aneroid cuff-pressure manometer is a simple, handheld instrument that should be utilized by following the manufacturer's guidelines (Fig. 3–19).

Measuring Cuff Volume

The measurement of cuff volume is another mechanism advocated to prevent complications related to excessive C/T pressure. The premise for continuous recording of cuff volume is that a gradually increasing volume alerts the clinician to tracheal dilation. Troubleshooting actions may then be taken, or the possibility of extubation can be pursued more actively.

The cuff should first be inflated by either the MLT or the MOV technique. Cuff volume is then determined by fully deflating the cuff. Problems with this procedure include the disruption of mechanical ventilation, especially of the maintenance of PEEP, and the potential for aspiration of oral secretions pooled on top of the cuff. This procedure may therefore not be tolerated by patients receiving full ventilatory support. The potential for aspiration is reduced by suctioning the secretions pooled on top of the cuff at *any* time a cuff is let down. The institution of a sigh breath while the cuff is inflated to minimal leak may

Box 3-2   Measurement of Cuff Pressures With a Sphygmomanometer

1. Attach a three-way stopcock to the manometer tubing, a 10 cc syringe, and the pilot balloon. Ensure that the stopcock is turned off to the balloon to prevent the escape of air.
2. Prime the manometer tubing with enough air so that the pressure reads 10 mm Hg. Failure to prime the tubing will cause some air from the cuff to fill the dead space of the tubing without registering pressure on the manometer. The 10 mm Hg pressure will serve as the baseline pressure.
3. Turn the stopcock so that it is open from the cuff to the manometer (off to the syringe). Measure the pressure reading on the manometer.
4. Obtain the actual cuff pressure with the following formula:

    Manometer reading $-$ 10 mm Hg = Cuff pressure

5. Convert millimeters of mercury to centimeters of H_2O with the following formula:

    $$mm\ Hg \times 1.36 = cm\ H_2O$$

    where 1 mm Hg = 1.36 cm H_2O, or 1 cm H_2O = 0.74 mm Hg

NOTE: If the volume in the cuff is increased or decreased with use of the 10 cc syringe (to achieve MOV or MLT), another pressure reading must be obtained. Even 0.5 cc of volume can make a significant difference in cuff pressure.

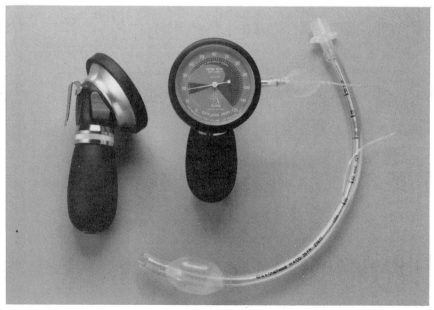

FIGURE 3-19 Aneroid pressure manometer. The bulb is squeezed to inflate the cuff. Depression of the thumb valve (shown in left view) allows for deflation. Movement of a very small volume of air is possible. (Courtesy of J.T. Posey Company, Arcadia, Calif.)

move the secretions cephalad and also assist in their removal before cuff deflation.

Special Cuffs

In the attempt to alleviate problems associated with excessive or changing
cuff pressures, the foam-filled cuff evolved (Fig. 3–20). The foam-filled cuff
(FOME-CUF, Bivona, Inc., Gary, Ind.) allows for maintenance of low cuff pressures and adapts to a change in pressures, which can occur in air transport, in the
operating room when nitrous oxide (which diffuses across the cuff) is used, and
during positive-pressure ventilation.

Before insertion, the foam-filled cuff must be collapsed by active aspiration of
all air. The collapse of the pilot port confirms that the cuff is in a collapsed state.
Plugging the pilot port with its attached stopper maintains the collapsed state.
After insertion, the inflation line is left open and the cuff self-inflates to ambient airway pressure. Because the natural tendency of the foam in the cuff is to
expand, pressure in the cuff actually decreases as the volume in the foam cuff increases. Stretching of the trachea and the possibility of resultant injury are reduced. However, failure to recognize the paradoxical mechanism of inflation of
the foam cuff, accompanied by injection of air into the cuff, may result in exces-
sively high pressures.

The FOME-CUF device is a dynamic open system. It may be left open to at-

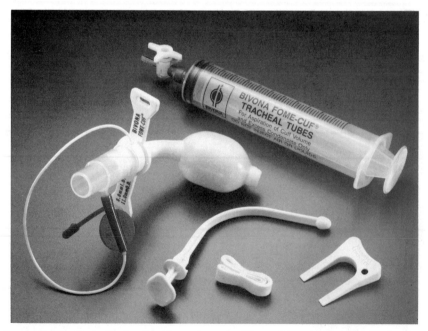

Figure 3-20 Foam-filled cuff tracheostomy tube. The cuff is actively deflated before insertion. The cuff then passively inflates to ambient pressure if left open to air. The pilot
balloon shown here is attached to the nipple of the Sideport AutoControl airway connector. See text for explanation. (Courtesy of Bivona Medical Technologies, Gary, Ind.)

mospheric pressure or to ventilatory system pressure. The cuff is typically left open to atmospheric pressure during spontaneous respiration or high-frequency ventilation. Connecting the inflation line to a side-port adapter placed between the airway and the ventilator ciruitry allows the cuff to inflate and deflate with cycling of the ventilator, ensuring a seal at peak inspiratory pressure. Typical applications of this setup include positive-pressure ventilation, except at high frequency and during anesthesia.

Air-filled cuffs require periodic assessment of cuff pressure, whereas the manufacturer of the FOME-CUF recommends periodic measurement of the *volume* of air in the cuff. If the volume of air in the cuff is *decreasing,* the foam is more fully expanded and the clinician is alerted to the possibility of tracheal dilation.

Managing Air Leaks

Air loss may be:
- From around the cuff as a result of patient position changes
- From the cuff itself
- From a faulty one-way valve on the pilot balloon
- From a cracked or broken air inflation line

If it is determined that the leak is due to position changes, then repositioning the patient's head should correct the problem. If the leak is from the cuff or from a cracked or broken inflation line (often at the point of attachment to the airway), then call for assistance in reintubation. In the interim, if the patient is symptomatic, the methods of supporting ventilation include increasing the tidal volume delivered by the ventilator to compensate for the gas escaping through the upper airway, and increasing the FIO_2 to 1.0 to ensure adequate oxygenation. If the patient remains unstable, call for assistance and prepare for reintubation.

A leak may also occur because of a broken inflation line at the point where the pilot balloon attaches. Temporary repair may be achieved by cutting off the one-way valve–pilot balloon housing, inserting a 20-gauge intravenous catheter into the tubing, and attaching a three-way stopcock. Cuff inflation may then be maintained, thereby avoiding emergency reintubation.

Leaks in the one-way valve often occur because the valve has become stuck in the open position, allowing air to escape. To prevent further air loss, attach a Luer-Lok syringe, or a stopcock turned off to the cuff, to the end of the valve. It should be noted that inserting a syringe into the valve with excessive force may result in a jammed or cracked valve.

Air leak may also be due to a misplaced endotracheal or tracheostomy tube. Before the tube is repositioned, any secretions that have collected above the cuff should be suctioned from the oropharynx. The cuff is then deflated and, with assistance, the tube is repositioned and stabilized.

SPECIAL CONCERNS

Self-extubation

The two most frequent methods by which self-extubation is accomplished is (1) by using the tongue and (2) by leaning forward and downward to the restrained hands and then manually removing the tube. Even the most vigilant caregivers may sometimes find themselves with a patient who has intentionally removed his or her airway. Conditions that place the patient at a high risk for self-extubation are as follows: patients with head truma or with drugs or alcohol on board; change of shift, when patients may not have a direct caregiver in their room or nearby to observe them as closely; the night shift, because there are fewer personnel to observe and interrupt an attempted self-extubation; and delay of patients who are ready for extubation but must wait "for the doctor's order, for the arterial blood gas values to come back," and so on. The best approach to the problem is to implement preventive measures (Table 3–5).

Laryngeal and Tracheal Injury

The primary sites of injury from artificial airways are the larynx and the trachea. Two major mechanisms are mainly responsible for airway damage: *tube movement*, which causes abrasion, and *pressure*, which causes necrosis. Duration of intubation also appears to play a significant role in glottic injury. Preventive measures should be implemented throughout the period of intubation in an effort to reduce the incidence of complications. Areas to focus on are head movement, tube size, cuff pressures, and duration of intubation.

Head motion, especially flexion and extension, should be kept to a minimum because it results in significant movement of the tube in the airway and therefore

TABLE 3–5 Self or Unplanned Extubation: Preventive Measures

Measure	Rationale
Vigilant monitoring of all intubated patients	Interception of self-extubation attempt
Application of soft restraints to all intubated patients	Safety measure used until it can be ascertained that patient thoroughly understands airway's importance and demonstrates no periods of confusion or agitation
Use of "mitts" and restraint vests as necessary	Wrist restraints insufficient to prevent patient from leaning forward and grasping at airway
Positioning of ventilator circuitry and equipment attached to it (e.g., in-line suction apparatus) up and over patient's shoulder	Deterrence of airway removal by pulling on its extensions
Nasal or orogastric tube not taped to ETT	Deterrence of airway removal by pulling on equipment secured to it
ETT securely taped around patient's head	Greater stabilization provided than by taping only to the cheeks
ETT harness used to secure tube in high-risk patient (particularly helpful in patients who "tongue" at their tube)	Provision of greater stability than tape provides—if applied properly (Some models also provide bite block, making it more difficult to maneuver tube with tongue.)
Generous administration of sedation and analgesics, particularly to patient with tenuous respiratory status	Control of patient in environment that may be perceived as intolerable
Timely removal of ETT from patient ready for extubation	Avoidance of delay, which could lead to frustration and eventual intervention by patient

abrasive injury. Some patients may require sedation for effective reduction of excessive head movement. A tube of the apropriate size should be used in an effort to reduce the injury larger tubes cause. Generally, this calls for a size 7.0 to 7.5 in female patients and an 8.0 to 8.5 in male patients. Excessive cuff-to-tracheal wall pressure may result in necrotic injury to the tissue; therefore the cuff must be monitored and managed conscientiously.

Duration of intubation is another factor that appears to play a significant role in glottic injury. Consideration should be given to tracheostomy after 10 days of intubation because the incidence of glottic injury rises after this period. However, the question of when to perform a tracheostomy on a patient requiring prolonged intubation has no simple answer applicable to all patients. In patients in whom injury risk has been reduced, endotracheal intubation may be maintained for weeks. Others may benefit from early tracheostomy, such as patients who will obviously require prolonged intubation for secretion management and prevention of aspiration (e.g., severely neurologically depressed patients). The benefits of tracheostomy must be weighed against its complications (i.e., hemorrhage, infection, tension pneumothorax, vascular erosion, tracheal stenosis after decannulation), which can be more serious than the complications of endotracheal intubation.

The most frequent injuries above the glottis are hematomas, edema, and lacerations of the epiglottis during intubation attempts. As a result, it is not uncommon for the laryngeal reflexes (cough, gag, swallow) to be blunted for a period after intubation or for the patient to have hoarseness. The vast majority of these injuries heal without sequelae.

Injuries at the level of the glottis are the most serious of the complications of intubation. Vocal cord erythema, edema, abrasions, and ulcerations occur most commonly at the point where the endotracheal tube makes contact with the vocal cords. Because the endotracheal tube lies in the posterior portion of the glottis, at the site of the arytenoid cartilages and the posterior commissure, these sites are most commonly injured. The most common early symptom of injury are hoarseness and possibly stridor after extubation. Chronic fibrosis and granuloma formation may occur with healing and result in impaired vocal cord function and loss of airway patency. Injury to the recurrent laryngeal nerve may result in permanent paralysis, but this complication is uncommon. Persistent hoarseness, cough especially when associated with liquid oral intake, and dyspnea after extubation could indicate laryngeal ulceration, granuloma formation, or motor paresis. The patient should be monitored for possible aspiration or upper airway obstruction. A swallowing evaluation may be indicated. In many institutions, speech therapy consultations serve as the mechanism to attain an evaluation of the effectiveness of the patient's swallow function. Instruction may then be provided on exercises to improve the effectiveness of glottic closure, methods of swallowing to reduce the incidence of aspiration (e.g., chin tuck), and food consistencies that may best be tolerated by the patient.

Tracheal mucosa and cartilage injury occur most commonly at the point of contact with the artificial airway cuff and where the tip of the tube contacts the tracheal wall. Two factors are primarily responsible: high cuff–to–tracheal wall pressure and mechanical motion. The two most common injuries are (1) tracheomalacia, or dilation of the trachea, which is seen at the level of the cuff, and (2) tracheal stenosis, which occurs with healing. Stenosis may occur at any point along the length of mucosal contact with the artificial airway.

Management of the patient's airway is a significant part of the total care of the patient-ventilator system. The prevention of adverse sequelae of the use of an artificial airway should serve as an outcome goal for practitioners caring for patients supported by mechanical ventilation. It is extremely rewarding when a patient who has had prolonged ventilatory support undergoes successful extubation/decannulation. How unfortunate it is, however, when this event is tainted by potentially preventable chronic morbidity for the patient.

Mouth Care

Meticulous mouth care should be performed in the intubated patient to prevent inoculation of the respiratory tract with oral pathogens. Before the procedure, ensure that the cuff is appropriately inflated. The teeth, tongue, and palate should be cleaned with toothpaste and a toothbrush or a sponge-tipped swab. Rinse the mouth with tap water, a weak mouthwash solution, or, if halitosis is a problem, a tap water and hydrogen peroxide solution because of its bactericidal effects. A blunt-tipped syringe may be held in one hand for irrigation and a suction catheter in the other hand for aspiration. In some cases the patient may be able to assist by swishing and then expectorating the mouth rinse.

REMOVAL OF THE ARTIFICIAL AIRWAY
Extubation

When the indications for intubation have resolved and the patient is stable, extubation may be performed. Begin by explaining the procedure to the patient. Suction the patient one final time through the artificial airway and translaryngeally to remove secretions that may have pooled on top of the cuff. The tape is removed, the patient is instructed to take a deep breath, and the cuff deflated. Immediately the patient is told to forcefully exhale or cough while the tube is removed in one swift movement. If the patient cannot cooperate to time exhalation with tube removal, a positive pressure breath should be delivered with a manual resuscitation bag. The rationale for patient exhalation during extubation is to force secretions remaining above the cuff up into the oropharynx during extubation, reducing the potential for aspiration. The patient should then be asked to cough and speak as assessment of these functions is performed. Supplemental, humidified oxygen may be required. If the patient develops signs of upper airway obstruction, cool mist or racemic epinephrine nebulization is indicated to reduce edema. Observe the patient closely for obstruction.

Decannulation

Decannulation is not an exact science. In general, there are two methods: immediate decannulation and gradual decannulation. For the immediate procedure, after determination that the indications for tracheostomy have been resolved and the patient is stable, the tracheostomy tube is removed and the patient immediately begins using the natural airway for gas exchange and secretion removal. In the gradual procedure, the tracheostomy tube is replaced at intervals by a tube of a smaller size (downsizing). This allows for gradual closure of the stoma, a transition period toward reuse by the patient of the natural airway for gas exchange and secretion removal, and assessment by the caregiver of the adequacy of these functions before tube removal. A tracheostomy button may be used after the tube is removed. After decannulation has been performed, the stoma is covered with a dry dressing. If air loss is a problem, then the stoma may be covered with petrolatum-impregnated gauze and then dry gauze. Stomal dressings should be changed twice a day and the site assessed for healing and complications.

RECOMMENDED READINGS

Bishop, M.J. (1989). Mechanisms of laryngotracheal injury following prolonged tracheal intubation. *Chest, 96*(1), 185–186.

Bivona, Inc. (1991). *FOME-CUF Users Manual.* Gary, Ind: Bivona, Inc.

Crabtree Goodnough, S.K. (1988). Reducing tracheal injury and aspiration. *Dimensions of Critical Care Nursing* 7(6), 324–332.

Grassmick, B.K., and Bander, J. (1993). Long-term airway management. In R.W. Carlson and M.A. Geheb (Eds.). *Principles and Practice of Medical Intensive Care* (pp. 967–977). Philadelphia: W.B. Saunders.

Hoffman, L.A. (1994). Timing of tracheotomy: What is the best approach? *Resp Care* 39(4), 378–385.

Kersten, L.D. (1989). *Comprehensive Respiratory Nursing: A Decision-making Approach.* Philadelphia: W.B. Saunders.

Manzano, J.L., et al. (1993). Verbal communication of ventilator-dependent patients. *Crit Care Med* 21(4), 512–517.

Marsh, H.M., Gillespie, D.J., and Baumgartner, A.E. (1989). Timing of tracheostomy in the critically ill patient. *Chest* 96(1), 190–193.

Mason, M., and Watkins, C. (1992). Protocol for use of the Passy-Muir tracheostomy speaking valves. *Eur Respir J* 5(suppl 15), 148s.

Plevak, D.J., and Ward, J.J. (1991). Airway management. In G.G. Burton, J.E. Hodgkin, and J.J. Ward (Eds.). *Respiratory Care: A Guide to Clinical Practice.* Philadelphia: J.B. Lippincott, 449–504.

Plummer, A.L., and Gracey, D.R. (1989). Consensus conference on artificial airways in patients receiving mechanical ventilation. *Chest, 96*(1), 178–180.

4

Administration of Oxygen, Humidification, and Aerosol Therapy

OXYGEN THERAPY

The delivery of supplemental oxygen may be necessary for the correction or prevention of hypoxemia. As shown in Chapter 2, in room air the fraction of inspired oxygen (FIO_2) is 0.21. That is, of all the air that one inspires, 21% consists of oxygen molecules. Therefore, *supplemental O_2 administration* is the delivery of any oxygen concentration greater than 21%.

Indications

The need for supplemental oxygen should be determined through evaluation of the patient's arterial blood gas and clinical assessment findings (Table 4–1). In general, indications for oxygen therapy include the following:
- Correction of hypoxemia, thereby decreasing the work of breathing and the myocardial workload it imposes, and promotion of adequate oxygen delivery to the tissues. The correction of hypoxemia, in and of itself, will not ensure the sufficient delivery of oxygenated blood to the tissues. A competent cardiovascular system is also necessary for carrying the adequately oxygenated blood to the tissues.
- Improvement of oxygenation in patients with decreased O_2 carrying capacity (e.g., those with anemia, sickle cell disease).
- Promotion of the reabsorption of air in body cavities (e.g., pneumocephalus, small pneumothorax).

Oxygen as a Drug

The administration of oxygen should be done with as much care and attention as the practitioner uses when administering any other drug. Oxygen, like most drugs, has safe dose ranges, adverse physiologic effects, and toxic manifestations that are associated with higher doses and prolonged use. For correction of hypoxemia, enough oxygen should be administered to saturate the hemoglobin 92% or better. This will safely achieve a PaO_2 of about 60 to 70 mm Hg. Administering additional supplemental oxygen, once the hemoglobin is fully saturated (99% to 100%), places the patient at risk of having toxic effects of this drug.

TABLE 4–1   Signs and Symptoms of Hypoxemia

System	Mild to Moderate	Severe
Central nervous system	Confusion, agitation, combativeness	Lethargy and obtunded mental status
Cardiac	Tachycardia, ectopy Hypertension	Bradycardia Hypotension
Respiratory	Dyspnea, tachypnea, shallow respirations, labored breathing	Increasing dyspnea and tachypnea, possible bradypnea or agonal respirations
Arterial blood gas	PaO_2: 60–80 mm Hg	PaO_2 < 60 mm Hg
Skin	Cool, clammy	Cyanosis

Complications Associated With Oxygen Use

HYPOVENTILATION AND CARBON DIOXIDE NARCOSIS

Oxygen-induced hypoventilation may occur because of suppression of the hypoxic respiratory drive. Normally, carbon dioxide is the primary stimulant driving the respiratory system. However, in patients with chronic hypercapnia ($PaCO_2$ >45 mm Hg), the central nervous system response to an elevated CO_2 level becomes blunted and hypoxemia becomes the major ventilatory stimulus. Administration of oxygen-enriched gas to these individuals may result in hypoventilation, hypercapnia, and possibly apnea. Under these circumstances, oxygen should be administered in low concentrations (<30%) while the patient is observed for signs of respiratory depression. If oxygenation remains inadequate and respiratory depression occurs, then mechanical ventilation is necessary.

ABSORPTION ATELECTASIS

Absorption atelectasis occurs when the alveoli collapse because the gas within them is absorbed into the bloodstream. Nitrogen, a relatively insoluble gas, normally maintains a residual volume within the alveolus. During the breathing of high concentrations of oxygen, nitrogen may be replaced, or "washed out" of the alveolus. When the alveolar oxygen is then absorbed into the pulmonary capillary, the alveolus partially to totally collapses. Absorption atelectasis is more likely to occur in areas where ventilation is decreased, such as in airways that are distal to partial obstruction, because the oxygen is absorbed into the blood at a faster rate than it is replaced.

PULMONARY OXYGEN TOXICITY

The exposure of the pulmonary tissues to a high oxygen tension can lead to pathologic parenchymal changes. The degree of injury is related to the duration of exposure and to the oxygen tension of the inspired air, not to the PaO_2. Generally, an FIO_2 of >0.5 is considered toxic. The first signs of O_2 toxicity are due to the irritant effect of oxygen and reflect an acute tracheobronchitis. After only a few hours of breathing 100% oxygen, mucociliary function is depressed and clearance of mucus is impaired. Within 6 hours of the administration of 100% O_2, nonproductive cough, substernal pain, and nasal stuffiness may develop.

Symptoms such as malaise, nausea, anorexia, and headache may be reported. These changes are reversible on discontinuation of oxygen therapy.

More prolonged exposure to high oxygen tension may lead to changes in the lung that mimic adult respiratory distress syndrome. Disruption of the endothelial lining of the pulmonary microcirculation results in leakage of proteinaceous fluid. An exudate consisting of edema, hemorrhage, and white blood cells forms in the lung. The damage to the lung may progress to cell death. The function of the pulmonary macrophage is also depressed, rendering the patient more susceptible to infection. The tissue injury in the lung caused by hyperoxia is generally agreed to be due to the production of biochemically reactive, oxygen-derived free radicals that overwhelm the body's antioxidant defenses. Termination of exposure to toxic levels of oxygen allows cellular repair to begin; the repair may also result in varying degrees of pulmonary fibrosis, however.

Avoiding the use of high concentrations of oxygen for prolonged periods is the key to avoiding pulmonary injury from high oxygen tension. The lowest FIO_2 capable of generating a sufficient oxygen saturation serves as the best guide to oxygen therapy titration.

RETROLENTAL FIBROPLASIA

Administration of excessive amounts of oxygen to premature infants may result in constriction of the immature retinal vessels, endothelial cell damage, retinal detachment, and possible blindness. The amount of injury that occurs is related to the PaO_2; therefore it is recommended that the PaO_2 be maintained in the 60 to 90 mm Hg range in neonates.

OXYGEN DELIVERY SYSTEMS

Many devices for administering supplemental oxygen are available. These devices are classified into two general categories: *low-flow systems* and *high-flow systems*. Whether a system is low or high flow does not determine its capability of delivering low versus high concentrations of oxygen. When choosing the appropriate technique for delivering supplemental oxygen, one must consider the device's advantages and disadvantages, the FIO_2 limits of the device, and its appropriateness for a particular patient (see Box 4–1).

Box 4–1   Oxygen Delivery Systems

Low-Flow Systems	*High-Flow Systems*
Nasal cannula	Venturi masks
Simple face mask	
Partial rebreathing mask	LARGE-VOLUME AEROSOL SYSTEMS
Nonrebreathing mask	High-humidity face mask
	High-humidity face tent
	High-humidity tracheostomy mask/collar
	High-humidity T piece (or "blow-by")

Low-Flow Systems

Low-flow systems, by definition, do not provide all the gas necessary to meet the patient's total minute ventilation. These systems require that the patient entrain, or draw in, room air while gas enriched with oxygen is also inspired from a reservoir. The reservoir of oxygen may be in the nasopharyngeal or oropharyngeal cavities, a mask, or a reservoir bag. With these systems, the FIO_2 delivered to the patient can only be estimated because the humidity, temperature, and actual FIO_2 cannot be precisely controlled. The FIO_2 is determined not only by the amount of oxygen delivered to the patient but also by the ventilatory pattern and thus by the amount of air the patient entrains. Low-flow delivery systems include the nasal cannula, simple face mask, partial rebreathing mask, and nonrebreathing mask.

NASAL CANNULA

Description and Technique. Made of lightweight green or white plastic, the nasal cannula consists of tubing and two prongs that fit into the nose (Fig. 4–1). To apply the device, direct the prongs inward, following the curvature of the nasal passages. Hook the tubing behind the patient's ears and adjust the strap under the chin. Correct use of a nasal cannula requires that the nose be free of obstruction and the cannula and prongs are correctly positioned. Mouth breathing is believed not to preclude the use of the nasal cannula unless there is complete obstruction of the nares, because oxygen will be drawn in from the anatomic reservoirs: the nasopharynx and oropharynx. However, more research is needed in this area. The nasal cannula is capable of delivering an FIO_2 ranging from 0.24 to 0.44, depending on the amount of flow (measured in liters) (Table 4–2). The maximal flow rate is 6 L/min because higher flow rates, while not affording an appreciably higher FIO_2, cause crusting of secretions, drying of the nasal mucosa, and epistaxis.

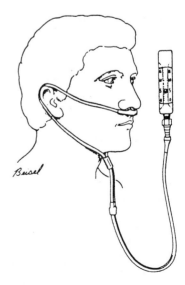

FIGURE 4–1 Nasal cannula in place, attached to an oxygen flowmeter. (Reprinted with permission from Kofke, WA: Postoperative respiratory care techniques. Part III. Weaning from mechanical ventilation and oxygen therapy. *Curr Rev PACN* 1992; 13:161.)

TABLE 4–2 Estimated F_{IO_2} With Low-Flow Oxygen Delivery Devices*

100% O_2 Flow Rate (L/min)	F_{IO_2}
Nasal Cannula	
1	0.24
2	0.28
3	0.32
4	0.36
5	0.40
6	0.44
Simple Oxygen Mask	
5–6	0.40
6–7	0.50
7–8	0.60
Partial Rebreather Mask†	
7	0.65
8–15	0.70–0.80
Nonrebreathing Mask	
Set to Prevent Collapse of Bag	0.85–1.0

*Exact F_{IO_2} delivered varies with changes in tidal volume, respiratory rate, minute ventilation, and ventilatory pattern.
†Flow rate should be set so that reservoir bag only partially collapses on inspiration.

Advantages
- Inexpensive
- Well tolerated, comfortable
- Patient can eat and drink
- May be used with patients who have chronic obstructive pulmonary disease
- May be used with humidity

Disadvantages
- May cause pressure sores around ears and nose
- May dry and irritate nasal mucosa

SIMPLE FACE MASK

Description and Technique. The placing of a mask over the patient's face increases the size of the oxygen reservoir beyond the limits of the anatomic reservoir; therefore a higher F_{IO_2} can be delivered. The oxygen flow must be run at a sufficient rate, usually 5 L/min or greater, to prevent collection, and thus rebreathing, of exhaled gases high in carbon dioxide. Flow rates greater than 10 L/min, however, do not appreciably increase the F_{IO_2} because the reservoir within the mask is filled.

The simple face mask (Fig. 4–2) has vent holes on the sides for the entrainment of room air and the release of exhaled gases. It has no valves or reservoir bag. Apply the mask securely over the patient's mouth, nose, and chin. Press the flexible metal pieces over the bridge of the nose to create a seal for prevention of gas loss. Adjust the strap around the patient's head and instruct the patient in the importance of wearing the mask as applied. Intermittently clean the inside of the mask and remove accumulated water, particularly when humid-

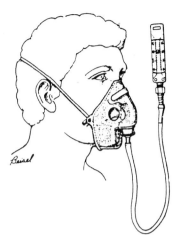

FIGURE 4-2 Simple face mask attached to an oxygen flowmeter. (Reprinted with permission from Kofke, WA: Postoperative respiratory care techniques. Part III. Weaning from mechanical ventilation and oxygen therapy. *Curr Rev PACN* 1992; 13:161.)

ity is used. Assess the skin for areas of pressure. Switch to a nasal cannula at mealtime.

Advantages
- Simple, lightweight
- Can be used with humidity
- Delivery of FIO_2 up to 0.60

Disadvantages
- May be considered confining by some patients, who may feel the need to remove the mask to speak
- Limitation of access to patient's face for expectoration of secretions and other needs
- Difficulty obtaining correct application when nasogastric or orogastric tube is in place
- Uncomfortable when facial trauma or burns are present
- May cause drying or irritation of the eyes

PARTIAL REBREATHING MASK

Description and Technique. The design of the partial rebreathing mask is similar to that of the simple face mask, with the addition of an oxygen reservoir bag (Fig. 4–3). Increasing the oxygen reservoir beyond the size of the anatomic reservoir allows the delivery of an FIO_2 greater than 0.60. The mask should fit snugly, and the oxygen flow rate should be adjusted so that the bag deflates by only about one third on inspiration. During inspiration the patient draws air from the mask, from the bag, and through the holes in the side of the mask. During expiration the first one third of exhaled gases will flow back into the reservoir bag. This portion of exhaled gases comes from the anatomic dead space; therefore it is still rich in oxygen, humidified, and warmed, and it contains little CO_2. If oxygen flow to the system is high enough to keep the bag from deflating more than one third its volume during inhalation, then exhaled CO_2 will not accumulate in the reservoir bag. On the next breath the patient will inspire part of the previously exhaled gas, along with 100% oxygen from the source. The bag is not a reservoir for CO_2, a common misconception associated with the name *partial rebreather.*

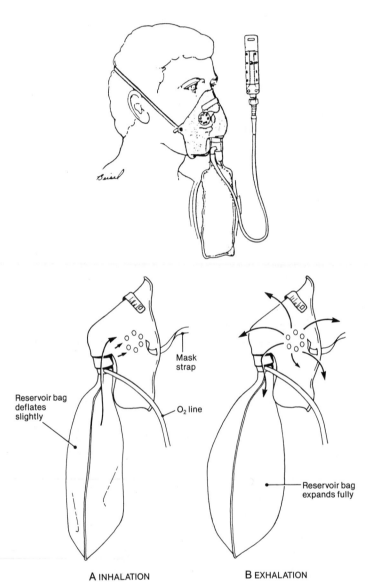

A INHALATION   **B** EXHALATION

FIGURE 4–3 (*Top*) Partial rebreathing mask correctly in place and attached to an oxygen flowmeter. (*Bottom*) Arrows indicate the direction of gas movement on (*A*) inhalation and (*B*) exhalation. (*Top* reprinted with permission from Kofke, WA: Postoperative respiratory care techniques. Part III. Weaning from mechanical ventilation and oxygen therapy. *Curr Rev PACN* 1992; 13:161. *Bottom* from Kersten, LD: *Comprehensive Respiratory Nursing: A Decision-making Approach*. Philadelphia: WB Saunders, 1989.)

Advantages
- FIO_2 >0.60 is delivered in moderate to severe hypoxia.
- Exhaled oxygen from the anatomic dead space is conserved.

Disadvantages
- Insufficient flow rate may lead to rebreathing of CO_2.
- Mask over mouth may lead to feelings of claustrophobia in patients with severe hypoxemia.
- Mask prevents access to mouth for eating, drinking, expectorating.
- Flow rate of 15 L/min may be insufficient to meet minute ventilation needs of severely dyspneic patients.
- High oxygen flow rates may cause drying and irritation to the eyes.

NONREBREATHING MASK

Description and Technique. Nonrebreathing masks, like the partial rebreather, have a reservoir bag, but they also have one-way valves between the reservoir bag and the mask and over the exhalation ports of the mask (Fig. 4–4). The purpose of these valves is to prevent exhaled gases from entering the bag and the entrainment of room air, respectively. On inspiration, the side port valves close and the valve between the bag and mask connection opens, allowing for inspiration of 100% O_2. On expiration, the exhalation port valves open and the valve between the bag and mask closes, promoting the release of exhaled gases into the room and preventing their entry into the bag.

The flow rate should be set to prevent the reservoir bag from collapsing on inspiration. If the flow rate is set properly and if a tight fit is achieved, then theoretically the delivered FIO_2 is 1.0. However, in reality, the FIO_2 is usually nearer to 0.8 to 0.9, because a tight fit is seldom achieved and room air is pulled in around the mask. In some institutions one of the side port flaps is removed as a safety measure, so that in the event of inadvertent discontinuation of the oxygen source the patient can still inspire room air. This action will also decrease the delivered FIO_2 because, when the valve is removed, more room air entrainment occurs.

Advantage
- Delivery of >80% oxygen to severely hypoxemic patient when an individual skilled in intubation is not available or it is desirable to defer intubation

Disadvantages
- Uncomfortable if tight fit, with possible feelings of claustrophobia
- Limited access to mouth for eating, drinking, expectorating
- Possible sticking of valves
- Eye irritation from high flow rates of oxygen and improper fit at the nose

High-Flow Systems

High-flow systems are those in which the flow of gases is sufficient to meet all of the patient's minute ventilation requirements. These devices either have fixed air-oxygen entrainment ratios or reservoirs/flow rates that are adequate to provide all of the patient's inspired volume. In general, for delivery of a consistent FIO_2 to a patient with a variable (deep, irregular, shallow) ventilatory pattern, a high-flow system should be used. The FIO_2 remains fairly constant and is not affected by the patient's ventilatory pattern. Temperature and humidity can also be

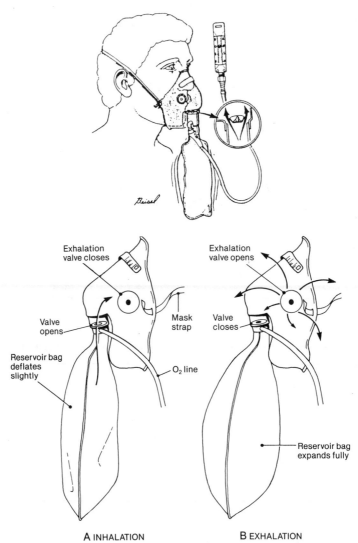

Figure 4–4 (*Top*) Nonrebreathing mask correctly in place and attached to an oxygen flow meter. (*Bottom*) Arrows indiate the direction of gas movement on (A) inhalation and (B) exhalation. (*Top* reprinted with permission from Kofke, WA: Postoperative respiratory care techniques. Part III. Weaning from mechanical ventilation and oxygen therapy. *Curr Rev PACN* 1992; 13:161. *Bottom* from Kersten, LD: *Comprehensive Respiratory Nursing: A Decision-making Approach*. Philadelphia: WB Saunders, 1989.)

controlled. High-flow delivery systems include Venturi masks and large-volume aerosol systems, which include the high-humidity face mask, high-humidity face tent, high-humidity tracheostomy collar or mask, and high-humidity T piece. The application of mechanical ventilation fits the definition of a high-flow system; however, it is placed in a class of its own.

VENTURI MASK

Description and Technique. The Venturi, or Venti, mask appears much like a simple face mask; however, it has a jet adapter placed between the mask and the tubing to the oxygen source. The jet adapters come in various sizes (and are often color coded) corresponding to various FIO_2 values. The Venturi mask operates on the Bernoulli principle of air entrainment (Fig. 4–5). As gas flows under pressure at a rapid flow rate through the narrowed orifice of the jet adapter, an area of subatmospheric pressure develops lateral to the small opening. This creates a "jet drag" that leads to the entrainment of room air through side ports located on the adapter. The FIO_2 is modified either by altering the size of the side ports or by altering the jet orifice diameter, both of which affect the amount of air entrained. The appropriate flow rate is usually inscribed on the jet adapter. Large volumes of air are entrained with the Venturi mask; volumes of oxygen-enriched gas (with a stable FIO_2), sufficient to meet even large minute ventilation needs, are therefore delivered with this device (Table 4–3).

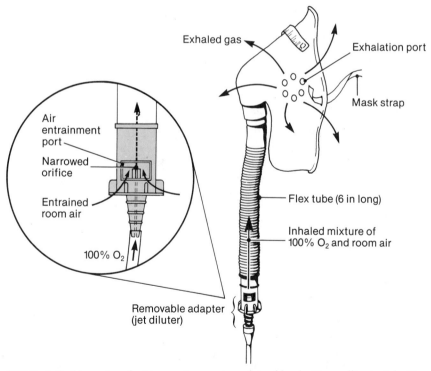

Exhaled gas

Exhalation port

Mask strap

Air entrainment port

Narrowed orifice

Entrained room air

Flex tube (6 in long)

Inhaled mixture of 100% O_2 and room air

100% O_2

Removable adapter (jet diluter)

FIGURE 4–5 Venturi mask. Air entrainment is explained by the Bernoulli principle. Gas flowing under pressure at a rapid flow rate through the narrowed orifice of the Venturi adapter creates an area of subatmospheric pressure laterally. A "jet drag" pulls (entrains) room air through side ports located on the adapter. FIO_2 is increased by either decreasing the size of the side ports or increasing the size of the jet orifice, both of which decrease the amount of room air entrained. (Modified from Kersten, LD: *Comprehensive Respiratory Nursing: A Decision-making Approach.* Philadelphia: WB Saunders, 1989.)

TABLE 4–3 Venturi Devices (Mask and Nebulizer) Delivered F_{IO_2}, Flow Settings, and Air-Oxygen Entrainment Ratios*

F_{IO_2}	Flow Rate (L/min)	Air: O_2 Entrainment Ratio	Total Liter Gas Flow (L/min)
0.24	4	25:1	104
0.28	6	10:1	66
0.35	8	5:1	48
0.40	8	3:1	32
0.60	12	1:1	Twice O_2 flow

*Flow rate settings and exact total number of liters of gas flow may vary slightly between products of different manufacturers. Consistency may also vary because products are generally plastic and are mass produced.

Advantages
• Delivery of a very predictable F_{IO_2}
• Useful in patients to whom delivery of excessive oxygen could depress the respiratory drive
Disadvantages
• Limited access to patient's mouth for eating, drinking, and expectorating
• Claustrophobic feeling generated by the mask
• Irritation to the eyes because of high flow rates

Large-Volume Aerosol Systems

The addition of humidity to the inspired gases is indicated to hydrate retained secretions and improve the function of the normal mucociliary escalator (see Humidification/Nebulization, below). High-flow devices, used for administering humidified supplemental oxygen to patients who have an artificial airway, are the T-piece and the tracheostomy mask/collar. If the patient is breathing through the natural airway, the high-humidity face mask and the high-humidity face tent may be applied. Humidity may be added when various low-flow systems are used; however, the four systems described above are the only high-flow systems to which humidity may be applied.

With each of the following systems, after correct assembly and before application of the device, the F_{IO_2} must be chosen and the oxygen flow rate adjusted to ensure that it is operating like a high-flow system (i.e., that all of the patient's ventilatory needs are being met by the system). The desired F_{IO_2} is chosen by adjusting the air entrainment port on the nebulizer (Fig. 4–6). The initial flow rate is then set at 10 L/min. To ensure that the patient's entire minute ventilation needs are being met by the device, adjust the flow rate so that a constant mist can be seen coming from the extension tubing on the T-piece, from the exhalation port on the tracheostomy collar, from the exhalation ports on the face mask, and from over the top of the face tent. If the patient's ventilatory needs are high, and one flowmeter with nebulizer is therefore inadequate to deliver sufficient flow rates and support a constant mist, then utilize two. Use of a second nebulizer can be achieved by using a "wye" adapter.

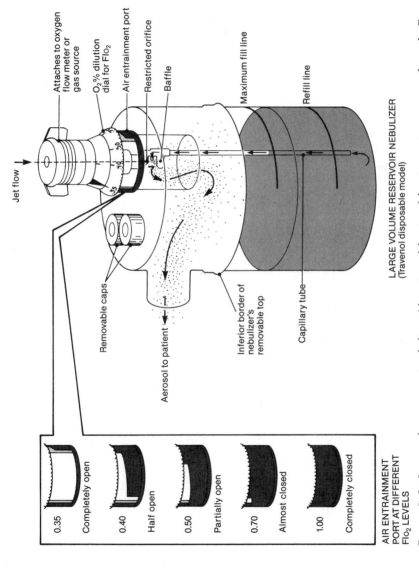

FIGURE 4–6 Large-volume reservoir nebulizer. Alteration of the size of the air entrainment port adjusts the FiO_2. (From Kersten, LD: *Comprehensive Respiratory Nursing: A Decision-making Approach.* Philadelphia: WB Saunders, 1989.)

Jet flow

Attaches to oxygen flow meter or gas source

O_2 % dilution dial for FiO_2

Air entrainment port

Restricted orifice

Baffle

Maximum fill line

Refill line

Removable caps

Aerosol to patient

Inferior border of nebulizer's removable top

Capillary tube

LARGE VOLUME RESERVOIR NEBULIZER
(Travenol disposable model)

AIR ENTRAINMENT PORT AT DIFFERENT FiO_2 LEVELS

0.35 Completely open

0.40 Half open

0.50 Partially open

0.70 Almost closed

1.00 Completely closed

HIGH-HUMIDITY T-PIECE (OR "BLOW-BY")

Description and Technique. The high-humidity T-piece attaches to the endotracheal or tracheostomy tube to provide oxygen and humidification to a patient who is not using a mechanical ventilator. Corrugated tubing coming from the nebulizer attaches to one end of the T-piece. An extension (reservoir) of corrugated tubing is attached to the other end of the T-piece. The entire setup is connected to the patient's artificial airway (Fig. 4–7). The desired FIO_2, ranging from 0.28 to 1.0, is chosen by adjusting the air entrainment port on the nebulizer. The initial flow rate is set at 10 L/min. To ensure that the patient's entire minute ventilation needs are being met by the device, adjust the flow rate so that a constant mist can be seen coming from the extension piece on the T-tube.

Advantages
- High humidity prevents airway drying and helps to thin the secretions.
- Device is light in weight.
- Precise FIO_2 can be delivered.

Disadvantages
- Tubing can become heavy with accumulated water and pull on the airway.
- When patient is changing body positions, accumulated water may accidentally drain into the patient's airway.
- Failure to properly regulate flow rate creates a low-flow system.

HIGH-HUMIDITY TRACHEOSTOMY MASK (TRACHEOSTOMY COLLAR)

Description and Technique. The tracheostomy mask, also known as the tracheostomy collar, is a clear mask designed to fit over a tracheostomy tube or a laryngectomy tube. The hole in the anterior portion of the collar-shaped mask is

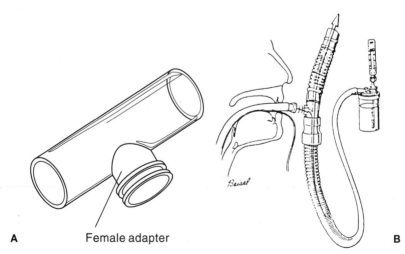

A Female adapter **B**

FIGURE 4–7 The T-piece, or T-tube, is connected to an endotracheal or tracheostomy tube to provide humidifed oxygen. Use of a nebulizer provides humidity in an aerosol form. (*Bottom* reprinted with permission from Kofke, WA: Postoperative respiratory care techniques. Part III. Weaning from mechanical ventilation and oxygen therapy. *Curr Rev PACN* 1992; 13:161.)

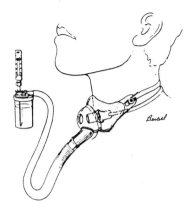

FIGURE 4–8 The high-humidity tracheostomy mask, or collar, fits over a tracheostomy or laryngectomy tube. The hole in the front of the mask is for exhalation. (Reprinted with permission from Kofke, WA: Postoperative respiratory care techniques. Part III. Weaning from mechanical ventilation and oxygen therapy. *Curr Rev PACN* 1992; 13:161.)

the exhalation port. It should be applied to the patient with the large-bore oxygen tubing connection at the bottom and the neck strap adjusted to ensure a snug fit (Fig. 4–8).

The desired FIO$_2$, ranging from 0.28 to 1.0, is chosen by adjusting the air entrainment port on the nebulizer. The initial flow rate is set at 10 L/min. To ensure that the patient's entire minute ventilation needs are being met by the device, adjust the flow rate so that a constant mist can be seen from the exhalation port.

Advantages
- High humidity prevents airway drying and helps to thin the secretions.
- Device is lightweight and comfortable.
- Precise FIO$_2$ can be delivered.

Disadvantages
- Secretions can accumulate in the tracheostomy collar.
- Tubing can become heavy with accumulated water, dislodging collar from proper position and thus compromising accurate FIO$_2$ delivery.
- When patient is changing body positions, accumulated water may accidentally drain into the patient's airway.
- Failure to properly regulate flow rate creates a low-flow system.

HIGH-HUMIDITY FACE MASK
Description and Technique. The high-humidity face mask is similar in design to the simple face mask. Differences are that the high-humidity face mask is attached to a wide-bore oxygen tubing and nebulizer and that the exhalation ports are larger to accommodate larger aerosol particles and high water output. The mask should be applied as described previously in the discussion of the simple face mask. After the mask is applied, the FIO$_2$ is chosen by adjusting the dial at the top of the nebulizer. The initial flow rate is set at 10 L/min. To ensure that the patient's entire minute ventilation needs are being met by the device, adjust the flow rate so that a constant mist can be seen coming from the mask's side ports.

Advantages
- High humidity prevents airway drying and helps to thin the secretions.
- Delivery of FIO$_2$ is more precise than with a simple face mask.

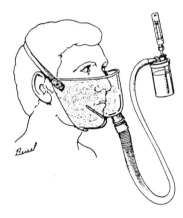

Figure 4-9 High-humidity face tent. (Reprinted with permission from Kofke, WA: Postoperative respiratory care techniques. Part III. Weaning from mechanical ventilation and oxygen therapy. *Curr Rev PACN* 1992; 13:161.)

Disadvantages
- Mask is confining.
- Access to mouth for eating, drinking, expectoration is limited.
- Mask becomes uncomfortable as inside of mask and face rapidly become wet.
- Rushing air and gurgling water, collected in tubing, become noisy.
- Failure to regulate flow rate properly creates a low-flow system.

High-Humidity Face Tent
Description and Technique. The face tent is a shell-shaped device that fits under the patient's chin, hugging the jaw, with the top arching over the patient's face (Fig. 4–9). The FIO_2 of the delivered gases is set by adjusting the air entrainment port on the nebulizer (range, 0.28 to 1.0). The initial flow rate on the nebulizer should be set at 10 L/min and then adjusted as necessary to produce a visible mist.

The volume of gas supplied by this device should meet the patient's entire minute ventilation needs; therefore it fits the criteria for categorization of a high-flow system. Theoretically a precise FIO_2 can be delivered by this device; however, because of the openness of the face tent and the ease with which it slips out of place, room air may be breathed at varying amounts, diluting the desired FIO_2.

Advantages
- High humidity prevents airway drying and helps to thin the secretions.
- Face tent is more comfortable than the simple or high-humidity face masks for the patient who has facial trauma or burns or who has undergone facial surgery.

Disadvantages
- Face tent is difficult to keep in place.
- Delivery of precisely prescribed FIO_2 is difficult.

MANUAL RESUSCITATION BAGS

Description

Manual resuscitation bags (MRBs) (Fig. 4–10) are used to provide oxygen and positive-pressure ventilation to a sealed airway such as a mask, endotracheal

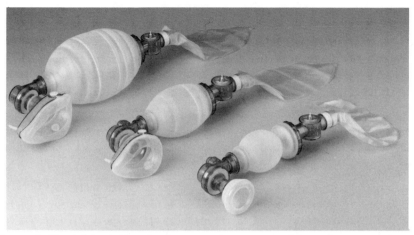

FIGURE 4–10 Adult, child, and infant manual resuscitation bags with oxygen reservoir. (Laerdal™ silicone resuscitators courtesy of Laerdal Medical Corporation, Armonk, N.Y.)

tube, or tracheostomy tube. MRBs consist of a self-inflating bag; an oxygen inlet valve, ideally capable of accepting an oxygen flow of 15 L/min; a nonrebreathing valve(s), which directs the flow of oxygen-enriched gas to the patient and prevents exhaled gases from entering the bag; in pediatric models, a pressure relief valve that opens when proximal airway pressure exceeds a specified amount; and a standard-size (15 mm) adapter that enables the system to attach to a mask or directly to an artificial airway. Additional accessories include oxygen reservoirs and positive end-expiratory pressure (PEEP) valves.

When the bag is squeeezed to create inhalation, positive pressure opens the nonrebreathing valve, allowing the flow of oxygen from the bag into the mask or artificial airway and into the patient. If inspiratory pressures are high, a pop-off valve, if present, will be activated. The pressure-release valve should be capable of being deactivated for adequate ventilation in patients with high airway resistance or low pulmonary compliance. On exhalation, the exhaled gases close the nonrebreathing valve and open a passage to the atmosphere, through which they escape.

MRBs are indicated for both oxygenation and ventilation of patients who have inadequate or absent spontaneous respirations in an arrest situation, who are being transported between departments or institutions (in the absence of a transport ventilator), and who require preoxygenation and ventilation between passes of a suction catheter.

MRBs provide positive-pressure ventilation and, because of the resistance to inspiration created by the nonrebreathing valve, are not intended to provide assisted ventilation in spontaneously breathing patients. The spontaneously breathing patient would have to be capable of generating sufficient negative pressure to open the valve and draw in the oxygen-enriched gas. Furthermore, when the MRB is used with a mask and spontaneous respirations resume, simply holding the setup loosely over the patient's mouth and intermittently squeezing the bag will not provide sufficient oxygen-enriched gas. CO_2 may also be rebreathed because it collects in the mask. In a scenario of reliable and adequate spontaneous respiratory efforts, a tight-fitting mask is more appropriate than a MRB.

When spontaneous respirations are present and the use of a MRB is still indicated, the operator must ensure the simultaneous compression of the squeeze bag with the patient's inspiratory effort. Failure to synchronize manual ventilation with the patient's spontaneous effort may result in patient discomfort, complaints of dyspnea, and gastric distention (when the MRB is being used with a mask).

Factors that determine the FIO_2 delivered by a MRB include the oxygen flow rate, the ventilation rate and tidal volume, and whether an oxygen reservoir is present. MRBs may be used with or without supplemental oxygen. In general, a higher FIO_2 is delivered when the oxygen flow rate is high (15 L/min) and the tidal volume and ventilatory rate are lower. Theoretically, 100% oxygen should be delivered when an oxygen reservoir is in place. Bench studies reveal variable performance in regard to the fraction of delivered oxygen. The FIO_2 values range from 50% to 94% in currently available models. For adequate patient oxygenation, the bag must be capable of delivering adequate oxygen and set up to do so, and a PEEP valve should be used if the PEEP is already 5 cm H_2O or greater. The PEEP valves may be built in or attachable and should be capable of generating PEEP up to 12 cm H_2O.

Volume delivery capability is affected by squeeze bag volume, whether one hand or two are used to compress the bag, hand size, and whether a complete seal has been achieved at the MRB-patient interface. Volume delivery may also be affected eventually by operator fatigue.

Technique

MRB to Mask

When using a bag-valve-mask (BVM) setup, employ a clear mask, if available, to visualize the airway and detect the presence of any vomitus or secretions that could be aspirated. The operator should be positioned at the head of the patient. An oral airway should be placed in the unconscious person to assist in maintaining a patent airway. For more optimal airway patency, use the head-tilt position if not contraindicated. The mask is applied over the mouth and nose and is held securely in place by the thumb and forefinger placed in a C-shaped position on the top of the mask; the third, fourth, and fifth fingers are hooked under the edge of the mandible (Fig. 4–11). Firm pressure must be used to achieve a tight seal while ensuring that the fingers on the jawline are not exerting excessive pressure on the soft tissue under the jaw. The bag is then compressed while a tight seal is maintained, and the chest is observed for adequate respiratory excursion. Sufficient time for exhalation and BVM refill should be allowed before delivery of the next breath.

BVM ventilation is a difficult technique to master and should be performed only by those trained in the skill. Maintaining a seal and a patent airway is challenging, because some of the tidal volume is often lost through leaks around the mask. Performance of the technique by two persons, one to hold the mask in position and the other to compress the bag, may provide more optimal results.

MRB to Artificial Airway

The MRB can be attached to an ETT or tracheostomy tube through the use of a standard-size (15 mm) adapter. The bag may then be squeezed using a one- or two-handed technique. Compression of the bag with two hands has been

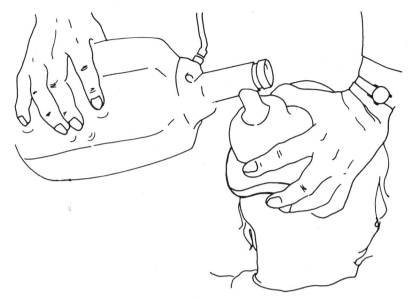

FIGURE 4-11 Technique of bag-valve-mask (BVM) ventilation. (From Wade, JF: *Comprehensive Respiratory Care*. St. Louis: CV Mosby, 1982.)

shown to deliver more optimal volumes. Use of only one hand may be necessary when only one operator is present and the second hand is needed to hold a sterile suction catheter or the airway so that excessive movement and irritation can be avoided.

HUMIDIFICATION/NEBULIZATION

Recall from Chapter 1 that the nasal passages are remarkably efficient at humidifying all inspired gases. By the time air reaches the subglottic space, it is 98% to 100% humidified. Supplemental oxygen, however, is a dry gas. Its administration can lead to the drying of the respiratory passages, dehydration and thickening of the mucus in the airways, and therefore a decrease in the efficiency of the mucociliary system. Ciliary activity may be further retarded when oxygen concentrations are high. For maintenance of the normal function of the mucociliary system, it is generally agreed that supplemental, inspired medical gases should be humidified when administered at flow rates greater than 4 L/min. Humidity, therefore, should be added to supplemental gases when the amount of humidity in that gas is less than normal. This principle *always* applies when the natural airway is bypassed by an endotracheal or tracheostomy tube, to prevent desiccation of the airways.

The administration of aerosol, or high humidity, is recommended when secretions are thick and secretion retention, mucus plugging, or crusting is a problem. Individual patient evaluation is required, however, because further irritation of the airways can occur when high humidity is delivered in certain disease states, such as bronchitis and cystic fibrosis. Conversely, inflammatory processes in the upper airway, such as tracheobronchitis, or postextubation laryngeal

---

Box 4-2   Definitions of Common Terms

Humidification: water evaporated in gas; water in its *gaseous* (vapor) form
Aerosol: suspension of liquid or solid *particles* (water, medications) in gas
Nebulizer: a system that produces aerosol particles that are then carried
  into the airways with the delivered gases

---

edema may benefit from the application of humidity. Humidity is also useful in the treatment of asthma, in which high flow rates of dry oxygen may exacerbate the disease. High humidity is also beneficial after inhalation anesthesia, when ciliary and surfactant activities are depressed.

Humidification can be provided without heating the inspired gases; however, raising the temperature increases the capacity for humidification. Heating of gases delivered into the airways may also serve the dual purpose of efficiently re-warming hypothermic patients. This principle is most often applied in the post-operative and emergency room arenas. High-flow gases delivered into the tra-chea by T-piece, tracheostomy collar, or mechanical ventilator generally should be heated.

In this chapter the principles of humidification and aerosol systems, as they relate to the prophylactic humidification of supplemental oxygen therapy and the therapeutic use of aerosol medication administration, will be reviewed. See Box 4-2.

Humidification Devices

BUBBLE THROUGH HUMIDIFIER

Description. The bubble-through or diffusion head humidifier (Fig. 4–12) is used with the nasal cannula, simple face mask, and reservoir masks. Bubble-

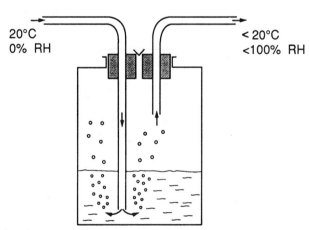

20°C
0% RH

< 20°C
<100% RH

FIGURE 4–12 The bubble-through or diffusion head humidifier saturates gas with water vapor; it does not generate an aerosol. See text for uses. (From Shelly, MP: Inspired gas conditioning. *Resp Care* 1992;37:1074.)

through humidifiers vary in design. In the least efficient form gas is simply forced down a tube to the base of the water reservoir. In a more efficient form a diffuser at the end of the tube breaks the gas into bubbles, thereby increasing the surface area of gas and water, which promotes evaporation. The size of the bubbles varies with the design of the diffuser. The smaller the bubbles, the greater the content of water in the delivered gas because of the increase in the gas-water interface. Other factors that affect the amount of humidity are the water level and the flow rate of gas. Maximal gas-water contact is provided when the column of water through which the bubbles must pass is tall. Therefore the water level should be checked frequently. Higher flow rates cool the water, decreasing its evaporative capacity and reducing contact time. Heating a bubble humidifier is not practical because the gases cool before reaching the patient, and any additional humidity gained is then lost again through condensation.

General Principles: Bubble-Through Humidifier

- Sterile water should be used in humidifiers to prevent nosocomial infection.
- Prevent blockage of small-bore O_2 delivery tubing by water that has spilled over into the tubing from the bubbling action within the humidifier.
- Devices have a positive-pressure release valve on the top. If the small-bore tubing becomes kinked or compressed, back pressure will be released through this valve. When the valve is activated, a whistling sound is emitted, alerting the practitioner to investigation and corrective action so that O_2 flow to the patient can be resumed.

HEATED HUMIDIFIERS

Description. Heated humidifiers are most often used when gases are being delivered via an artificial airway and a mechanical ventilator. Heating the water causes a larger number of water molecules to gain sufficient kinetic energy to enter the gaseous state; therefore the water vapor content of the inspired air is increased. There are three basic designs—cascade (bubble through), pass over, and pass-over wick—which allow the patient's entire inspiratory volume to be heated and humidified (Fig. 4–13).

Cascade Humidifier. In the cascade bubble-through humidifier, gas travels to the bottom of the cascade of water and is forced through a grid or mesh, creating fine bubbles. Thus the principles of cascade humidification are similar to those of bubble-through humidification. In addition, as the gas flow emerges from under the water, it is directed across the surface of the water. This increases contact time and has the effect of increasing evaporation and humidification. The gas is then delivered to the patient by large-bore, corrugated tubing.

Pass-Over Humidifier. The pass-over humidifier has a simple design, and its name explains the principle of operation. In this humidifier, gas passes over a heated water bath. Rising water vapor enters the gas, which is then transported to the patient.

Pass-Over Wick Humidifier. In the pass-over wick humidifier, some material, such as paper or composite material, is partially submerged in the water. This material absorbs water and serves as the wick. Gases are humidified as they circulate around or through the saturated wick.

General Principles: Heated Humidifiers

- A thermometer, preferably one of an in-line design, should be used to determine that the desired temperature has been reached and not exceeded. A reading slightly less than body temperature is appropriate. Overheated

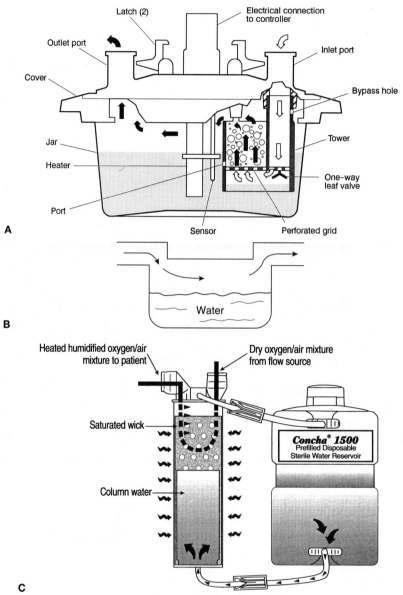

Figure 4-13 The three basic designs of heated mainstream humidifiers: (A) cascade (bubble through), (B) pass over, and (C) pass-over wick. See text for details. (A provided by Puritan-Bennett Corporation, Carlsbad, Calif. C provided courtesy of Hudson Respiratory Care, Inc., Temecula, Calif.)

water should be drained and replaced because it can cause airway burns. Heed all temperature alarms.

- When a heating unit is described as servo-controlled, a microprocessor is working with the thermometer to maintain a constant temperature. Ensure that the temperature probe is appropriately applied and functioning.
- Accumulated water in the tubing should be emptied periodically and discarded. It should *never* be allowed to drain back into the humidifier or into the patient, because it may be contaminated with bacteria. Excessive condensate also increases the FIO_2 delivered.
- Water in the tubing increases resistance to gas flow and will reduce delivered tidal volume during use of pressure modes of ventilation and increase pressure in volume modes.
- Refill the reservoir's water level every 2 to 4 hours as needed to ensure maximal humidification. Some models have a continuous water-feed system. Be sure to install it correctly, because overflowing water could flood the inspiratory circuit and be aspirated by the patient.
- Assess the patient for sputum character, breath sounds, and patency of artificial airway to determine whether there is adequate humidification.

HEAT AND MOISTURE EXCHANGERS

Heat and moisture exchangers (HMEs) are devices that fit between the airway and the ventilatory circuitry. They are commonly referred to as artificial noses. The principle behind the HME is a simple one. Exhaled gases pass through the HME, where water condenses on the inner surfaces and heat is retained. The retained heat and moisture are then added to the next inspired breath.

Some of the materials used in HMEs are sponge, corrugated paper, felt, stainless-steel screen, porous plastic foam, and ceramic. The larger the surface area within the HME, the more heat and moisture can be exchanged; however, deadspace volume (rebreathed gases) also increases. In patients with high minute ventilation demands, this increased dead space may be intolerable. As retained humidity increases in the HME, so does flow resistance increase and thus the work of breathing; therefore its use should be restricted in patients with respiratory muscle weakness or in patients who are difficult to wean. Since the effectiveness of the HME depends on how much heat and moisture are in the patient's exhaled gases, it should not be used on patients who are dehydrated, have hypothermia, or have thick, tenacious secretions.

HMEs are simple to use, are cost-effective, and provide freedom from potential electrical or thermal injury. There is also reduced concern that the patient will become overhydrated or will have condensate in the ventilator tubing inadvertently "dumped" into the airway during turning. The device should be firmly attached in place to avoid gas leakage at the connections and should be changed every 24 hours, or more often if mucus becomes trapped in the element.

AEROSOL THERAPY (NEBULIZERS)

Aerosol therapy is widely used in respiratory care even though much research is needed and controversy surrounds its administration. This section will review the indications and generally accepted methods of administration of both large- and small-volume aerosol therapy.

Large-Volume Aerosol Delivery Systems (Nebulizers)

Large-volume aerosol delivery systems are used therapeutically to humidify inspired medical gases. Two systems, the jet and the ultrasonic nebulizer, are used to increase the moisture content of gases administered by the high-humidity face mask, face tent, T-piece, or tracheostomy collar. Some confusion arises as a result of the use of the term "high humidity" in association with these systems, because in reality an aerosol is delivered to the patient, as well as humidity. Aerosol therapy delivers water *particles*, not just water *vapor* into the airways. The categories of nebulizers, jet and ultrasonic, describe the technique by which the aerosol is physically produced (Fig. 4–14). Aerosols may be cooled or heated.

JET NEBULIZER

The jet nebulizer is pneumatically driven, using the Venturi principle to create an aerosol. Gases from the flowmeter, delivered under high pressure, are passed through a jet. A capillary tube, with one end immersed under the liquid, intersects with the jet. Air pressure around the jet decreases, drawing water into the capillary tube. Water exits the capillary tube at the site of the jet flow and is shattered into small particles. This spray is further fragmented as it is blown against a baffle. A baffle, which may be a sphere, plate, or rod, for example, further reduces the size of the particles as they collide with it. After contact with the baffle, the aerosol is then delivered to the patient. The smaller the particle size, the greater its depth of penetration into the lung.

The orifice at the top of the nebulizer, which determines how much air will be entrained, is adjusted to achieve the desired FIO_2. The higher the FIO_2, the less mixing of room air is desired and thus the narrower is the opening. Aerosol content will also decrease as the amount of entrained air decreases. Jet nebulizers may be heated or cooled.

ULTRASONIC NEBULIZER

The ultrasonic nebulizer, which is electrically driven, uses high-frequency sound waves to create an aerosol mist by vibrating the solution. It may be used for continuous therapy but is primarily used for intermittent therapy. Ultrasonic nebulizers are used much less frequently than jet nebulizers, primarily because the latter devices are much simpler and there is less potential for equipment problems.

General Principles: Aerosol Therapy
- The patient's face should be dried periodically as a comfort measure.
- Aerosols may induce bronchoconstriction in patients with hypersensitive airways, such as those with asthma or cystic fibrosis. Consider using a humidification system in these patients.
- Bacterial contamination of the water may occur. Use strict hand-washing procedures, do not allow water in the tubing to drain back into the nebulizer, and use only sterile water or physiologic saline solution.
- Keep tubing free of excessive water, which increases the delivered FIO_2.
- Overheated water should be drained and replaced because it can cause airway burns. Ensure that the water level does not drop below the indicated level.
- In the pediatric population, fluid overload may be a problem. Monitor fluid balance.

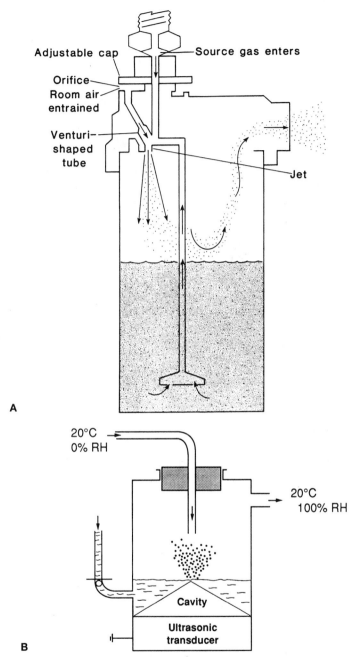

FIGURE 4-14 Nebulizers produce aerosols that may be cooled or heated. (A) Oxygen is forced through a small-lumen cannula in the *jet nebulizer*. This creates subatmospheric pressure at the top of a capillary tube, drawing water upward in the tube. The water is hit by the jet stream and then forced into a baffle, which breaks the aerosol into even finer particles. (B) The *ultrasonic nebulizer* creates a cavity of high-frequency sound waves that vibrate the solution, creating an aerosol geyser. (A from Kacmarek, RM, and Stoller, JK: *Current Respiratory Care*. Toronto: BC Decker, 1988. B from Shelly, MP: Inspired gas conditioning. *Resp Care* 1992;37:1075.)

Small-Volume Aerosol Delivery Systems (Nebulizers)

Small-volume aerosol systems are used for the administration of medications. Advantages of the aerosol versus the parenteral route of administration are that smaller doses are required, there is a rapid therapeutic effect because of direct administration of drug into the area in need of treatment, administration techniques are simple, and the use of the aerosol route is associated with fewer systemic side effects. Three types of small-volume aerosol delivery systems will be discussed: small-volume jet nebulizers, metered-dose inhalers, and dry-powder inhalers.

The effectiveness of an aerosol is determined by its ability to deposit a drug in the lung. Factors that determine drug deposition are the size of the aerosol particles and the amount produced, airway characteristics (size, geometry), and the patient's ventilatory pattern. The larger the particle produced by the delivery device, the more proximal the deposition in the airway. The diameter of the airway affects aerosol delivery in that the size of the airway is positively correlated to aerosol deposition. As bronchodilators are administered and the airway dilates, more drug may be deposited with subsequent inhalations. Artificial airways significantly reduce the amount of drug deposited in the lungs and, when in place, will therefore affect the dosages used. The patient's ventilatory pattern, which enhances drug deposition, is a slow, steady inhalation (occasionally to inspiratory capacity), followed by breath holding at end-inspiration to allow for particle settling. Larger inspiratory volumes will generally result in more aerosol delivery to the lung. If the patient requires mechanical ventilation, the sigh and end-inspiratory pause features, if not contraindicated, may be activated during an aerosol treatment.

Small-Volume Nebulizers

Small-volume nebulizers (SVNs) operate by the same principle as the large-volume jet nebulizer: the Venturi principle and the Bernoulli effect. SVNs are simple devices powered by portable compressors or hospital gas supplies (Fig. 4–15). SVNs are used in three ways: as handheld devices, incorporated into the breathing circuit of intermittent positive-pressure breathing (IPPB) machines, or placed in the circuitry of a mechanical ventilator. With the advent of disposable respiratory therapy supplies, the incidence of contamination of SVNs has decreased.

After the drug is placed in the nebulizer, it may be diluted to a larger volume with normal saline solution. Many SVN drugs are now available in unit dose vials. The gas flow rate is set at 6 L/min to achieve maximal drug delivery. The treatment should continue until no more aerosol can be produced. In all SVN designs, some of the solution remains after the treatment is completed. This is known as the dead volume and represents the solution that adheres to the inside of the SVN. The amount of dead volume may be diminished by intermittently tapping the sides of the nebulizer throughout the treatment so that the droplets on the walls of the nebulizer will fall to the bottom and be renebulized.

Multiple factors must be taken into consideration when an SVN is placed in mechanical ventilator circuitry. The SVN should be placed in the inspiratory limb. If a loss of volume in the circuitry occurs, then the point where the nebulizer is attached should be assessed as the potential cause of a circuit leak. Nebulized drug will be deposited both in the artificial airway and in the ventilator cir-

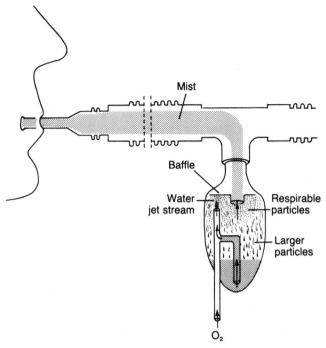

FIGURE 4-15   Typical design of a small-volume jet nebulizer. See text for explanation. (From Luce, JM, Pierson, DJ, and Tyler, ML: *Intensive Respiratory Care*. Philadelphia: WB Saunders, 1993.)

cuitry; therefore the drug doses need to be increased. Deposition of drug in the artificial airway increases as airway radius becomes smaller. Initially the dosage may be doubled, with further titration determined by carefully monitored, objective patient responses. To improve drug deposition, the patient needs to take a large breath periodically. It is recommended that, unless contraindicated, the patient undergoing mechanical ventilation and receiving an SVN should receive four to eight breaths per minute of tidal volumes (VTs) of 8 to 12 ml/kg. This slow rate, large VT pattern of ventilation will promote favorable drug dispersion. Continuous positive airway pressure (CPAP) should therefore be changed to synchronized intermittent mandatory ventilation (SIMV) or assist/control (A/C). Patients who are using pressure support ventilation (PSV) and receiving medication through a continuous-flow SVN must overcome the increased pressure gradient created by the SVN to trigger the ventilator. The patient's respiratory rate should be carefully monitored; if it drops, the PSV trigger sensitivity should be increased or an SIMV backup rate added.

METERED-DOSE INHALERS

The metered-dose inhaler (MDI) is a small canister that contains medication and an inert gas propellant. A mouthpiece is attached when the MDI is used by spontaneously breathing patients (Fig. 4–16). It may be used with or without an adjunct known as a spacer (see below). When activated, the MDI delivers a

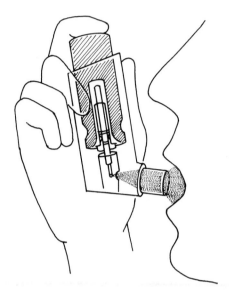

FIGURE 4-16 A metered-dose inhaler. (From Luce, JM, Pierson, DJ, and Tyler, ML: *Intensive Respiratory Care*. Philadelphia: WB Saunders, 1993.)

single dose of drug. The canister may contain hundreds of such doses. The gas propellants are chlorofluorocarbons, which are known to contribute to ozone layer depletion and global warming and therefore will be banned worldwide by the year 2000. Drug companies are presently researching compounds that could be used as new propellants, and new techniques that could be used as alternatives to the MDI may be seen in the future.

The MDI is portable, requires no compressed gas source, is less expensive than the SVN, and is associated with less risk of equipment contamination. In many institutions all patients supported by mechanical ventilation receive their aerosol therapy by MDI unless the drug needed does not come in an MDI. Choice of MDI over SVN in the spontaneously breathing patient is dependent on the patient's being able to coordinate the timing of activation of the device with proper inhalation. However, the use of a spacer (see below) may eliminate this indication for use of an MDI.

The techniques for MDI administration are outlined for the spontaneously breathing patient (Box 4–3) and for the patient undergoing mechanical ventilation (Box 4–4). The timing from inhalation to activation of the MDI is crucial to the success of drug delivery to the lungs. After exhalation to functional residual capacity, the MDI should be activated during a slow, deep inhalation, followed by at least a 4-second breath hold. For the patient using a ventilator, the best ventilatory pattern for optimal drug deposition is not known.

For the spontaneously breathing patient, two types of placement of the mouthpiece at the time of actuation are recommended: (1) between the lips with the mouth open and (2) 4 cm from the open mouth. Consensus as to the optimal method has not been reached. The rationale for placing the mouthpiece at a distance from the lips is that when the lips are closed, the majority of the drug is thought to be deposited in the oropharynx.

Box 4–3 Technique for Administration of Metered-Dose Inhaler (MDI) in Spontaneously Breathing Patients

1. Shake the vial 15 to 20 times after warming it to room temperature.
2. Hold the MDI upright, either between the lips with the mouth open or 4 cm in front of the open mouth.* If a spacer is being used, hold the MDI between the lips.
3. Exhale completely to resting level (functional residual capacity).
4. Begin to inhale slowly and deeply, and activate the MDI. Continue inhaling to total lung capacity.
5. Hold breath for 4 to 10 seconds.
6. Wait 3 to 10 minutes before repeating steps 2 to 5 for each additional puff ordered.
7. After completion of the treatment, rinse mouth and gargle as necessary to remove drug deposited in the mouth and oropharynx.

---

*Controversy exists over proper placement of the MDI mouthpiece; see text for explanation.

Spacers. *Spacers* are adjuncts for use with the MDI to eliminate the need for precise timing of inspiration to activation; they promote steady inspiratory flow and reduce large-particle deposition in the mouth or artificial airway, because these particles are deposited in the spacer. In patients using an MDI through their natural airway, the deposition of less drug in the mouth reduces systemic absorption of swallowed drug, oral irritation, and bad taste. The spacer fits between the MDI and the mouth or into the ventilator circuitry (Fig. 4–17). The drug is activated into the spacer, followed by inspiration. Spacers are indicated for individuals unable to time activation and inspiration properly and for all patients undergoing mechanical ventilation, because the spacers promote delivery of optimal-size particles. Some commercial spacers used with the natural

---

Box 4–4 Technique for Administration of Metered-Dose Inhaler (MDI) During Mechanical Ventilation

1. Assemble MDI adapter and place in ventilator circuitry.
2. Adjust ventilator to deliver tidal volumes of 12 to 15 cc/kg unless contraindicated. Alternatively, use the sigh feature unless contraindicated.
3. Shake the vial 15 to 20 times after warming it to room temperature.
4. Place MDI in circuit adapter and activate MDI immediately at the start of a ventilator-delivered inspiration. If a spacer is used, activate the MDI several seconds before the start of inspiration or at end-exhalation, whichever is most practical.
5. If not contraindicated, apply a 2- to 3-second end-inspiratory pause.
6. Wait 1 minute between puffs and assess the patient for therapeutic and adverse effects.
7. Ensure that all ventilator settings are returned to pretreatment settings.

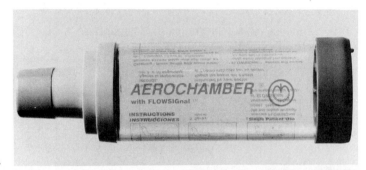

A

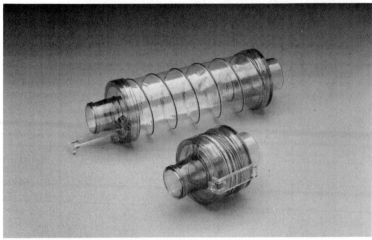

B

FIGURE 4-17 Spacers are adjuncts used with the metered-dose inhaler. They are available for (A) spontaneously breathing patients or (B) as a device that fits into the circuitry of the mechanical ventilator. (Courtesy of Monaghan Medical Corporation, Plattsburgh, N.Y.)

airway promote slow, steady inspiratory flow by whistling if inspiration is too rapid.

DRY POWDER INHALERS

Dry powder inhalers (DPIs) are available for only a limited number of drugs. The drug is placed in the inhaler in its powder form, usually contained within a gelatin capsule. When the inhaler is activated, the capsule is pierced. The DPI is breath activated; inspiration draws the powder into the lungs. Advantages of the DPI over the MDI are that problems with exact timing of inspiration are eliminated and chlorofluorocarbons are not required. Disadvantages include a requirement of higher inspiratory flow rates than with the MDI or SVN, an association with heavy oropharyngeal deposition, a limited number of drugs available in DPI form, a limited number of doses provided, clumping of the drugs when they become moist, an association with a greater incidence of bronchospasm (especially in persons with asthma), and their inability to be used in ventilatory circuits.

RECOMMENDED READINGS

American Association for Respiratory Care (1991). Aerosol Consensus Statement— 1991. *Respir Care* 36(9), 916–921.

AARC Aerosol Guidelines Committee (1992). AARC clinical practice guidelines: Selection of aerosol delivery device. *Respir Care* 37(8), 891–897.

AARC Mechanical Ventilation Guidelines Committee (1992). AARC clinical practice guidelines: Humidification during mechanical ventilation. *Respir Care*, 37(8), 887–890.

Beers, M.F., and Fisher, A.B. (1993). Oxygen toxicity. In R.W. Carlson and M.A. Geheb (Eds.). *Principles and Practice of Medical Intensive Care* (pp. 949–957). Philadelphia: W.B. Saunders.

Bolgiano, C.S., Bunting, K., and Shoenberger, M.M. (1990). Administering oxygen therapy: What you need to know. *Nursing* (June), 47–51.

Brown, L.H. (1990). Pulmonary oxygen toxicity. *Focus on Critical Care* 17(1), 68–75.

Ebert, J., Adams, A.B., and Green-Eide, B. (1992). An evaluation of MDI spacers and adapters: Their effect on the respirable volume of medication. *Respir Care* 37(8), 862–868.

Emergency Cardiac Care Committee and Subcomittees, American Heart Association (1992). Adult advanced cardiac life support. Part III. Guidelines for cardiopulmonary resuscitation and emergency cardiac care. *JAMA* 268(16), 2199–2241.

Fisher, A.B. (1980). Oxygen therapy: Side effects and toxicity. Proceedings of the Conference on the Scientific Basis of Inhospital Respiratory Therapy. *Am Rev Respir Dis* 122, 61–69.

Hess, D. (1991). Aerosol bronchodilator delivery during mechanical ventilation: Nebulizer or inhaler? *Chest* 100(4), 1103–1104.

Kacmarek, R.M. (1992). Humidity and aerosol therapy. In D.J. Pierson and R.M. Kacmarek (Eds.). *Foundation of Respiratory Care* (pp. 793–824). New York: Churchill Livingstone.

Kacmarek, R.M., and Hess, D. (1991). The interface between patient and aerosol generator. *Respir Care* 36(9), 952–976.

Kissoon, N., et al. (1991). Evaluation of performance characteristics of disposable bagvalve resuscitators. *Crit Care Med* 19(1), 102–107.

Kofke, W.A. (1992). Postoperative respiratory care techniques. Part III. Weaning from mechanical ventilation and oxygen therapy. *Curr Rev PACN* 13(21), 161–168.

Levitzky, M.G., Cairo, J.M., Hall, S.M. (1990). *Introduction to Respiratory Care.* Philadelphia: W.B. Saunders.

Lieberman, D.E. (1992). Respiratory care in the post-anesthesia care unit. *Curr Rev PACN* 14(10), 77–84.

McCabe, S.M., and Smeltzer, S.C. (1993). Comparison of tidal volumes obtained by one-handed and two-handed ventilation techniques. *Am J Crit Care* 2(6), 467–473.

Miracle, V.A., and Allnutt, D.R. (1990). Using a manual resuscitator correctly. *Nursing* (May), 49–51.

Newman, S.P. (1991). Aerosol generators and delivery systems. *Respir Care* 36(9), 939–951.

Ryerson, G.G., and Block, A.J. (1991). Oxygen as a drug: Clinical properties, benefits, modes, and hazards of administration. In G.G. Burton, J.E. Hodgkin, and J.J. Ward (Eds.). *Respiratory Care: A Guide to Clinical Practice* (pp. 319–339). 3rd ed. Philadelphia: J.B. Lippincott.

Stemp, L.I. (1992). Manual resuscitators and spontaneous ventilation: An evaluation [Letter to the Editor]. *Crit Care Med* 20, 1496.

Ward, J.W., and Helmholz, H.F. (1991). Applied humidity and aerosol therapy. In G.G. Burton, J.E. Hodgkin, and J.J. Ward (Eds.) *Respiratory Care: A Guide to Clinical Practice* (pp. 355–396). 3rd ed. Philadelphia: J.B. Lippincott.

Lung Expansion Therapy and Bronchial Hygiene

The provision of supplemental oxygen is often necessary to ensure the adequacy of oxygenation. Oxygen alone should be viewed as only supportive therapy. For the patient to return to an optimal state of oxygenation, without supplemental oxygen, the underlying abnormality must be treated with appropriately chosen bronchial hygiene techniques. The two basic goals of the therapies discussed in this chapter are to expand the lung, thus opening and stabilizing the alveoli, and to clear the alveoli and airways of secretions.

LUNG EXPANSION THERAPY

Atelectasis

Atelectasis occurs in many hospitalized patients, particularly in the intensive care unit, where they may not breathe deeply enough or sigh often enough and bed rest may be prolonged. Atelectasis develops because of failure to expand the lung adequately or because of absorption of air distal to congested airways. When the volume of air in the lung is decreased, pulmonary compliance decreases and the work of breathing necessary to expand the lung increases. If the patient is weak and unable to generate the work necessary to expand the lung, the tidal volume decreases, blood gases further deteriorate, and the atelectatic process worsens.

Atelectasis is classified as either microatelectasis or macroatelectasis. The former cannot be seen on x-ray film but is physiologically evident by a widened alveolar-to-arterial oxygen difference (A-a gradient) or a below-normal PaO_2. Macroatelectasis is both radiographically and physiologically evident. The goal of lung expansion therapy, which includes maneuvers that promote larger-than-tidal (closer to inspiratory capacity) inspirations is to prevent, decrease, or correct alveolar collapse and atelectasis.

Deep Breathing

Description. Deep breathing is a simple and yet very effective lung expansion technique. It is indicated for any patient who is at risk of having atelectasis and who can participate in conscious control of ventilation.

Technique. Place the patient in an upright position or, if the patient is in a side-lying position, support the arms, head, and flexed legs with pillows. Instruct the patient to inhale slowly and deeply. To promote diaphragmatic breathing, teach the patient to gently push out the belly during inspiration. For some patients, it is useful to place a hand on their upper abdomen while making a conscious effort to push outward on their hand during inspiration. The deeply inspired breath should be held for several seconds, which may promote collateral ventilation. Exhalation is passive. The patient should be instructed to take 8 to 10 deep breaths per hour while awake and may be motivated to do so if the benefits of this simple respiratory exercise are explained.

Incentive Spirometry

Description. Incentive spirometry (IS) provides patients with a visual cue as to how well they are performing their deep-breathing exercises and therefore may serve as a motivator or provide an "incentive" to their performance. IS is indicated to prevent or correct atelectasis particularly in the postoperative patient. The visual cue provided to the patient varies according to the type of spirometer. Some spirometers have balls that rise to the top of one or more chambers, whereas others have bellows that contract as the patient inspires. One type of IS allows for the determination of the actual volume that the patient is inspiring. This type is known as a volume spirometer, as opposed to a flow spirometer (Fig. 5–1).

Technique. Assist the patient to an upright position. Instruct the patient to fully exhale, insert the mouthpiece firmly between closed lips, and inhale slowly and as deeply as possible (to inspiratory capacity). The breath should be held for 2 to 3 seconds and then the mouthpiece removed from the mouth for exhalation. The patient may rest 30 to 60 seconds between breaths to prevent hyperventilation, respiratory alkalosis, and dizziness. The maneuver should be repeated 6 to 10 times per hour, which mimics the average number of sighs a person usually makes.

If possible, the patient should be coached in the use of the IS preoperatively. Preoperative technique and volumes then serve as a reference for comparison of postoperative performance. IS is cost-effective because after the staff teaches the patient to use the IS and observes a successful demonstration, the patient can perform the exercise independently. Observing the patient performing the IS

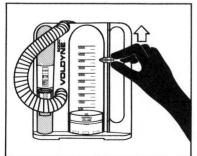
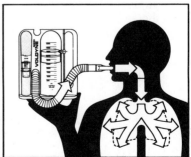

FIGURE 5–1 The volumetric incentive spirometer provides visual feedback of the inspired volume. (A) The inspiratory goal is marked by the clinician. (B) The patient may then independently perform IS, working to raise the piston to the prescribed level. (Courtesy of Sherwood Medical, St. Louis, Mo.)

twice daily will serve as encouragement and allow for determination of performance, reinforcement of the goal, and further instruction as necessary.

Positioning and Mobilization

Regular turning is beneficial in reducing atelectasis in the bedridden patient. Areas of the lung in the most dependent regions have the smallest resting volume, and thus the greatest tendency to collapse, particularly at reduced inspiratory volumes. The airways are smallest in the dependent regions in all body positions because of the effect of gravitational forces on the lung. Gravity pulls on the lung as it "hangs" in the thorax. Because of this gravitational pull, and because the intrapleural pressure is the most negative, the airways in the uppermost region are expanded to the greatest extent. This is true regardless of body position: supine, upright, lateral decubitus, or prone. Blood flow is also gravity dependent in nature and therefore is always greatest in the most dependent regions, tending to compress the alveoli. For a more detailed explanation of the distribution of ventilation and perfusion in the lung, see Chapter 2.

Changing the patient's body position may be used prophylactically and therapeutically. Regularly turning and changing of the patient's body position will vary the position of the lung and assist in the prevention of atelectasis. For patients who already have atelectasis, placing them in a position with the atelectatic area uppermost may promote reexpansion of the lung.

Mobilization of the patient to a sitting position or, even better, to ambulation is most beneficial in expanding the lung. In the upright and ambulatory positions, the compression of the abdomen on the diaphragm and thus the lung bases is eliminated and the lung volumes improve.

The reader is strongly encouraged to refer to Chapter 2 to review the effect of body position on ventilation-perfusion matching. Topics of discussion include the clinical significance of postural variation on gas exchange and the therapeutic application of patient positioning to improve oxygenation.

Intermittent Positive-Pressure Breathing

Description. Intermittent positive-pressure breathing (IPPB) assists in inflation of the lungs through the application of positive pressure on inspiration. IPPB is indicated for the reversal of atelectasis when deep breathing, IS, and coughing therapies have not been successful. The patient must be spontaneously breathing to initiate an inspiratory effort, which triggers the IPPB machine to deliver the positive-pressure breath. It may be delivered by mouthpiece or mask, or through a tracheostomy with the use of an adapter. IPPB promotes lung expansion and improved cough because the patient obtains a larger inspiratory volume than might be taken independently. The work of breathing decreases and ventilation-perfusion matching improves as the lung is expanded and secretion removal is enhanced. Substantial controversy exists over the theoretic advantages of IPPB because the benefits described above have not been consistently reproduced in clinical studies. Aerosol medications such as bronchodilators and mucokinetics may also be administered during IPPB; however, medication administration alone should not be considered an indication for IPPB because it is more expensive and probably no more effective than handheld nebulizers administered with thorough patient instruction.

The use of IPPB is contraindicated (1) in patients with untreated pneumothorax, because the positive pressure may force additional air into the pleural space, (2) in patients who have recently undergone tracheal or pulmonary surgery or pulmonary biopsy, because pressure application to the affected area may cause rupture of the site and pneumothorax, and (3) in the hemodynamically unstable patient, because the positive pressure in the thorax may further decrease venous return and impede cardiac output. Hypotension may be particularly pronounced in the patient with hypovolemia. IPPB is also contraindicated in patients who are unable to cooperate, because the therapy may be ineffective and gastric distention may occur secondary to air being forced into the esophagus.

Technique. To initiate the treatment, assist the patient to an upright position. If supplemental oxygen was being administered before IPPB, the same FIO_2 should be delivered during the treatment. The patient forms a seal around the mouthpiece and inhales, triggering the IPPB machine. The sensitivity should be set at 1 to 2 cm H_2O so that the patient will not need to exert excessive negative pressure to trigger a breath. Air and oxygen then flow into the lungs under positive pressure. At the height of inspiration the patient should hold the breath for 3 to 5 seconds, particularly if medications are being administered, because an inspiratory pause will improve their distribution. The patient then exhales passively through the mouthpiece so that exhaled volumes can be registered. The amount of pressure used during the treatment depends on the *volumes exhaled,* which should be 12 to 15 cc/kg, or 20% larger than pre-IPPB inspiratory capacity. Typical pressures used during IPPB range from 15 to 20 cm H_2O; however, use of much higher pressures has been reported. Treatments may be given as often as every 2 hours. Each treatment, which typically lasts no longer than 20 minutes, should provide for 6 to 10 breaths per minute.

Complications from IPPB include the following:

- Hyperventilation when the patient is not properly coached and breathes too rapidly
- Hypotension caused by decreased venous return
- Patient discomfort, emesis, and gastric dilation, which create pressure on the diaphragm and may lead to the development of an ileus
- Nosocomial infection caused by bacterial contamination of poorly managed equipment
- Secretion impaction caused by the positive pressure, especially when IPPB is applied to the patient in the upright position
- Pneumothorax and pneumomediastinum as a result of high volumes and pressure

Hypoxemia, CO_2 retention, and acute ventilatory failure should not be viewed as indications for IPPB but, rather, for mechanical ventilation. Improvements in the patient with IPPB tend to be transient, and application is costly because it requires the constant attendance of a respiratory practitioner. Perhaps the interpreted success of IPPB in some patients is due not to the treatment itself but to the fact that pulmonary toileting is receiving concentrated attention.

Continuous Positive Airway Pressure Treatments

CONTINUOUS POSITIVE AIRWAY PRESSURE MASK

Description. The continuous positive airway pressure (CPAP) mask applies a specified amount of positive pressure into the airways in an effort to open the alveoli, improve functional residual capacity, and thereby improve oxygenation. The therapeutic effects of positive pressure occur during exhalation. When the patient expires, it is against the resistance of positive pressure, which creates back pressure in the lungs, promoting alveolar recruitment and improving alveolar stability.

The use of CPAP is indicated for the spontaneously breathing patient with hypoxemia caused by atelectasis. It may be used continuously or applied as a periodic treatment. It is particularly useful when efforts are directed toward avoiding intubation and preventing reintubation in the patient who has recently undergone extubation. When CPAP is used intermittently as a treatment, both the duration of the CPAP treatment and the amount of CPAP applied should be documented. CPAP is contraindicated in patients with recent tracheal or esophageal surgery.

Technique. For application of a CPAP mask, a flow generator is connected to an oxygen source and the flow adjusted to the desired FIO_2 with the use of an oxygen analyzer. A humidification system is connected to the flow generator and tubing. Another piece of tubing connects the humidification system to the oxygen inlet valve on the CPAP mask. The appropriate positive end-expiratory pressure (PEEP) valve is then applied on the bottom port of the mask. The valves generally come in expiratory resistances ranging from 2.5 to 20 cm H_2O, increasing in increments of 2.5 cm H_2O. A head strap is used to attach the system snugly to the patient's face. The flexible head-strap pieces are adjusted by securing the holes in the strap to prongs on the mask (Fig. 5–2). The mask should not be applied until flow has been established. The fit of some mask models may be further adjusted by inflation of a cushion seal on the mask.

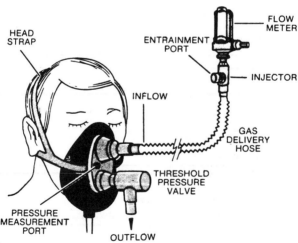

Figure 5–2 The CPAP mask fits snugly around the patient's face. Positive pressure, which is applied during expiration, promotes alveolar recruitment and stability, increases the functional residual capacity, and thereby improves oxygenation. See text for further explanation. (From Smith, RA: Mask and nasal continuous positive airway pressure. In RM Kacmarek and JK Stoller [Eds.]: *Current Respiratory Care*. Toronto: BC Decker, 1988.)

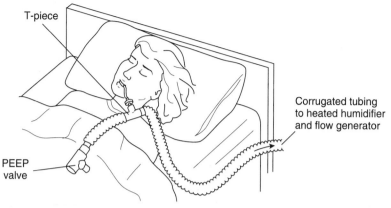

T-piece

Corrugated tubing
to heated humidifier
and flow generator

PEEP
valve

FIGURE 5-3 CPAP created by a PEEP valve placed in the expiratory line of a spontaneously breathing patient with an artificial airway.

Advantages of mask CPAP include the application of positive pressure without the use of a ventilator. It may avert the need for intubation and mechanical ventilation, with all the potential complications, and does not require as much patient effort or cooperation as active deep breathing or incentive spirometry.

Disadvantages and potential complications of mask CPAP include the following:

- Possible gastric insufflation and possible vomiting with aspiration, which may be prevented by using gastric decompression (patient should be told to indicate whether nausea is occurring)
- Discomfort, erythema, and possible skin breakdown around mask pressure points (nose, cheeks, chin) (use soft, inflatable seal masks to reduce problem)
- Feeling of being confined or feeling of claustrophobia, particularly when patient's mentation is impaired by hypoxemia
- Decreased cardiac output and hypotension in acute myocardial infarction, untreated pneumothorax, and hypovolemia, because the positive pressure in the thorax reduces venous return and thus cardiac output
- Possible CO_2 retention because of an increase in dead space if the positive pressure overdistends the normal alveoli
- Possible pneumothorax, with increased risk in patients with bullous lung disease

CPAP BY TRACHEAL TUBE WITH A PEEP VALVE

Description. CPAP may be administered to spontaneously breathing patients with an endotracheal or tracheostomy tube without the use of a ventilator. It is indicated to promote alveolar recruitment and reverse atelectasis, thereby increasing functional residual capacity and improving oxygenation. The patient breathes against a prescribed expiratory resistance ranging from 2.5 to 12.5 cm H_2O, which is created by a PEEP valve placed in the expiratory line (Fig. 5-3).

Technique. The CPAP setup includes a flow generator connected to the oxygen source, which is adjusted until the desired FIO_2 is achieved. Corrugated oxygen tubing extends from the flow generator to the humidification system and from the humidifier to a T-piece attached to the patient's airway. A reservoir of extension tubing is attached to the opposite end of the T-piece, and the PEEP valve is placed on the end of the reservoir tube.

The *advantage* of CPAP by endotracheal or tracheostomy tube using a PEEP valve is application of positive pressure without the use of a ventilator and its concomitant risks. *Disadvantages and complications* include the following:

- Decreased cardiac output and hypotension in patients with cardiac dysfunction or hypovolemia, because the positive pressure in the thorax reduces venous return and thus cardiac output
- Possible CO_2 retention, caused by an increase in dead space if positive pressure overdistends normal alveoli
- Possible pneumothorax, a risk that is increased in patients with bullous lung disease.

SECRETION REMOVAL TECHNIQUES

Cough

Coughing is a normal protective pulmonary reflex (see Chapter 1). It is first-line therapy—the most important therapy for the removal of retained secretions. An effective cough requires the development of intraabdominal and intrathoracic pressure, followed by a rapid expiratory flow. The cough maneuver begins with a larger-than-tidal breath. The glottis is then closed and the thoracic and abdominal muscles contract, building intrapleural and intrapulmonic pressures to maximum levels. As the glottis is suddenly opened, the air in the lungs is rapidly exhaled, moving material in the airways forward to the pharynx, where it can be either expectorated or swallowed.

Ineffective cough may be due to several factors. The cough reflex may be blunted because of central nervous system abnormalities, or the irritant receptors may lack responsiveness, as may occur with prolonged intubation. The patient may suppress coughing because of pain, particularly after abdominal or thoracic surgery or trauma. The expiratory muscles of the thorax and/or abdomen may be weakened because of disuse or sedation or may be paralyzed by spinal cord injury so that an effective cough cannot be generated. When a patient is intubated, the glottis cannot close; therefore the development of increased intrathoracic pressure and thus effective forced expiratory flow is impaired. When the patient's cough is ineffective, encouragement and coaching are often necessary. Coughing is required only when secretions are present. The effectiveness of the cough may be judged by sputum production and improvement in breath sounds.

COUGH COACHING AND PREPARATION

The patient should be assisted to a position that is conducive to optimal cough. The most effective cough is produced in a sitting position, with the trunk flexed slightly forward so that the abdominal muscles can contract and the abdominal contents are pushed up against the diaphragm. The patient who is in bed can achieve optimal muscle contraction either by sitting in the Fowler's position with the knees drawn up or by lying on one side with the knees drawn up. The patient with a surgical incision can also be instructed in methods to splint the incision, such as hugging a pillow or pressing a small blanket against the surgical area. Both maneuvers can help to stabilize the thoracic or abdominal wall and lessen the strain placed on the incision line.

An effective method of pain control should be implemented to promote patient cooperation and compliance with coughing. Many methods of pain control are available and should be administered with the goal of controlling the pain while not suppressing the respiratory drive or reflexes. Pain medication may be administered orally, intravenously, epidurally, or in sustained-release topical patches. In many cases, patient-controlled analgesia may be instituted, allowing the patient an active part in the pain control regimen.

COUGH TECHNIQUES

It is a common misperception that if the patient cannot mobilize secretions when instructed to breathe deeply and cough, then more advanced and costly techniques, such as postural drainage and percussion, suctioning, and bronchoscopy, are indicated. However, several cough methods can be tried with the patient to achieve the goal of sputum production.

With all cough techniques, instruct the patient to begin by slowly taking in a deep breath to allow the inspired air to reach the distal airways. The breath should then be held for several seconds, allowing collateral flow to assist in inflating airways that are below functional residual capacity. After coughing, the next breath should be taken through the nose to prevent sucking partially mobilized secretions back down into the airways.

Controlled Cough. The controlled, or voluntary, cough begins with a slow, deep breath held for several seconds. Forceful coughing using the abdominal muscles is then done two or three times in succession during exhalation. Coughing requires effort and can be tiring. Successive coughing may mobilize secretions even in weak patients unable to produce one large, forceful exhalation. The maneuver may be repeated as necessary, with rest between efforts using slow, deep breathing.

Huff Cough. Huffing is similar to the voluntary cough but modified in that the glottis remains open. After taking in a slow, deep breath and holding it for several seconds, the patient holds the glottis open while forcefully exhaling by making the sound *huh*. Because the glottis is held opened, high airway pressures are not produced, and yet secretions are propelled forward in the airways because rapid flow rates are produced. Less airway collapse occurs in huff coughing because airway pressures are lower. This technique is therefore useful in patients with chronic obstructive pulmonary disease and in those with hyperreactive airways.

Quad (Assisted) Cough. The quad, or assisted, cough is used in patients with neuromuscular disease that has rendered the abdominal muscles nonfunctional and in patients with diaphragmatic abnormalities. In either case the patient is unable to generate sufficient expiratory force for effective coughing. After taking a slow, deep breath, the patient is manually assisted to cough during an expiratory effort. The caregiver offering the assistance places the palm of the hand flat on the patient's abdomen, just under the xiphoid process, and pushes inward and upward on the diaphragm just as the patient exhales. Alternatively, if abdominal compression is contraindicated, the caregiver's hands may be placed on the patient's lateral rib cage and quickly pressed inward with each cough (a maneuver called rib springing). For the patient whose respiratory effort also prohibits sufficient inhalation, hyperinflation with a manual resuscitation bag may improve inspiratory volume and thus expiratory flow.

Suctioning

Suctioning of the airway is probably one of the most common procedures performed in the intensive care setting by nurses, respiratory therapists, and appropriately trained technicians. The purpose of suctioning is secretion removal. This goal should be obtained while patient discomfort and adverse hemodynamic effects are minimized and hypoxemia related to suctioning is prevented. Suctioning should be performed when needed, not on a routine basis, because of the potential trauma to the airway and induction of suctioning-related complications. The need for suctioning is determined by auscultation of the breath sounds, visual inspection of the airway for the presence of secretions, and/or an increase in peak inspiratory pressure unexplained by other factors that increase airway resistance. Though suctioning may be performed nasopharyngeally, this section will focus on the technique of endotracheal suctioning (ETS).

Potential complications of the ETS procedure include cardiac dysrhythmias, hypoxemia, cardiac arrest, vagal stimulation, mucosal trauma, atelectasis, infection, and increased intracranial pressure. The cardiac complications may stem from procedure-induced hypoxemia or from tracheal stimulation. Tracheal stimulation may result in tachycardia and hypertension because of increased sympathetic nervous system (SNS) activity. In individuals who have lost SNS control (spinal cord injury above the first thoracic vertebra [T1]), bradycardia may result because vagal activity is unopposed.

It is reasonable that a patient with a marginal oxygenation status will tolerate ETS less well than a patient with an optimal baseline PaO_2. Prevention of ETS-induced hypoxemia is paramount; therefore several techniques targeted toward its elimination will be addressed in this section. When intrapulmonary pressure becomes negative, because of suction application and the removal of gases from the lung, atelectasis may occur. In patients with increased ICP there is a stepwise increase in ICP with each pass of the suction catheter; therefore the number of passes should be minimal and guided by monitoring of cerebrovascular status. Mucosal trauma is influenced by the vigor with which ETS is performed and also by mucosal invagination into the catheter end or side holes. The result is defoliation of ciliated epithelium from the mucosa, which impairs mucociliary function, causes edema, and possibly results in small hemorrhagic areas, as evidenced by blood streaking in the aspirate. Mechanisms for reducing tracheal trauma are discussed in the sections Suction Catheter Design and Endotracheal Suctioning Technique, below.

SUCTION CATHETER DESIGN

Suction catheters are generally for single use and are made of polyvinylchloride. This clear material makes it easier to inspect the aspirated secretions for quantity, color, and character. They are easy to insert into the endotracheal tube (ETT), thereby eliminating the need for lubrication, which would increase catheter manipulation and the opportunity for contamination.

Suction Catheter Size. The diameter of the suction catheter should be no greater than approximately half of the diameter of the ETT to allow gases to flow around the catheter during suctioning. Generally a size 14 French (range, 12 to 16) suction catheter is used in adults. The 14 French catheter has a 4 mm outer diameter and therefore can be used with a tube 8.0 mm or larger. A catheter that is too small will make secretion removal difficult, especially if secretions are

thick. The clinician will then be tempted to pass the suction catheter more often, which may lead to patient discomfort or procedure-related complications.
The catheter should be of sufficient length to extend approximately 2 inches
(5 cm) beyond the end of the endotracheal tube.

Tip Design. The catheter should have more than one eye at the tip of the
catheter for greater contact with secretions during their removal. Catheters with
only one eye have been associated with increased mucosal trauma from adher-
ence. The quest to develop a catheter that results in reduced mucosal trauma has
resulted in the availability of catheters with two eyes, four eyes, beveled tips,
blunt tips, and "mushroom" tips. A more important factor in reducing tracheal
injury is probably ETS technique—the intensity with which the procedure is
performed, and the onset and duration of the application of negative pressure
(see Endotracheal Suctioning Technique, below).

CLOSED TRACHEAL SUCTION SYSTEMS

Open suctioning involves disconnecting the patient from the ventilator to
insert the suction catheter. A closed tracheal suction system (CTSS) allows
the catheter to be advanced into the airway without disconnection from the
ventilator. A CTSS consists of a suction catheter housed in a plastic sheath,
an adapter that attaches to the ventilator circuitry and allows the system to
remain continuously attached, an irrigation port for tracheal lavage solution
instillation and for rinsing the catheter after use, and a thumb-activated suction control valve (Fig. 5–4). After insertion of the catheter into the ETT
and the performance of suctioning, the catheter is withdrawn back into the
plastic sleeve. Proported advantages of maintaining a closed system include reduction in the potential for environmental contamination, maintenance of
positive-pressure ventilation and PEEP, and continuation of oxygen supply.
Concerns related to use of the CTSS include infection control, effectiveness, creation of excess negative pressure from application of suction in a closed
system, and cost.

There is no doubt that there is less potential for environmental contamination with the CTSS. This is a distinct advantage, especially in conditions spread
by airborne particles, such as tuberculosis. The maintenance of positive-pressure
ventilation and PEEP is particularly advantageous in patients who are sensitive
to its discontinuation, such as those with apnea or high levels of PEEP. For
prevention of suction-related hypoxemia, patients must still undergo hyperoxygenation before, during, and after ETS with a CTSS. The closed system is
maintained by performing hyperoxygenation with the ventilator, either by activating the 100% O_2 for suctioning feature, if available, or by adjusting the FIO_2
manually. The addition of hyperinflation will further reduce the incidence of
hypoxemia.

When the CTSS is used properly, there is no increase in the incidence of
nosocomial pneumonia. The catheter must be properly rinsed after each use, and
the entire system should be changed every 24 hours. Some caregivers believe that
they cannot remove secretions as effectively with the CTSS because they do not
vigorously manually ventilate the patient, which they believe loosens secretions
and stimulates cough. With the CTSS, cough can still be stimulated with the
catheter or with instillation of normal saline solution. The purpose of manually
ventilating the patient with open suctioning is hyperinflation. With the CTSS
hyperinflation should be performed with the ventilator.

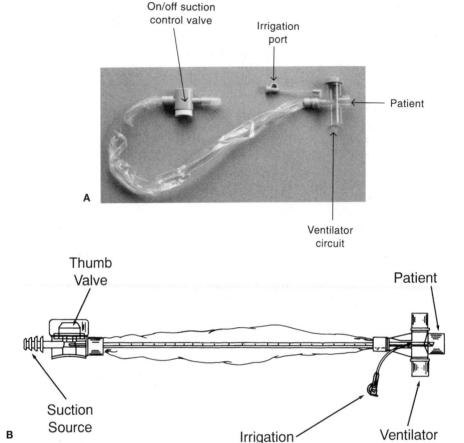

FIGURE 5-4 Closed tracheal suction systems. (A) Ballard Trach Care. (B) Concord/Portex Steri-Cath. (A, Courtesy of Ballard Medical Products, Draper, Utah. B, Courtesy of SIMS Concord/Portex, Smiths Industries Medical Systems, Keene, N.H.)

Suction effectiveness is improved by appropriately setting the suction regulator and by *straight* withdrawal of the catheter to prevent kinking at the airway connection or at the suction control valve. Additional practical tips regarding the use of the CTSS are that gloves must always be worn (even though the system is closed) and the catheter must be fully withdrawn until the black mark is visible in the sheath. Partial occlusion of the airway with the catheter, when it is not properly withdrawn into its sheath, results in increased airway resistance and elevated peak airway pressures.

Suctioning in a closed system may result in negative airway pressures when suction flow rates exceed ventilator flow rates. This negative pressure may result in a loss of PEEP, reduction in oxygen supply to the lungs, atelectasis, and hypoxemia. These adverse effects are more likely to occur in the control mode of ventilation and at low ventilator flow rates (e.g., 25 L/min). More research is needed in this area.

Cost-effectiveness is a paramount concern in all health care settings. The CTSS costs more than a single open-system suction catheter set, and therefore if the patient only infrequently undergoes suctioning or requires only short-term ventilation (e.g., for rapid weaning postoperatively), a CTSS is not warranted. The CTSS has been shown to be cost-effective if the patient requires frequent suctioning. Savings may also be realized in lost charges because of the once-a-day charge, the saving of personnel time because it is not necessary to gather and set up supplies for each suctioning procedure, and the reduction in infection. It is recommended that institutions develop a set of indications for use of the CTSS to avoid its arbitrary use on all patients.

ENDOTRACHEAL SUCTIONING TECHNIQUE

Aseptic technique is imperative during ETS. The hands should be washed both before and after the procedure, and sterile gloves and a sterile suction catheter must be used. It is advisable that eye protection for the clinician be routine. Universal precautions should be adhered to during ETS.

The amount of negative pressure produced by the suction source should be adjusted to 100 to 150 mm Hg, but recommendations in the literature vary. To adjust the suction level, turn the suction source on, occlude the end of the suction tubing, and adjust the vacuum regulator until the dial reads between 100 and 150 mm Hg. As the vacuum regulator is adjusted from 40 to 200 mm Hg, suction flows generally vary from 10 to 30 L/min. Suctioning research has yet to define the ideal suction flow rate for secretion recovery. Furthermore, there is no simple method widely available for measuring suction flow.

Begin the procedure by preoxygenating the patient with 100% oxygen and performing hyperinflation with 3 to 5 breaths. Insert the catheter gently until resistance is met, and then, to prevent the suction catheter from grabbing the mucosa, withdraw the catheter approximately 1 cm before applying suction. The greatest degree of tracheal trauma has been shown to occur at the point where the suction catheter meets tissue resistance, especially if suction is applied at this point. No suction should be applied during insertion of the catheter into the airway. The duration of suction application affects the degree of suction-related hypoxemia, presumably because oxygen is also withdrawn from the lungs, along with secretions. Suction application should be limited to 10 seconds and may be continuous or intermittent. Results of research on continuous versus intermittent suction are inconclusive because of the variation in catheters used and the amount of suction applied. Both methods have been shown to be damaging to the tracheal epithelium. Continuous suction may improve secretion removal but also increases the amount of air drawn from the patient's lungs, especially in a CTSS. Intermittent suction is recommended whenever the catheter may make contact with the mucosa, which occurs to a greater extent in nasopharyngeal suctioning. While the catheter is being removed, it should be twirled between the thumb and fingers so that the eyes of the catheter are exposed to a larger surface area and therefore remove more secretions.

Perform hyperoxygenation and hyperinflation (see below) between passes of the suction catheter. The amount of elapsed time between catheter passes depends on the patient's recovery, as evidenced by cardiopulmonary monitoring, but should minimally be 20 to 30 seconds. The catheter may be cleared of thick secretions with sterile water or normal saline solution between passes of the suction catheter. Most suction catheter kits contain a disposable, expandable cup that can be used for this purpose.

After the suctioning procedure is completed, the catheter is rinsed and may then be used to suction the patient's oral cavity and pharynx to remove any excess saliva and oropharyngeal secretions that have pooled on top of the ETT cuff. After the suction catheter is disconnected, the suction tubing should also be cleared of secretions with the remaining sterile solution or water. Finally, dispose of all supplies properly.

Hyperinflation. Hyperinflation is the delivery of breaths that are 150% of the normal tidal volume. Hyperinflation may be performed with a manual resuscitator bag (MRB) or the ventilator. When a MRB is used, the patient must be disconnected from the ventilator, which results in the loss of positive-pressure ventilation and PEEP. The volumes delivered with a MRB vary between individuals because of hand size and use of a one- versus two-handed technique. Rarely can an individual actually deliver hyperinflation volumes with a MRB when performing the procedure without an assistant. Use of one hand may result in volumes that are actually smaller than ventilator volumes. Alternating between suctioning and bagging may also result in contamination of the suction catheter. Use of a bag may possibly improve the mobilization of secretions as well as the clinician's feel for the secretions in the airway. The rate of ventilation may be varied to meet the patient's inspiratory efforts, which may be increased because of the ETS procedure.

Ventilator hyperinflation is performed by activating the sigh feature. The use of a ventilator may be superior because the delivered volume and flow are precisely controlled and PEEP is maintained. The sigh feature should be used cautiously in patients with high peak airway pressures and tracheobronchial disruption, large pleural air leaks, or recent pulmonary surgery.

Hyperinflation has been associated with increases in mean arterial pressure and mean airway pressure (possibly due to technique). Because hyperinflation may have adverse effects in some patient populations, its use should be assessed on a case-by-case basis.

Hyperoxygenation. A universal finding in studies is that hyperoxygenation before and after suctioning is the most critical variable in determining the postsuction PaO_2 and preventing hypoxemia during ETS. Hyperoxygenation may be performed with an MRB or the ventilator; however, no single technique for delivering 100% oxygen has been defined as the standard, and further research is needed.

To achieve hyperoxygenation with an MRB, one must be sure that the bag is capable of delivering 100% O_2 (Chapter 4). The highest FIO_2 concentrations are delivered in bags with reservoirs when the flow rate is set at 15 L/min and the rate of bag compression is adjusted to allow the reservoir to fill between breaths. Use of an MRB may be sufficient in patients with normal lung function but not in patients with abnormal lung function and dependence on a critical FIO_2 level.

Some ventilators have a 100% O_2 button to aid in the hyperoxygenation of patients before, during, and even after ETS. Factors to be aware of in regard to this ventilator feature are as follows: (1) all ventilators have a washout volume, the internal volume of the ventilator that must be flushed out before the delivered FIO_2 is actually 100%, and (2) the amount of time that the ventilator is going to deliver the 100% oxygen varies. These factors must be taken into consideration in determining when to initiate and when to terminate ETS or reactivate the 100% O_2 feature. If the FIO_2 must be turned up *manually*, a time delay occurs before 100% O_2 is delivered to the patient because of the ventilator washout volume. It is critical that the clinician remembers to turn the FIO_2 setting back down to the baseline level after the suctioning procedure is completed.

Hyperinflation Combined With Hyperoxygenation. In subjects with normal lung function, hyperoxygenation alone for three to five breaths may be sufficient to prevent hypoxemia related to ETS. Hyperinflation without hyperoxygenation is not an acceptable practice with critically ill patients because improved ventilation alone will not prevent suction-related hypoxemia. The combination of hyperinflation and hyperoxygenation with three to five breaths before ETS, between passes of the suction catheter, and after ETS consistently produces the greatest increase in PaO_2 in suctioning studies.

Normal Saline Instillation. The introduction of small amounts of sterile normal saline solution, usually 10 ml or less, is referred to as tracheal instillation or lavage. Generally, normal saline instillation (NSI) is performed to loosen thick secretions and make their passage through the suction catheter easier, and to stimulate cough. Whether more secretions are removed using NSI is unknown. The aspiration of the lavage fluid itself may lead the practitioner to believe that an increased volume of secretions has been removed.

In regard to the distribution of NSI, research shows that it does not affect secretions beyond the main-stem bronchi. Normal saline solution that is not removed with the suction catheter may flow deeper into the airways; however, as a lavage technique, NSI is probably very poor. Bronchoalveolar lavage, along with bronchoscopy, is a superior technique (see the Bronchoscopy section, below). Normal saline solution that migrates into the airways may actually increase intrapulmonary shunt and worsen oxygenation; however, these adverse effects have not been found consistently in research on NSI. Because the suction catheter itself induces cough, NSI is not routinely recommended for this purpose. As a vigorous stimulant of cough, NSI may be deleterious in some patient populations, such as patients with increased intracranial pressure. It may be indicated in patients with thick secretions until more effective methods of secretion hydration, such as systemic hydration and adequate humidification of inspired gases, can be implemented. More research is needed on the efficacy of NSI as a pulmonary hygiene technique.

Patient Monitoring During ETS. Continuous arterial saturation with a pulse oximeter is the optimal method of assessing the potential for hypoxemia during ETS. In the intensive care unit, all patients have cardiac monitors to allow assessment of heart rate, rhythm, and hemodynamic pressure effects of ETS. Continuous monitoring of mixed venous oxygen saturation allows assessment of the balance between oxygen supply and demand during ETS. Suctioning stimulates the sympathetic nervous system. Oxygen consumption may increase and mixed venous oxygen saturation ($S\overline{v}O_2$) may decrease despite increases in arterial oxygen saturation (SaO_2), especially in patients with a high oxygen demand or diminished cardiac reserve at baseline. Visual inspection of the patient for color and psychologic tolerance should be performed throughout the procedure.

Box 5–1 Chest Physiotherapy: Therapeutic Considerations

---

1. Before chest physiotherapy (CPT) is started, the patient should be positioned comfortably. Support may be provided by pillows, blankets, rolled towels, foam wedges, or other available supplies.
2. The patient should be maintained on the same amount of supplemental oxygen received before postural drainage. The FIO_2 may be increased if a particular position adversely affects oxygenation. If oxygenation remains decreased, the position should be modified or the therapy aborted.
3. The patient should take slow, deep breaths throughout the therapy.
4. Premedicate the patient with pain medication as necessary.
5. Coughing and/or suctioning should be used throughout the treatment as necessary to remove mobilized secretions.
6. Tube feedings and/or oral intake should be held for 30 minutes to 1 hour before the treatment is initiated.
7. Appropriate monitoring as determined by the patient's severity of illness and relative stability should be instituted. Monitor the neurologic, cardiovascular, and respiratory systems for evidence of cardiorespiratory compromise.
8. Examine the secretions produced for color, consistency, texture, odor, and amount.
9. Evaluate the effectiveness of the CPT through assessment of the following: chest x-ray film, work of breathing, dyspnea, breath sounds, sputum production, lung volumes, PaO_2, and measures of intrapulmonary shunt.

Chest Physiotherapy

Chest physiotherapy (CPT) encompasses the techniques of postural drainage, percussion, and vibration. Coughing or suctioning should always accompany CPT so that the mobilized secretions can be expelled. CPT may be performed by nurses, respiratory therapists, physical therapists, or other appropriately trained personnel. The purposes of these procedures are to prevent the accumulation of secretions, to mobilize retained secretions, to reduce airway obstruction, and to reduce impaired oxygenation from intrapulmonary shunt by improving ventilation. CPT is indicated when the mucociliary escalator and the cough mechanism have been inadequate in removing pulmonary secretions and exudate. Normal airway clearance mechanisms may be deemed inadequate when there is lack of improvement in the following assessment findings: chest x-ray film, work of breathing and dyspnea, breath sounds, sputum production, lung volumes, PaO_2, and intrapulmonary shunt (Box 5–1).

Specific indications for CPT encompass a number of clinical problems. Postural drainage, along with the manual techniques of percussion and vibration, is beneficial in disease processes in which sputum production is large or its removal is impeded. In these patients, secretion retention persists despite deep breathing and coughing. Radiologic evidence of obstructive atelectasis caused by mucous plugging of airways (segmental collapse), aspiration, or lung abscess further confirms the need for these therapies. Patients who are on prolonged bed rest, are paralyzed, or unconscious, have neuromuscular disease, have an inhalation injury or multiple-system trauma, or have undergone abdominal or thoracic surgery should be evaluated for CPT.

POSTURAL DRAINAGE

Postural drainage (PD) is the technique of using various body positions to promote the flow of secretions toward the larger airways, where the secretions can then be coughed up or suctioned out. PD takes advantage of the effect of gravity on the flow of mucus. Various body positions, based on an understanding of normal pulmonary anatomy, are used to promote drainage of specific lobar segments (Fig. 5–5). The affected area is placed in the most upright position in an

LOWER LOBES
_____

Posterior basal segment   Elevate feet 30 degrees

Prone position; 3 to 4 pillows under hips or head down

Percuss/vibrate lower ribs

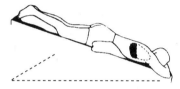

Lateral basal segment   Elevate feet 30 degrees, have client lie on side. Percuss and vibrate lower ribs

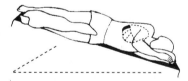

Superior segment   Have client lie on stomach with pillow under stomach

Percuss/vibrate between shoulders and lower ribs.

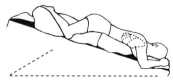

FIGURE 5–5 Body positions used for postural drainage. Chair-seated positions may be achieved in the bed when the patient is critically ill. Postural drainage may be performed in conjunction with percussion or vibration. (From Weilitz, PM: *Pocket Guide to Respiratory Care*. St. Louis: Mosby–Year Book, 1991.)

Continued on following page.

Anterior basal segment — Have client lie on back with knees flexed. Elevate foot of bed 30 degrees. Percuss/vibrate over lower ribs.

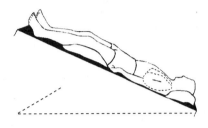

Right middle lobe (medial and lateral segments)

Have client lie on left side.

Place pillow at back.

Rotate ¼ turn back.

Elevate foot of bed 15 degrees.

Percuss/vibrate over nipple area.

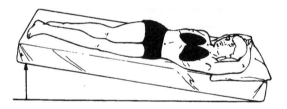

Lingula

Have client lie on right side.

Place pillow at back.

Rotate ¼ turn back.

Elevate foot of bed 15 degrees.

Percuss/vibrate over left nipple.

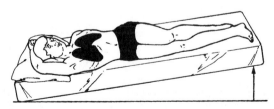

Figure 5–5 *Continued*

UPPER LOBES

Anterior apical segment   Have client sit up in chair, then lean back. Percuss/vibrate at shoulders. Extend fingers over collarbone.

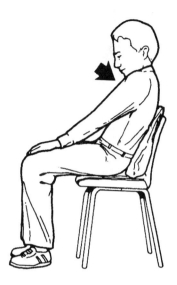

Posterior apical segment   Have client sit up in chair, then lean forward over pillow. Percuss/vibrate at shoulders.

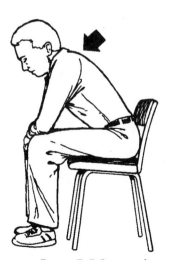

Figure 5–5 *Continued*

Continued on following page.

Left upper lobe posterior segment	Have client lie on right side, then rotate forward, leaning over pillow. Percuss/vibrate over left shoulder.

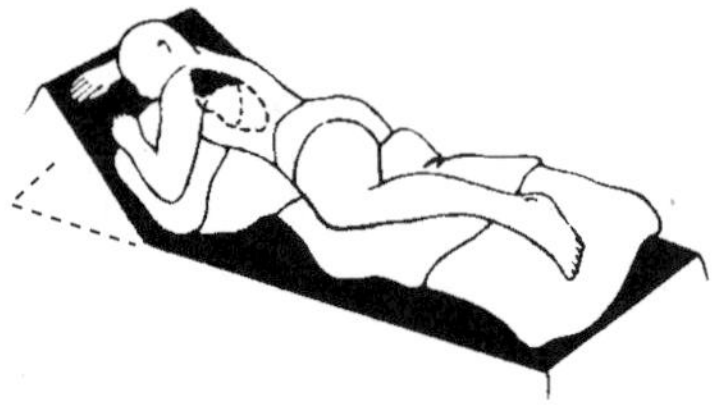

Right upper lobe posterior segment	Have client lie on left side, rotating turn forward onto pillow for support. Bed should be flat. Percuss/vibrate over right shoulder blade.

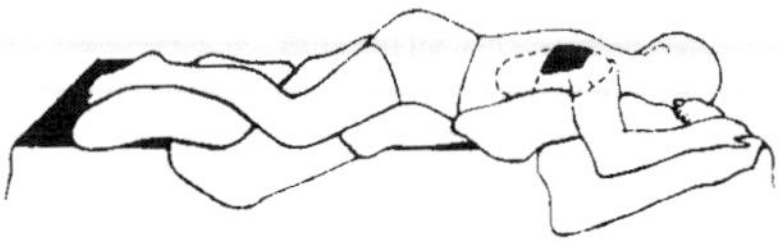

Anterior segment	Have client lie flat on back. Percuss/vibrate just below collarbone.

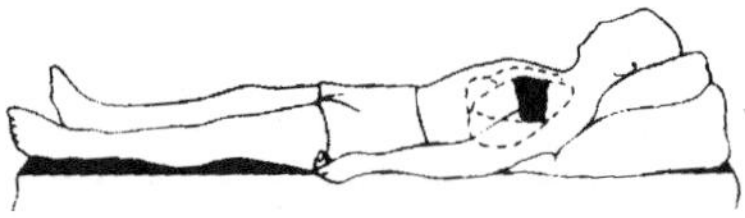

FIGURE 5–5 *Continued*

effort to promote drainage of the lung segment by achieving an optimal gravitational effect on mucous flow. The position to be used with a specific patient is determined by x-ray and auscultatory findings. Positions may need to be modified as indicated by deteriorating neurologic, cardiac, or pulmonary assessment data, by position contraindications secondary to trauma or surgery, or by the presence of tubes or drains.

The length of time that a position should be maintained is variable and depends on a balance between achievement of therapeutic effect and patient tolerance. Intermittently the patient should be assisted to cough or suctioned to remove the mobilized secretions. Mobilized secretions have been known to gravitate into nondiseased lung segments, necessitating therapy in these areas as well.

PERCUSSION

Percussion is a manual technique used in conjunction with postural drainage to promote the advancement of secretions toward the larger airways. Percussion is performed by rhythmically and alternately clapping cupped hands (Fig. 5–6) over the relevant area of lung. The cupping of the hands creates a cushion of air, which reduces the force of impact. The action should produce a hollow popping sound, not a slapping one. The shoulders and elbows remain relaxed so that the rhythmic movement is generated from the wrists. The effect is the transmission of energy waves through the chest, which shakes and vibrates secretions, loosening them, thus aiding in their removal.

Percussion should be performed directly on the chest wall and not over a towel or other covering, as some clinicians advocate. The use of a covering requires that greater force be applied to achieve the same effect, and the air cushion is lost in the covering. Furthermore, anatomic landmarks are not visible, nor is the presence of erythema, petechiae, subcutaneous emphysema, or other indicators that the therapy should be discontinued or altered. Precautionary factors that need to be considered before the initiation of postural drainage with percussion are outlined in Table 5–1.

VIBRATION

Chest vibration is used in conjunction with postural drainage. It may be used as an alternative to percussion, particularly around surgical incisions, where it may be more comfortable. It is performed by placing the flat of the hands over the chest wall of the affected lung area and vibrating the hands quickly during the *expiratory* phase of the respiratory cycle (Fig. 5–7). The vibration is superficial and creates an oscillatory movement that is reflected to the deep tissues, thereby assisting in the loosening of mucus and promoting its flow. The procedure should follow a maximal inspiration, which can be facilitated in the patient supported by mechanical ventilation with the delivery of a large breath with a manual resuscitator bag or sighing the patient with the ventilator. If the procedure is performed correctly, the patient will have spurts of exhaled air. Mechan-

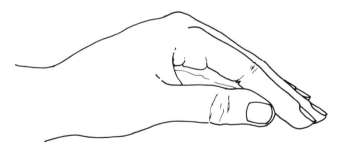

FIGURE 5–6 Cupped position of the hand used for percussion. The thumb and index finger are pinched together; the fingers are then extended, held together, and flexed at a 90° angle to the palm of the hand. Incorrect hand position results in a slapping sound, whereas correct hand position results in a hollow, popping sound. (From Wade, JF: *Comprehensive Respiratory Care: Physiology and Technique.* St. Louis: CV Mosby, 1982.)

TABLE 5-1 Chest Physiotherapy: Precautionary Factors

Precaution	Rationale
Recent MI and CHF, dysrhythmias	HR and BP may rise, increasing myocardial oxygen demand. Head-down position increases central blood volume, which may not be tolerated in CHF. Restrict to patients who can be monitored closely.
Recent craniotomy or head trauma	Administer CPT (including use of varying degrees of Trendelenburg position) cautiously and only with appropriate monitoring of ICP and CPP. Administer sedation and maintain neck alignment. Restrict to patients with clear benefit and modify therapy as necessary. Head-down position is contraindicated in unrepaired cerebral aneurysm.
Unstable spine injuries or recent spinal surgery	Placing the entire bed in the head-down position while maintaining spinal alignment may be used. Care must be taken not to put stress on recent spinal fusions. Use must be individualized.
Hypoxemia that worsens with body position changes, extreme dyspnea	Monitor patients closely with continuous real-time monitoring (e.g., pulse oximetry). Modify positions as necessary.
Lung abscess	Postural drainage and percussion are therapies of choice. Discontinue if frank hemoptysis occurs. Have suction available to prevent asphyxiation from rapid dislodgment of a large volume of pus. There is risk of "spillover" of contaminated material into uncontaminated area, with consequent spread of infection.
Pulmonary contusion	May assist in clearing blood and thus reducing this potential bacterial growth medium. Contraindicated in concomitant coagulopathy.
Frank hemoptysis (active or recent)	Percussion and vibration are contraindicated because they may worsen bleeding and dislodge clots. CPT may be given cautiously in conditions where modest blood streaking is present.
Rib fracture and flail chest, osteoporosis	May be performed by an experienced therapist while monitoring for rib shift or any other motion. When properly performed, percussion may apply less pressure than coughing or lying on the injury. Positive-pressure ventilation may promote internal stabilization of the area.
Subcutaneous emphysema	Monitor for and report any increase in subcutaneous air. When no chest tubes are present, CPT should be held until pneumothorax is ruled out.
Asthma and/or bronchospasm	An inhaled bronchodilator may be given 10 to 20 minutes before CPT.
Chest tubes, vascular lines, artificial airways, incisions	Extreme care must be used not to dislodge lines, drains, or airways. Administer gentle percussion or vibration around incisions and chest tubes.
Tube feedings	Gastric tube feedings should be held for 1 hour before CPT. Small bowel (duodenal/jejunal) feedings may continue if there is no gastric reflux.

MI = Myocardial infarction; CHF = congestive heart failure; HR = heart rate; BP = blood pressure; ICP = intracranial pressure; CPP = cerebral perfusion pressure.

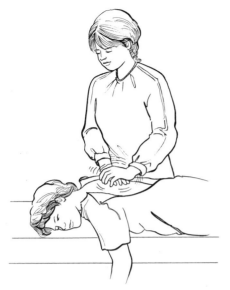

FIGURE 5-7 Chest vibration.

ical vibrators, which were originally introduced for home care, are available, but they show no clear advantage over manual vibration.

Bronchoscopy

The bronchoscope may be used for therapeutic as well as diagnostic purposes. There are two types of bronchoscopes: rigid and flexible. The use of the rigid bronchoscope is limited to the operating room under general anesthesia. The flexible bronchoscope is used in the intensive care setting by the intensivist, surgeon, or pulmonologist because it has many advantages over the rigid scope. This section is limited to discussion of the flexible bronchoscope.

The bronchoscope consists of a rigid hand piece and a flexible extension that averages 55 to 60 cm long. The hand piece contains a viewfinder lens, a thumb lever for flexion and extension of the tip, a finger-activated suction valve, an instrument port, and a site where suction is connected (Fig. 5–8). Visualization of the airways is provided by fiberoptics. The bronchoscope must also be connected to a light source. The bronchoscopy procedure may be performed nasally, orally, or through an endotracheal or tracheostomy tube. The flexible scope provides much greater visualization than the rigid one because it can be advanced to the third or fourth divisions of the segmental bronchi. The bronchoscope is portable, and the procedure can be easily performed at the patient's bedside, which eliminates the risks inherent in transporting the patient. A portable cart, set up with all the necessary procedural supplies, improves efficiency.

Therapeutic indications for bronchoscopy include removal of aspirated foreign bodies, especially those beyond the reach of a rigid bronchoscope; secretion retention not responsive to other therapies, including CPT, because the bronchoscope can be used to aspirate thick secretions or an abscess; and facilitation of endotracheal intubation. Endotracheal intubation is performed by inserting the bronchoscope through the endotracheal tube, advancing the bronchoscope

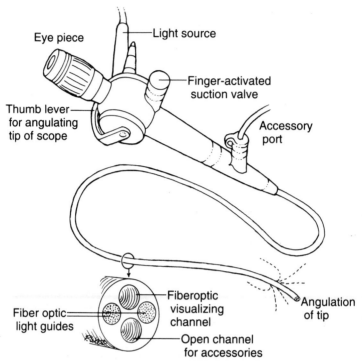

Eye piece

Light source

Finger-activated
suction valve

Thumb lever
for angulating
tip of scope

Accessory
port

Fiber optic
light guides

Fiberoptic
visualizing
channel

Angulation
of tip

Open channel
for accessories

Figure 5-8 Component parts of the flexible fiberoptic bronchoscope. (From Johnson, NT, and Pierson, DJ: Pulmonary diagnostic procedures. In DJ Pierson and RM Kacmarek [Eds.]: *Foundations of Respiratory Care*. New York: Churchill Livingstone, 1992.)

through the glottic opening, and then passing the endotracheal tube over the bronchoscope. *Diagnostic indications* for bronchoscopy include acquisition of specimens, biopsy in distal airways, and inspection of the airways, such as in the presence of a mass, a tracheobronchial injury, or hemoptysis.

Bronchoscopy Procedure

During the bronchoscopy procedure, all members of the team should wear a mask, eye protection, and gloves. Protective gowns may also be worn. Prepare the patient who is taking food by mouth by withholding their diet for 6 hours. If the patient is receiving gastric, duodenal, or jejunal tube feedings, hold them for 1 hour and, as an extra precautionary measure, aspirate the stomach contents (if a gastric tube is in place) before initiating the procedure. Instruct the patient on what to expect and how to cooperate with the procedure. Appropriate laboratory studies should be obtained, including coagulation studies if a biopsy is to be performed.

Prepare for the procedure by gathering all necessary supplies, including medications. Various drugs may be used, including a drying agent such as atropine or topical anesthetics such as 1%, 2%, or 4% lidocaine, cocaine, or cetacaine, which is a solution of benzocaine and tetracaine used to suppress the gag reflex in nonintubated patients. An analgesic or sedative such as meperidine, codeine, morphine, diazepam, or midazolam is also generally administered. Diazepam and midazolam have the additional benefit of providing the patient with amnesia of the event. Ensure that the patient has a reliable intravenous access for administration of medication or fluids should hypotension occur.

The patient should be monitored throughout and after the procedure to detect any complications early. Minimal monitoring should include pulse oximetry, electrocardiography, and monitoring of the heart rate and blood pressure. The individual performing the bronchoscopy may become absorbed in the procedure; therefore the assistant is responsible for monitoring the patient and informing the physician of any patient problems. After the procedure the patient should be monitored for successful recovery. If a biopsy was performed, the presence of increasingly bloody sputum may indicate bleeding.

Patients undergoing mechanical ventilation should receive 100% oxygen throughout the procedure, and in patients supported by PEEP a bronchoscopy adapter should be used to avoid loss of PEEP. Auto-PEEP may develop because of the resistance to exhalation created by the bronchoscope as it partially occludes the airway. The peak airway pressure alarms may need to be reset to a higher limit because airway pressure will rise as the bronchoscope creates an increased resistance to airflow. So that a lower peak airway pressure can be maintained during the procedure, the tidal volume and flow rate may be decreased while the respiratory rate is concurrently increased, thus maintaining a steady minute ventilation. Exhaled tidal volumes and minute ventilation should be monitored for their adequacy, and the tidal volume should be titrated to maintain a sufficient minute ventilation.

SPECIMENS

Various specimens may be obtained during the bronchoscopy procedure. Bronchial washings are the aspirate obtained as the scope is passed through the airways. They may or may not be sent for culture because they may be contaminated with upper airway flora. The physician may prevent contamination by not applying suction until the lower airways are reached.

A double-sheathed brush catheter is used for obtaining sterile bacterial cultures. The brush is enclosed in a sheath as it is advanced through the bronchoscope to the area in question. The brush is then advanced beyond the sheath to obtain the specimen. It is then withdrawn back into the protective sheath, and the whole thing is removed from the bronchoscope.

For bronchoalveolar lavage (BAL), the distal airway is occluded by wedging the bronchoscope tip in the airway and then instilling 20 to 30 ml aliquots of nonbacteriostatic normal saline solution. The fluid is then aspirated into a suction trap. Microbiologic tests are run on the aspirate. BAL is useful for determining the cause of lung infections.

Endobronchial biopsy may also be performed with a variety of needle or forceps appliances.

COMPLICATIONS

When bronchoscopy is performed by a skilled bronchoscopist and with appropriate monitoring, complications are rare. Complications that should be considered include bronchospasm, vasovagal response, postprocedure fever, bleeding, cardiac dysrhythmias, and pneumothorax caused by the development of excessive airway pressures or inadvertent pleural biopsy.

When bronchoscopy is performed on intubated patients, interference with ventilation may occur because the bronchoscope creates resistance to ventilation. A cuffed airway at least 8.0 mm (inside diameter) in size may result in less compromise in airflow and tidal volume. Use of a swivel bronchoscope adapter will allow mechanical ventilation to continue throughout the procedure. Hypoxemia and cardiac dysrhythmias may occur and may possibly be due to mechanical obstruction of the airway and/or increased intrapulmonary shunt caused by lavage solutions. Interventions directed toward preventing these complications include increasing the FIO_2, flow rate, or tidal volume, limiting the amount of lavage used, and limiting the duration of suction application.

RECOMMENDED READINGS

Ackerman, M.H. (1993). The effect of saline lavage prior to suctioning. *Am J Crit Care* 2(4), 326–330.

Bostik, J., and Wendelgass, S.T. (1987). Normal saline instillation as part of the suctioning procedure: Effects on PaO_2 and amount of secretions. *Heart Lung* 16(5), 532–538.

Brutinel, W.M., and Cortese, D.A. (1991). Bronchoscopy. In G.G. Burton, J.E. Hodgkin, and J.J. Ward (Eds.). *Respiratory Care: A Guide to Clinical Practice* (pp. 691–704). Philadelphia: J.B. Lippincott.

Campbell, R.S., and Branson, R.D. (1992). How ventilators provide temporary O_2 enrichment: What happens when you press the 100% suction button. *Respir Care* 37(8), 933–937.

Czarnik, R.E., et al. (1991). Differential effects of continuous versus intermittent suction on tracheal tissue. *Heart Lung* 20(2), 144–151.

Faling, L.J. (1991). Chest physical therapy. In G.G. Burton, J.E. Hodgkin, and J.J. Ward (Eds.). *Respiratory Care: A Guide to Clinical Practice* (pp. 625–654). Philadelphia: J.B. Lippincott.

Hanley, M.V., Rudd, T., and Butler, J. (1978). What happens to intratracheal saline instillations? [abstract]. *Am Rev Respir Dis* 117(suppl), 124.

Hertz, M.I., et al. (1991). Safety of bronchoalveolar lavage in the critically ill patient. *Crit Care Med* 19(12), 1526–1532.

Judson, M.A., and Sahn, S.A. (1994). Mobilization of secretions in ICU patients. *Respir Care* 39(3), 213–226.

Jung, R.C., and Gottlieb, L.S. (1976). Comparison of tracheobronchial suction catheters in humans: Visualization by fiberoptic bronchoscopy. *Chest* 69(2), 179–181.

Mackenzie, C.F., Imle, P.C., and Ciesla, N. (1989). *Chest Physiotherapy in the Intensive Care Unit.* Baltimore: Williams & Wilkins.

Mancinelli-Van Atta, J., and Beck, S.L. (1992). Preventing hypoxemia and hemodynamic compromise related to endotracheal suctioning. *Am J Crit Care* 1(3), 62–79.

McQuillan, K.A. (1987). The effects of the Trendelenburg position for postural drainage on cerebrovascular status in head-injured patients [abstract]. *Heart Lung* 16(3), 327.

Noll, M.N., Hix, C.D., and Scott, G. (1990). Closed tracheal suction systems: Effectiveness and nursing implications. *AACN Clinical Issues* 1(2), 318–328.

Smith, R.A. (1988). Mask and nasal continuous positive airway pressure. In R.M. Kacmarek and J.K. Stoller (Eds.). *Current Respiratory Care* (pp. 33–37). Toronto: B.C. Decker.

Stone, K.S. (1990). Ventilator versus manual resuscitation bag as the method for delivering hyperoxygenation before endotracheal suctioning. *AACN Clinical Issues* 1(2), 289–299.

Taggart, J.A., Dorinsky, N.L., and Sheahan, J.S. (1988). Airway pressures during closed system suctioning. *Heart Lung* 17(5), 536–542.

Tyler, M.L. (1982). Complications of positioning and chest physiotherapy. *Respir Care* 27(4), 458–466.

Mechanical Ventilation: Indications, Basic Principles of Ventilator Performance of the Respiratory Cycle, and Initiation

INDICATIONS FOR MECHANICAL VENTILATION

The primary indication for mechanical ventilation is impending or existing respiratory failure. Its use is also indicated after major surgery and for therapeutic hyperventilation in the presence of intracranial hypertension.

Acute Respiratory Failure

Respiratory failure is the absence of the normal homeostatic state of ventilation as it relates to acid-base status of the blood and the exchange of oxygen and carbon dioxide. Therefore the candidates for mechanical ventilation are those patients whose lungs can no longer provide an adequate exchange of gases. This inadequacy is reflected in the patient's blood gases. Following is an objective clinical definition of respiratory failure:

- A PaO_2 of <60 mm Hg on an FIO_2 of >0.5 (oxygenation)
- A $PaCO_2$ greater than 50 mm Hg, with a pH of 7.25 or less (ventilation)

It is difficult to place a threshold value on a failing oxygenation status because so many factors, such as age and previous history of lung disease, determine the acceptable PaO_2 in any individual patient. It is more helpful to look at the trend of the patient's PaO_2 with time and to determine whether a deterioration is signifying respiratory failure. The ventilatory values listed above warn of life-threatening respiratory acidosis and respiratory failure. Clues to the presence of respiratory failure include an increasing respiratory rate, a decreasing tidal volume, an increase in the work of breathing as evidenced by an increase in the use of the accessory muscles of ventilation and paradoxical breathing, and complaints of dyspnea.

To make appropriate therapeutic decisions the clinician should differentiate whether the patient has failure to ventilate, failure to oxygenate, or a combination of the two (Fig. 6–1). *Failure to ventilate*, also called ventilatory failure or hypercapnic or respiratory pump failure, occurs when ventilatory demand exceeds ventilatory supply. Ventilatory demand is the minute ventilation required to

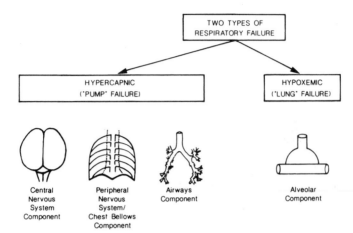

FIGURE 6-1 Acute respiratory failure may be divided into failure to oxygenate (hypoxemic failure) and failure to ventilate (hypercapnic failure). Hypercapnic failure may occur as a result of inability to sustain adequate ventilation by one or more of the three components of ventilation: the central nervous system, the peripheral nervous system innervating the muscles of ventilation, and the airways. Hypoxemic failure results from failure to adequately exchange gases at the alveolar level. (From Lanken, PN. Respiratory failure: An overview. In RW Carlson and MA Geheb [Eds.]: *Principles and Practice of Medical Intensive Care* [pp 754–763]. Philadelphia: WB Saunders, 1993.)

maintain a normal or baseline $PaCO_2$. Ventilatory supply is the maximal sustainable ventilation that a person can uphold without respiratory muscle fatigue. In disease, not only may ventilatory demand be increased but ventilatory supply may concurrently be markedly decreased, an imbalance that may result in respiratory failure (Fig. 6–2). The primary cause of *failure to oxygenate*, also known as hypoxemic respiratory failure, is physiologic shunt (Chapter 2). With shunt, the associated hypoxemia stimulates the respiratory drive, but because the ventilated oxygen is not interfacing with the pulmonary capillary, hypoxemia persists. Conservative measures such as the administration of supplemental oxygen may correct the hypoxemia; however, if it is not corrected, then a swift decision to intubate and mechanically ventilate must be made to prevent tissue hypoxia. Placing the patient on a ventilator allows for support of an increased ventilatory demand, the application of tidal volumes that will improve functional residual capacity, and the administration of therapies designed to improve oxygenation: high inspired oxygen concentrations and positive end-expiratory pressure (PEEP).

The decision to intubate and mechanically ventilate is based on sound clinical decision making after assessment of the patient's oxygenation, ventilation, and work of breathing. The decision is not an arbitrary one because of the complications associated with artificial airways and positive-pressure ventilation (see Chapter 8).

A classification of diseases that predispose a patient to respiratory failure is presented in Table 6–1. Such a classification is helpful because it offers insight into the pathophysiologic process underlying the failure and suggests suitable therapies. It must be remembered that the application of mechanical ventilation

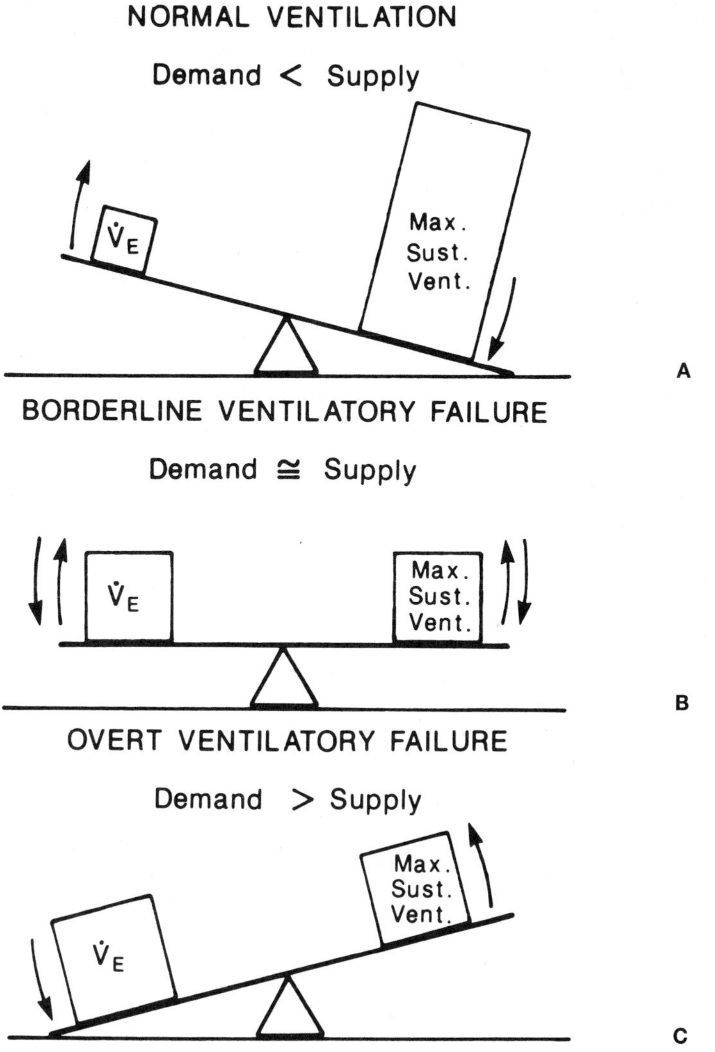

NORMAL VENTILATION

Demand < Supply

A

BORDERLINE VENTILATORY FAILURE

Demand ≅ Supply

B

OVERT VENTILATORY FAILURE

Demand > Supply

C

FIGURE 6–2 For maintenance of adequate gas exchange ventilatory supply, an individual's maximal sustainable ventilation must meet or exceed ventilatory demand, the individual's spontaneous minute ventilation ($\dot{V}E$). (A) The normal situation, in which maximal sustainable ventilation exceeds minute ventilation. Disease can lead to borderline respiratory failure (B) when maximal sustainable ventilation approximately equals minute ventilation needs. This state may be due to an increase in ventilatory demand or a decrease in supply or both. If demand exceeds supply, respiratory failure will ensue (C) and mechanical ventilatory support will become necessary. (From Lanken, PN. Respiratory failure: An overview. In RW Carlson and MA Geheb [Eds.]: *Principles and Practice of Medical Intensive Care* [pp 754–763]. Philadelphia: WB Saunders, 1993.)

Table 6-1 Categories of Intrapulmonary and Extrapulmonary Disorders Predisposing to Respiratory Failure

Category	Examples
Disorders of the CNS associated with a reduced drive to breathe	Overdose of respiratory depressant drugs such as sedatives and narcotics Cerebrovascular accident Cerebral trauma Subarachnoid hemorrhage
Disorders associated with neuromuscular function*	Guillain-Barré Multiple sclerosis Poliomyelitis Myasthenia gravis Spinal cord injury Electrolyte disorders (hypophosphatemia, hypomagnesemia)
Disorders associated with musculoskeletal and pleural functions	Kyphoscoliosis Flail chest Pleural effusion Pneumothorax Hemothorax

Disorders of the conducting airways	Upper airway obstruction
	  Epiglottitis
	  Obstructive sleep apnea
	Postextubation laryngeal edema
	Asthma
	Bronchospasm

Disorders of the gas exchanging units (alveoli and pulmonary capillaries)	Pulmonary contusion Pneumonia Pulmonary edema ARDS Aspiration Interstitial lung disease Near drowning Smoke inhalation

CNS = Central nervous system; ARDS = adult respiratory distress syndrome.
*Function of the peripheral nerves and muscles of ventilation.

does not correct the underlying disorder. It only supports the respiratory system until the appropriate therapies, such as bronchial hygiene and administration of antibiotics, can be applied to cure the underlying disease.

POSITIVE-PRESSURE VENTILATION

As a comparison of how respiration is altered when a mechanical ventilator is used, review of the mechanics of normal, spontaneous respiration is important. Recall from Chapter 2 that the physiology of spontaneous respiration requires that energy be expended to contract the muscles of respiration. The contraction of the respiratory muscles enlarges the thoracic cavity, which creates negative pressure within the chest and results in the flow of air, at atmospheric pressure, into the lungs. It would be ideal if mechanical ventilators could mimic the mechanics and physiology of spontaneous respiration while achieving the goals of adequate oxygenation and ventilation. Indeed, negative-pressure ventilators attempt to do so. However, almost all modern ventilators used in inpatient clinical settings are *positive*-pressure ventilators.

The positive-pressure ventilator uses a power source, known as the drive mechanism, to force air into the lungs during inspiration. Expiration occurs passively during positive-pressure ventilation. The patient may exhale to atmospheric pressure or to a set level of positive end-expiratory pressure (PEEP).

In spontaneous breathing, no conscious effort is required to pass through the phases of a respiratory cycle: "inspire, end inspiration, expire, begin a new inspiration." Imagine how tedious this would be! However, if a machine is to perform the respiratory cycle, it must be told, first, what the component phases of the respiratory cycle are and, second, how to carry out each of the phases as determined by the settings of the phase variables. Every ventilator has four basic phases that it must complete in providing a ventilatory cycle to the patient (Fig. 6–3):

1. Inspiration
2. Inspiratory-expiratory changeover
3. Expiration
4. Expiratory-inspiratory changeover

Within each phase are phase variables that are manipulated by the operator. They provide the ventilator with further information about how to carry out the phase. An example of a phase variable within the inspiratory phase is an end-inspiratory pause, and within the expiratory phase is the setting of PEEP. The following is a discussion of each of the four phases of ventilation in a positive-pressure ventilator. The phase variables are addressed in the Ventilator Settings section, below.

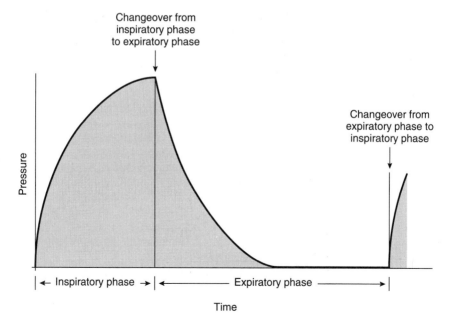

FIGURE 6–3 The four phases of the respiratory cycle on a ventilator. See text for explanation.

Inspiratory Phase

It is during the inspiratory phase that positive pressure is generated in order to create a pressure gradient that leads to lung inflation. The pressures within the airways, alveoli, and intrapleural spaces all become positive during inspiration, the exact opposite of what occurs during spontaneous inspiration (Fig. 6–4). This positive pressure causes the lungs to inflate and the thoracic cavity to expand.

How the positive pressure is generated is determined by the ventilator's drive mechanism. Discussion of drive mechanisms is useful for those purchasing ven-

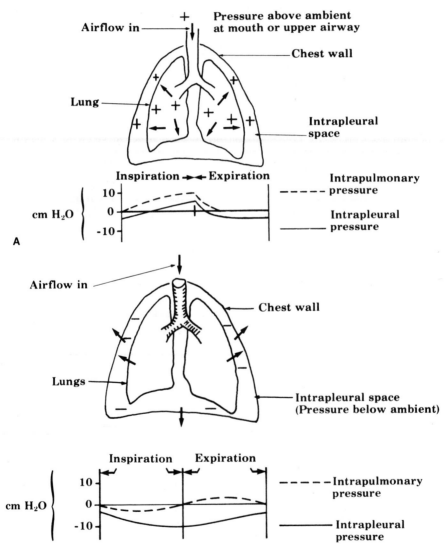

Figure 6-4 Comparison of the pressures within the thoracic cavity during positive-pressure ventilation (A) versus spontaneous respiration (B). (From Pilbeam, SP: *Mechanical Ventilation: Physiological and Clinical Applications*. St. Louis: Mosby–Year Book, 1992.)

tilators; however, it is not practical information that will impact the hourly, clinical decisions of the bedside practitioner. Therefore the most important thing to know about the inspiratory phase is that positive pressure is generated in the thoracic cavity. It is this positive pressure that causes most of the complications of mechanical ventilation, such as hemodynamic compromise and barotrauma (see Chapter 8).

Inspiratory-Expiratory Changeover

Ventilators are classified by the mechanism that cycles ventilation from the inspiratory phase to the expiratory phase. Most ventilators today are capable of functioning with up to three of the four cycling mechanisms: volume, flow, time, and pressure. It is important to begin to develop an understanding of the interrelationships among these four variables during mechanical ventilation of the patient. Whether the ventilator is functioning in a volume, flow, time, or pressure-cycled manner, the other factors need to be viewed as potential areas in which ventilation could be limited. One factor is controlled, and therefore it functions as the independent variable. The other factors are variable and need to be monitored, or appropriately adjusted, on the ventilator by the clinician (Table 6–2). This essential concept will become clearer with the following explanation of the four mechanisms that cycle the inspiratory-expiratory changeover.

VOLUME-CYCLED VENTILATION

In volume-cycled ventilation the ventilator cycles to end inspiration and begin expiration when a predetermined volume is delivered into the patient circuit. The time required to deliver the volume, the flow rate, and the pressure developed are variable. Once the predetermined volume and respiratory rate have been set on the ventilator, the inspiratory flow rate must be appropriately

TABLE 6–2 Mechanism of Cycling From Inspiration to Expiration on Positive-Pressure Ventilators

Cycling Mechanism	Controlled Variable (Independent Variable)	Variables to Monitor (M) or Adjust (A*) (Dependent Variables)
Volume	Tidal volume	Flow rate (A) Inspiratory time (A) Airway pressures (M)
Time	Inspiratory time	Flow rate (A) Tidal volume (M)† Airway pressure (M)
Pressure	Maximal airway pressure	Flow rate (A) Inspiratory time (M) Tidal volume (M)†
Flow	Flow rate	Inspiratory time (A or M) Tidal volume (M)† Airway pressure (A)

*Though a variable is adjusted, the implication is that it is also monitored on an ongoing basis so that appropriate adjustments can be made.
†In the use of any ventilatory cycling mechanism in which tidal volume is variable, frequent monitoring of the tidal volume is essential!

adjusted so that the tidal volume is delivered within the desired inspiratory time. The amount of pressure generated to deliver the prescribed tidal volume, the peak inspiratory pressure (PIP), will vary depending on compliance and resistance factors and must be closely monitored by the clinician. As compliance decreases or resistance increases, PIP will rise, because even under these circumstances the ventilator continues to deliver the committed volume.

TIME-CYCLED VENTILATION

In time-cycled ventilation, inspiration ends and expiration begins after a predetermined time interval has been reached. Cycling may be controlled by a simple timing mechanism or by setting the rate and adjusting the inspiratory/expiratory ratio, or percentage of inspiratory time. Both mechanisms tell the ventilator to cycle from inspiration to expiration after a preset amount of time has elapsed. When cycling occurs, the airway pressure attained, the inspiratory flow, and the tidal volume may all be variable on a breath-to-breath basis. In time-cycled ventilation the tidal volume is determined by gas flow rate multiplied by inspiratory time (Volume = Flow × Time). Because time is controlled, the flow rate must be adjusted to achieve the desired tidal volume before the ventilator cycles. Changes in airway resistance and pulmonary compliance will vary the airway pressure and may also reduce tidal volume unless the ventilator is capable of delivering constant flow under varying lung conditions.

PRESSURE-CYCLED VENTILATION

In pressure-cycled ventilation, inspiration ends and expiration begins when a predetermined maximal airway pressure limit is reached. The volume delivered, the flow rate, and the inspiratory time all vary on a breath-to-breath basis. The volume delivered is determined by the set cycling pressure, the flow rate, the patient's lung compliance, airway and circuit resistance to ventilation, and the integrity of the ventilator circuit. An initial cycling pressure is chosen while the exhaled tidal volume is monitored. Pressure is then adjusted until an acceptable tidal volume is achieved. Flow rate is adjusted while the respiratory rate is taken into consideration to achieve the desired inspiratory time. If the patient's lung characteristics deteriorate, the tidal volume will drop and the inspiratory time will shorten. Increasing the cycling pressure is the primary mechanism for correcting this problem. Increasing the flow rate may also help.

FLOW-CYCLED VENTILATION

In flow-cycled ventilation, inspiration ends and expiration begins when the flow rate decays to a predetermined percentage of its peak value. This critical flow rate where cycling occurs is the "terminal" flow rate. The volume in the lungs and the inspiratory time vary from breath to breath. The volume delivered to the patient's lungs is determined by a chosen generated pressure and by the compliance and resistance of the patient's lungs. At the start of inspiration the flow rate is maximum, but as the lungs fill with air, pressure within them increases and flow rate decreases (because of resistance to the flow). When the terminal flow rate is achieved, the ventilator cycles to the expiratory phase. Generated pressure is sustained throughout the inspiratory phase, unlike pressure cycling, in which it gradually rises and peaks at end-inspiration.

Flow cycling tends to be more comfortable for the patient than pressure cycling because in flow cycling the patient has a greater degree of control over the respiratory cycle. An example of a mode of ventilation that operates by these principles is flow-cycled, pressure-supported ventilation. The flow-cycled venti- lator is set up in the same manner as the pressure-cycled ventilator. An initial generated pressure is chosen while the exhaled tidal volume is monitored. Pres- sure is then adjusted until an acceptable tidal volume is achieved. Flow rate is ad- justed while the respiratory rate is taken into consideration, so that the tidal vol- ume is delivered in a comfortable inspiratory time. If the patient's lung compli- ance decreases or resistance increases, tidal volume will drop and the inspiratory time will shorten, which is exactly how pressure cycling responds under this con- dition. Compensation for a decreased tidal volume is accomplished by an in- crease in the generated pressure.

LIMITS TO INSPIRATION

A limit variable for inspiration is a target value for pressure, volume, or flow that cannot be exceeded. For example, a volume-cycled ventilator may have a pressure-limiting mechanism designed to prevent excessive airway pressures. This safety mechanism is in place in case a major change occurs in lung charac- teristics, such as tension pneumothorax, or in case the ventilator malfunctions. The pressure limit is usually set at 10 cm H_2O above peak inspiratory pressure. When the limit is reached, an audio or visual alarm (or both) gives a warning and the resulting volume is delivered but vented to the atmosphere. Thus the ventilator is still volume cycled but pressure limited. Another example is in the pressure support mode of ventilation, in which the breath is pressure limited but flow cycled. The limit variable must not be confused with the cycle variable. The limit variable has a maximal setting but does not cycle the ventilator from the inspiratory to the expiratory phase.

Expiration

The variable controlled during the expiratory time on the ventilator is known as the *baseline variable*. In all commonly used ventilators, pressure is the variable that is controlled during expiration. Exhalation occurs passively because of the elastic recoil of the lung during mechanical ventilation, but the patient passively exhales to a controlled baseline pressure. The end-expiratory pressure may be in equilibration with atmospheric pressure or may be above atmospheric pressure, which is known as PEEP (Fig. 6–5). In the latter case, some degree of positive pressure will always remain in the patient's chest at the end of exhalation. PEEP improves the functional residual capacity (FRC) by promoting the recruitment and stability of alveoli.

Some ventilator systems allow for the application of an expiratory retard, which is an increased resistance to flow during expiration. Expiratory retard was initially developed to mimic pursed-lip breathing, which is often observed in pa- tients with chronic obstructive pulmonary disease. Creating a resistance to expi- ratory flow prevents premature airway collapse and the trapping of gas in the lungs. An expiratory retard therefore promotes more complete emptying of the lungs, whereas PEEP increases the FRC.

Expiratory-Inspiratory Changeover

Once the expiratory phase has been completed, the changeover to the next inspiratory phase begins. This phase may be initiated by the patient or by the

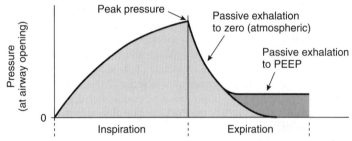

FIGURE 6-5 Expiration on a positive-pressure ventilator occurs passively because of the elastic recoil forces of the lung. Expiration occurs to a controlled *baseline* pressure, which may be zero (atmospheric), or to positive end-expiratory pressure (PEEP). (Modified from Pilbeam, SP: *Mechanical Ventilation: Physiological and Clinical Applications*. St. Louis: Mosby–Year Book, 1992.)

ventilator and is the basis of classifying modes of ventilation as assisted or controlled. The variable that is measured by the ventilator and that determines the initiation of a breath is known as the "trigger" variable. The most common trigger variables are time and pressure. When time is the trigger, the ventilator will trigger a breath after a preset time interval, which is determined by the respiratory frequency. When pressure is the trigger, the patient's spontaneous respiratory effort decreases the pressure within the inspiratory circuit and inspiration begins. The negative inspiratory effort that the patient must apply to initiate inspiration is known as the ventilator's *sensitivity*. Sensitivity, a ventilator setting controlled by the clinician, is discussed below in the Ventilator Settings section. The final way in which a ventilator can be triggered into the inspiratory phase is manually. This external cycling mechanism is activated by the clinician, all other cycling mechanisms are overridden, and a controlled breath is delivered.

VENTILATOR SETTINGS

Fraction of Inspired Oxygen Concentration (FIO_2)

When one is *initiating* mechanical ventilation for the patient in respiratory failure, it is best to err on the side of caution and to use a high FIO_2 (0.7 to 1.0) to ensure adequate tissue oxygenation. After an initial blood gas value is obtained, the FIO_2 may be decreased to achieve the goal of a clinically acceptable PaO_2 (>60 mm Hg) with an FIO_2 of 0.5 or less. A PaO_2 of 60 mm Hg or greater achieves an arterial saturation of 90% or greater under conditions of normal body temperature and pH. An FIO_2 of 0.5 or less minimizes oxygen toxicity. If an FIO_2 of >0.6 is necessary to maintain oxygenation, then the addition of PEEP should be considered.

Pulse oximetry should be considered for continuous monitoring of oxygenation and titration of the FIO_2. If blood gas values are used, it is common practice to wait 20 minutes after a ventilator change before obtaining the blood sample. Predictive equations for the selection of a satisfactory FIO_2 exist, but a trial-and-error approach (ideally with the use of a pulse oximeter) is probably just as useful. The reason is that both the patient's underlying disease process and the concurrently administered therapies affect the way individual patients respond to a change in FIO_2.

Use of correct terminology regarding the FIO_2 is to say that the patient is on an FIO_2 of 0.3 or 0.8, which acknowledges that the unit of measure, the FIO_2, is a fraction. Alternatively, one may say that the patient is on 30% or 80% oxygen. It is incorrect to say that the patient is on an FIO_2 of 30%, because this terminology mixes two units of measure.

Tidal Volume

Conventionally a tidal volume of 10 to 15 cc/kg is recommended for the patient supported by mechanical ventilation. Mechanical ventilator tidal volumes are larger than spontaneous tidal volumes (5 to 8 cc/kg) to prevent progressive alveolar collapse. It is known that atelectasis will develop in patients who breathe at a constant, normal tidal volume without intermittent deep sighs. This problem can be reversed through the intermittent application of sighs (volumes one and one-half times the tidal volume), formerly a common practice. The application of constantly larger-than-normal tidal volumes achieves the same goal and is the more common mechanism used today to prevent progressive alveolar collapse.

Smaller tidal volumes may be used when the lung is already hyperinflated, as in severe bronchospasm or in disease processes associated with a decrease in compliance. In the latter circumstance, large tidal volumes may result in an increase in PIP, predisposing the patient to barotrauma. In diffuse disease processes, such as adult respiratory distress syndrome, large tidal volumes are maldistributed to the areas of best compliance. The result is overdistention of the more healthy alveoli, which leads to an increase in physiologic dead space and a greater potential for barotrauma. It is advisable under these conditions to use tidal volumes <12 cc/kg and higher respiratory rates.

EXHALED TIDAL VOLUME

Regardless of mode of ventilation, the most accurate measure of the volume received by the patient is the exhaled tidal volume (EVT). For example, when pressure- or flow-cycled modes of ventilation are used, the generated pressure is set to determine the patient's tidal volume; however, as previously explained, the actual tidal volume may vary from breath to breath because of the patient's lung characteristics. Furthermore, when a volume-cycled mode of ventilation is used, the desired tidal volume is set on the ventilator, but it is misleading to believe that the patient's lungs will always receive this set tidal volume. Though the desired tidal volume is predetermined and set on the ventilator control panel, it is not guaranteed to be delivered to the patient. Some volume may be lost because of leaks in the ventilator circuitry, leaks around the airway, or a pleural air leak, or it may be lost as compressible volume in the ventilator circuitry. The volume actually received by the patient, in any mode of ventilation, must be confirmed by monitoring the EVT on the display panel of the ventilator. When the EVT deviates from the set tidal volume by 100 cc or more in an adult, then the practitioner must troubleshoot the system (see Chapter 8). The EVT data are displayed at different places on different ventilators. The bedside practitioner must become familiar with the location of this information so that trend monitoring can be carried out properly.

Tubing Compression and Compliance Volume

Gas flows not only into the patient when inspiration is initiated but also into the ventilator circuitry. Of course, the gas in the ventilator circuitry, the compressible volume, does not participate in gas exchange. The amount of compressible volume in the circuitry is a function of the space available, the compliance of the ventilator tubing, and the opposing pressure from the patient's lungs. Gases compress when they are under pressure, and flexible ventilator tubing expands. As the patient's pulmonary compliance decreases, a larger percentage of the desired tidal volume becomes compressible volume because the tubing expands under the greater opposing pressure. More gas is also compressed within the humidifier, connectors, water traps, and internal circuitry of the ventilator. It is important to note that at the end of inspiration this compressible volume flows out of the expiratory limb, along with the gases from the patient's lungs, and is interpreted by the ventilator as part of the exhaled tidal volume.

It is possible to calculate the compressed volume by using the ventilator tubing compliance, or compressibility, factor supplied by the manufacturer. Ventilator tubing compliance is variable, but most tubings have a compliance factor of 2 to 4 ml/cm H_2O. This means that for each centimeter H_2O of airway pressure, 2 to 4 cc of gas are compressed in the circuitry. It becomes clear that when the lungs are noncompliant and airway pressures rise, more volume is compressed in the circuit.

The compressible volume in any given patient should remain relatively constant from one breath to the next. Therefore, if the exhaled tidal volume and minute ventilation that the patient is receiving are sufficient to maintain an appropriate $PaCO_2$ and acid-base status, then the volume of gas compressed in the ventilator circuitry has little significance. Compressible volume may be reduced by ensuring that the humidifier's water level is kept high and the length of the circuitry is minimal.

Respiratory Rate

The respiratory rate (RR) set on the ventilator should generally be as near physiologic RRs as possible: 10 to 20 breaths/min. Frequent changes in the RR are often required and are based on observation of the patient's work of breathing and comfort and on assessment of the $PaCO_2$ and pH. Most patients, during initial use of a ventilator, require full ventilatory support. The RR at this time is selected on the basis of the tidal volume, so that the minute ventilation (RR × V_T = Minute ventilation) is sufficient to maintain a normal acid-base status. As the patient begins to participate in the ventilatory work, the ventilator RR may be decreased.

Slow rates may be useful in patients with obstructive pulmonary disease because, as the rate is decreased, more time is available for exhalation and less air trapping will occur. Fast rates may be useful in patients with noncompliant lungs who require ventilation with smaller tidal volumes to prevent barotrauma from increased airway pressures.

A common problem in the patient supported by mechanical ventilation is that they are overventilated, which leads to alkalosis. It is therefore desirable for patients to set their own RR by using a mode of ventilation that allows patient-initiated breaths. Depending on the patient's ability to partially support ventilation, a guaranteed number of breaths may be supplied while the patient is allowed to breathe over this rate. The patient then adjusts the RR and $PaCO_2$ levels and thus maintains a more normal acid-base status (eucapnia). In some modes of ventilation (pressure support and continuous positive airway pressure), when both the patient's respiratory drive and the ability to work are sufficient, no RR is set on the ventilator.

Sensitivity

The sensitivity setting on the ventilator has to do with the trigger variable. The trigger variable is the variable manipulated to begin the delivery of inspiratory flow. Inspiratory flow may be pressure-triggered in a demand flow system or flow-triggered in the flow-by system. Flow-triggered systems are relatively new and are not available on all ventilators, though this type of system shows great promise for increased future use. Pressure-triggering is widely employed and is the mechanism used for initiating inspiratory flow on most commonly used ventilators.

PRESSURE-TRIGGERING

In a demand flow, pressure-triggered system, the flow of gas begins when the demand for flow is indicated. On mandatory breaths the demand for flow is indicated when a set time interval is reached. However, for patient-initiated breaths the demand for flow is indicated when a pressure drop in the ventilator circuit is sensed. Therefore the *sensitivity setting* reflects the amount of pressure drop below baseline pressure that the patient must develop in the ventilator circuit, on inspiration, in order to initiate the flow of gas. Sensitivity is also known as "triggering effort." The sensitivity setting is generally 2 cm H_2O less than end-expiratory pressure, or -2 cm H_2O. Therefore, if PEEP is at 5 cm H_2O, then inspiratory flow begins when pressure in the circuit drops to 3 cm H_2O. If PEEP is not being used, inspiratory flow begins when the patient decreases circuit pressure to -2 cm H_2O. Sensitivity should be set to allow the patient to trigger the ventilator easily. If the patient must use great effort to initiate the flow of gases, or if there is a delay from the time of patient effort to the start of the flow of gases, then the inspiratory muscle work is increased.

A high sensitivity setting will decrease the amount of patient effort required to trigger the ventilator; that is, the ventilator will be more sensitive to negative inspiratory efforts. If sensitivity is set too high, ventilator self-cycling, or auto-cycling, will occur. In auto-cycling, the machine triggers one breath immediately after another, without regard to where the patient is in the respiratory cycle. If the sensitivity setting is too low, so that the ventilator is not sensitive enough to the patient, the patient must generate significant inspiratory effort to initiate the flow of gases; thus the patient's work of breathing must increase. The patient may demonstrate use of the accessory inspiratory muscles and complain of dyspnea and of being unable to "get enough air." The setting may be so inappropriately low that the patient is effectively "locked out" from initiating inspiratory flow. More-negative sensitivity settings are appropriate to prevent auto-cycling. Auto-cycling will occur when there is an air leak resulting in an inability to maintain the set baseline pressure (PEEP) (see Box 6–1).

Box 6–1   Sensitivity Setting

- Also known as "triggering effort"
- Normal setting: -2 cm H_2O (2 cm H_2O below baseline pressure)

Setting too low	Patient must generate more work to trigger the flow of gas.
	Patient may effectively become "locked out" from initiating gas flow.
Setting too high	Auto-cycling of the ventilator will occur.
	Patient/ventilator dyssynchrony will occur.

FLOW-TRIGGERING

Flow-triggering is an assist mechanism used to eliminate the imposed work of pressure-triggering a breath. Pressure-triggering the ventilator requires work to be performed by the patient. The patient works to create the negative pressure in the ventilator circuit and continues this work for a period (measured in milliseconds) known as the lag time. The lag time extends from the instant when the patient performs the triggering effort, through the time when the ventilator assist mechanism senses this effort and signals the demand valve to open, until finally the gases travel in the opposite direction to the patient's airway. The patient performs metabolic work during the lag time. With flow-triggering, the work associated with patient triggering and lag time is eliminated.

Flow-triggering, known as flow-by (FB), is not a mode of ventilation but a means of triggering a breath on the ventilator. The FB system may be used in conjunction with synchronized intermittent mandatory ventilation or continuous positive airway pressure and, in its upgraded version, with assist/control. With the FB system there is virtually no lag time between the instigation of inspiratory effort and the start of gas flow. Inspiratory flow is instantly available and is sufficient to meet the patient's needs; therefore the inspiratory work of breathing is decreased.

With FB a predetermined flow of gas, known as the *base flow*, travels through the inspiratory circuit and is continuously and immediately available to the patient, eliminating lag time. The base flow is set in liters per minute and is steadily maintained as the microprocessor control in the ventilator constantly monitors flow in both the inspiratory and expiratory limbs.

Flow sensitivity is an operator-chosen setting that represents how much the expiratory flow has to be decreased by the patient to trigger the ventilator to deliver fresh gas. As stated previously, in the flow-by system the base expiratory flow is constantly monitored. As the patient inspires, base expiratory flow decreases, signifying flow diversion from the exhalation circuit to the patient's lungs. This change in base flow is sensed by the ventilator and results in an increase in fresh gas flow before base flow is exhausted. Sufficient flow is maintained to meet the patient's immediate demand until the ventilator delivers the type of breath prescribed.

Flow sensitivity settings vary by ventilator manufacturer. In the Servo 300 (Siemens Elema Corp., Solna, Sweden) flow sensitivity can be set from 0.7 to

2.0 L/min. In the Puritan-Bennett 7200a (Puritan Bennett Corp., Carlsbad, Calif.) flow sensitivity can be set between a minimum of 1 L/min and a maximum of one-half the base flow.

Base flow settings may range from 5 to 20 L/min in the Puritan-Bennett 7200a, while in the Servo 300 the base flow is fixed at 2 L/min. In setting up the base flow, it is important to know that the patient's work of breathing is not decreased by the use of higher flows. A lower base flow is associated with less water rain-out and gas conservation. The flow sensitivity setting should be as low as possible to maximize ventilator responsiveness to the patient's inspiratory flow demands. High flow sensitivity settings reduce the ventilator's capacity to sense the patient's inspiratory demands. If the setting is too low, auto-cycling may result. Auto-cycling at very low flow sensitivity settings may even result from the beating of the heart as it squeezes the lungs and creates flow (cardiac oscillations). The sensing of cardiac oscillations may be noted by the ventilator RR being the same as the electrocardiogram rate. In FB, auto-cycling may be detected in two ways: (1) by observing "assist" or "spontaneous" lights flashing signifying an inspiratory effort, when they are not synchronous with any patient respiratory muscle activity, or (2) by observing a RR reading on the vent that is much higher than the patient's actual rate.

An example of settings that may be used in the FB system are a base flow setting of 5 L/min with a flow sensitivity of 3 L/min. This means that a volume of 5 L/min of fresh gas is continuously traveling in the ventilator circuit, and when the *net* flow reaches negative 3 L/min, the vent is triggered to increase the flow rate until it again achieves the base flow setting.

Higher base flow and sensitivity settings are needed when PEEP is being used and the patient has an air leak that is causing loss of PEEP. (Loss of PEEP is detected by observing the pressure manometer and seeing pressure fall below the set-PEEP with no inspiratory effort.) The ventilator cannot recognize the difference in base flow changes caused by patient inspiration versus changes caused by a leak. As a result, the flow sensitivity level may be reached and the ventilator auto-cycles. The problem is corrected by increasing base flow to maximum and then slowly increasing flow sensitivity until auto-cycling is eliminated. Therefore, higher base flow and flow sensitivity settings are used to compensate for leaks, maintain PEEP, and eliminate auto-cycle while still maintaining exquisite sensitivity to patient demands.

Flow Rate

Flow rate is the speed with which the tidal volume is delivered; it is measured in liters per minute. Generally an initial flow rate of 40 to 60 L/min satisfies the patient's inspiratory demands and achieves a desirable inspiratory-to-expiratory (I:E) ratio. The inspiratory flow rate is the chief determinant of inspiratory time and thus of the I:E ratio. Therefore the flow rate must be adjusted for each patient on the basis of the desired I:E ratio, the tidal volume, and the RR (see Relationships Among VT, Flow Rate, RR, and I:E Ratio, below). The tidal volume (VT) must be delivered within an appropriate, comfortable time, and flow must meet or exceed the patient's inspiratory flow demand; if not, the patient will experience "air hunger," the work of breathing will be increased, and patient-ventilator dyssynchrony will result.

Higher flow rates (>60 L/min) shorten inspiratory time, thereby lengthening expiratory time (decreased I:E ratio), which may be desirable in patients with chronic obstructive pulmonary disease (COPD) and air trapping. Increasing the flow rate may have the negative consequences of increasing the peak inspiratory pressure (PIP) and adversely affecting the distribution of gases because flow becomes more turbulent. Slower inspiratory flow rates (20 to 50 L/min) will prolong inspiratory time, improve the distribution of gases, and reduce PIP as a result of a more laminar flow. Most ventilators are capable of delivering flow rates up to a range of 120 to 180 L/min, which should meet the needs of any condition in which the minute ventilatory demands are high or when the lungs are noncompliant and high RR/small VT ventilation is needed (see Box 6–2).

FLOW WAVE PATTERNS

Modern ventilators are capable of delivering the flow of gases in variable configurations known as flow wave patterns. There are four categories of waveforms: square, sinusoidal, accelerating, and decelerating (Table 6–3). Some microprocessor-controlled ventilators can generate more flow patterns, which are basically modifications of the standard four. A flow pattern is chosen on the basis of the patient's disease process and the pattern's ability to promote optimal gas distribution and affect inspiratory pressures. In some modes of ventilation, the ventilator is committed to the delivery of gases in a specific flow pattern.

Little research has validated the advantages of one waveform over another. Some evidence shows that the use of the decelerating waveform improves the distribution of gas in patients who have a diffuse, nonhomogeneous disease process in which adjacent alveoli require differing inspiratory times for adequate filling. (These are known as alveoli with varying time constants; see Chapter 2.) When necessary higher inspiratory flows lead to an increase in the PIP, adjusting the flow wave pattern (i.e., switching from the square to the sinusoidal pattern) may reduce the PIP. Modification of the flow wave pattern in an effort to reduce PIP should be done while the caregiver remains at the bedside to evaluate the effect of any change in patient comfort and the desired parameters (i.e., PIP).

Inspiratory-to-Expiratory Ratio

The inspiratory-to-expiratory (I:E) ratio is the duration of inspiration in comparison with expiration. Generally the I:E ratio is set at 1:2; that is, 33% of the

---

Box 6–2   Flow Rate

Definition	Speed with which the tidal volume is delivered.
Average setting	40–60 L/min.
High flow rates	Decrease inspiratory time.
	Increase PIP (more turbulent flow).
	May lead to maldistribution of gas.
	Required for high minute ventilation demands.
Low flow rates	Increase inspiratory time.
	Decrease PIP (more laminar flow).
	May improve distribution of gases.

TABLE 6–3 Standard Mechanical Ventilator Flow Wave Patterns

Label	Flow Wave Pattern	Description
Square		Peak flow rate is delivered immediately at the onset of inspiration, maintained throughout the inspiratory phase, and abruptly terminated at the onset of expiration. Most commonly used flow wave pattern.
Sinusoidal		Inspiratory flow rate gradually accelerates to peak flow and then tapers off. Believed to mimic spontaneous inspiratory patterns. May increase PIP.
Accelerating (ascending ramp)		Flow gradually accelerates in a linear fashion to the set peak flow rate.
Decelerating (descending ramp)		Flow is at peak at onset of inspiration and gradually decelerates throughout inspiratory phase. Flow ceases and ventilator cycles to expiratory phase when flow decays to a percentage of peak flow, usually 25%. May improve the distribution of gases when there is inhomogeneity of alveolar ventilation. Decreases dead space, increases arterial oxygen tension, and reduces PIP.

PIP = Peak inspiratory pressure.

respiratory cycle is spent in inspiration and 66% in the expiratory phase. This setting is believed to mimic spontaneous respiration when lung function is normal. It is also generally used because (1) shorter inspiratory times contribute to dead-space ventilation by overexpanding the most compliant alveoli and (2) longer inspiratory times increase the mean airway pressure, which may lead to hemodynamic instability. An I:E ratio of 1:3 or 1:4 may be used to ventilate the lungs of an individual with COPD and air trapping because the longer expiratory time promotes more complete exhalation and air trapping is reduced.

When a ventilator is time cycled, the I:E ratio is manipulated directly, usually by adjusting the inspiratory time. For example, if the patient's RR is 12 breaths per minute, 60 is divided by 12 to ascertain that a period of 5 seconds is devoted to each respiratory cycle. If the desired I:E ratio is 1:2, then multiplying 5 by 0.33 (the percentage of time allowed for inspiration) will determine the inspiratory time of 1.7 seconds. In volume-cycled ventilators the I:E ratio is set by adjusting the peak inspiratory flow rate while taking into consideration the patient's RR and the need to deliver the VT in a comfortable time. A higher inspiratory flow rate shortens inspiratory time and allows more time for exhalation.

To lengthen the inspiratory time, decrease the flow rate. For example, if the patient's I:E ratio is 1:3 and the desired I:E ratio is 1:2, then the flow rate is decreased.

Consideration of the I:E ratio is important because the longer the inspiratory phase, the higher is the mean airway pressure (MAP) (Fig. 6–6). As the MAP increases, so does the potential for hemodynamic compromise. Positive-pressure ventilation may reduce cardiac output by three mechanisms: decreasing venous return, increasing right ventricular (RV) afterload, and reducing, as a result, RV systolic emptying and left ventricular compliance (because the interventricular septum is displaced by the increased RV end-systolic volume).

INVERSE I:E RATIOS

I:E ratios of 1:1, 2:1, 3:1, and 4:1 are called inverse I:E ratios. The use of an inverse I:E ratio is restricted to specific noncompliant lung conditions in which the disease process exhibits a nonhomogeneous distribution. An inverse I:E ratio is used to improve oxygenation. In noncompliant lungs, the short inspiratory time of a normal I:E ratio allows unstable alveoli to collapse during the relatively longer expiratory phase. The inspiratory effect of an inverse I:E ratio is to allow unstable lung units more time to fill and an equilibration of volume between the alveoli as a result of collateral ventilation. Dead space ventilation and the percentage of shunt both decrease because gas is more evenly distributed in the lung. The relatively compliant alveoli are not overdistended by gases that preferentially flow to them, as may occur during an inflation period of standard duration. The simultaneous shortening of the expiratory phase prevents unstable alveoli from collapsing, because the next inspiration begins before they reach closing volume (Fig. 6–7).

Inverse I:E ratio ventilation increases mean airway pressure (MAP) because of the prolonged inspiratory time, as shown previously in Figure 6–6. MAP is the average airway pressure over the entire respiratory cycle and is a key determinant of oxygenation. An increase in MAP results in an increase in alveolar stability and recruitment, an increase in the functional residual capacity ensues, and thus oxygenation improves. A higher MAP has the negative effect of creating more

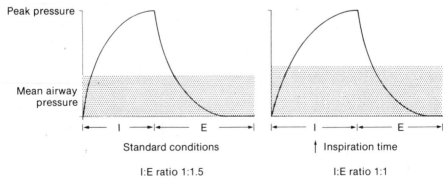

Figure 6–6 The effect of altering the I:E ratio on mean airway pressure (*shaded area*). As inspiratory time is lengthened, so is the amount of time that positive pressure is applied to the thorax; therefore the mean airway pressure rises. (Modified from Dupuis, YG: *Ventilators: Theory and Clinical Application*. St. Louis: CV Mosby, 1986.)

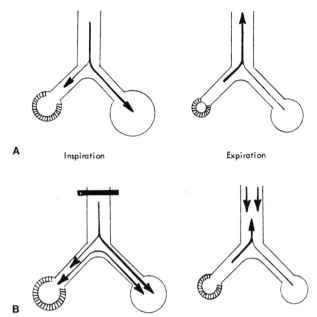

FIGURE 6-7 *Inspiratory* and *expiratory* effects of standard ventilation *(A)* and inverse-ratio ventilation *(B)* on the distribution of gases in lung units with varying time constants. *Shaded area* represents alveolus with decreased compliance (i.e., a longer time constant). *(A)* With a short inspiratory and longer expiratory time, noncompliant alveoli do not have time to fill during inspiration (shunt), whereas adjacent, compliant alveoli may become overdistended (dead space). On expiration, unstable alveoli collapse as they reach closing volume before the end of the expiratory phase. *(B)* Prolonging the inspiratory time allows noncompliant alveoli more time to fill and equilibration of gases between lung units of varying time constants. Reinflation after a shortened expiration causes gases to be trapped in the lung, which creates a PEEP-like effect promoting alveolar recruitment and stability. (From Gurevitch, MJ: Selection of the inspiratory:expiratory ratio. In RM Kacmarek and JK Stoller [Eds.]: *Current Respiratory Care.* Toronto: BC Decker, 1988.)

positive pressure in the thorax, which may lead to hemodynamic compromise by the mechanisms described above (see the Inspiratory-to-Expiratory Ratio section). Little overall improvement in the patient will be appreciated if arterial oxygenation improves but tissue oxygen delivery falls. Therefore the clinician must monitor tissue oxygen delivery (DO_2) closely, optimize all aspects of DO_2, and find the "ideal" I:E ratio for any given patient that improves *overall* oxygenation.

A phenomenon known as intrinsic PEEP, or auto-PEEP, occurs when the I:E ratio becomes an inverse ratio. Because the expiratory phase is shortened, the alveoli are not allowed to empty completely on expiration and gas is trapped in the lung. This trapped gas creates pressure in the alveoli that is known as auto-PEEP (Fig. 6–8). Auto-PEEP prevents end-expiratory alveolar collapse and adds a cumulative PEEP effect to the operator-chosen, or set-PEEP. The auto-PEEP plus the set-PEEP equals the total PEEP. Measurement of auto-PEEP requires the implementation of an end-expiratory pause (see Intrinsic PEEP section, below).

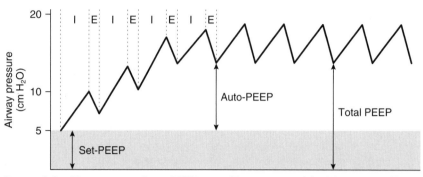

Figure 6-8 Phenomenon of auto-PEEP, caused by inversion of the I:E ratio. Insufficient expiratory time permits the trapping of gases in the lung. This trapped gas creates pressure, which is known as auto-PEEP.

Inverse I:E ratios are generally used with the pressure control mode of ventilation, but they may also be applied in the volume control mode by using an end-inspiratory pause or a slow inspiratory flow rate (Marcy and Marini, 1991).

Relationships Among V_T, Flow Rate, RR, and I:E Ratio

After an appreciation of the variables of V_T, flow rate, RR, and the I:E ratio is gained, it becomes evident that they are interrelated. For example, increasing the RR will affect the I:E ratio if the flow rate is not appropriately adjusted. To enhance understanding further, Figure 6–9 graphically depicts the relationships among these variables.

End-Inspiratory Pause

An end-inspiratory pause takes place when the lungs are held in an inflated state at a set pressure or volume, for a specified period (usually <2 seconds) at

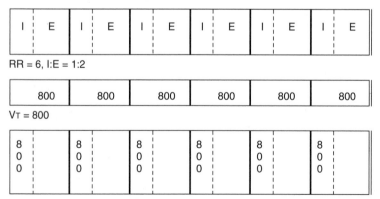

Figure 6-9 Relationships among tidal volume (V_T), flow rate, respiratory rate (RR), and the inspiratory-to-expiratory (I:E) ratio.

TABLE 6-4   Initial Ventilator Settings: Guidelines

Parameter	Initial Setting
Fraction of inspired O_2 (FIO_2)	0.7–1.0 (Err on side of caution; wean to 0.5 or less to prevent O_2 toxicity.)
Tidal volume (VT)	10–15 cc/kg
Respiratory rate (RR)	10–20 breaths per minute
Sensitivity	2 cm H_2O below baseline pressure
Flow rate	40–60 L/min (Adjust to deliver tidal volume in desired inspiratory time.)
Inspiratory-to-expiratory (I:E) ratio	1:2–1:3
Positive end-expiratory pressure (PEEP)	5 cm H_2O

the end of inspiration. This maneuver is called an inflation hold, inspiratory plateau, or end-inspiratory pause. The purpose is to increase the amount of time allowed for distribution of inhaled gases. As the volume of gas is momentarily held in the lungs, areas of dead-space ventilation and shunt may decrease as volume is redistributed to relatively less ventilated alveoli. In addition, the longer the lungs are held in an inflated state, the longer the end-inspiratory pause continues to increase the MAP. Increasing the MAP improves oxygenation but may also lead to reduction in venous return and in cardiac output.

A second purpose of an end-inspiratory pause is to allow for the monitoring of compliance and resistance. The pause is instituted at the peak of inspiration. The airway pressure dial will then drop to the plateau pressure. The difference between peak and plateau pressures is due to resistance to gas flow in the airways. The plateau pressure reflects pressure within the alveoli. It is also used to calculate static pulmonary compliance (see Chapter 2).

Sigh

All human beings sigh about 10 times per hour. The purpose of the sigh is to counteract small airway closure, which can occur when tidal volumes are monotonous. Sigh breaths delivered by the ventilator are usually set at 1.5 times the tidal volume of machine-cycled breaths and are given an average of 10 times per hour. A single sigh may be delivered, or sigh breaths may be given in multiples. Sighs should not be used when supraphysiologic tidal volumes (10 to 15 cc/kg) or PEEP are being used. Under either of these conditions the addition of a sigh may cause excessive peak airway pressures and possible barotrauma to the lungs. Guidelines for initial ventilator settings are given in Table 6–4.

POSITIVE END-EXPIRATORY PRESSURE

Positive end-expiratory pressure (PEEP) is the application of a constant, positive pressure in the airways so that, at end-expiration, the pressure is never allowed to return to atmospheric pressure. PEEP is measured in centimeters of H_2O. Typical settings for PEEP range from 5 to 20 cm H_2O. The positive pressure is actually applied throughout the ventilatory cycle, but it is used for its physiologic effects at end-expiration. By exerting positive pressure at end-expiration, PEEP recruits atelectatic alveoli, internally splints and distends already patent alveoli, counteracts alveolar and small-airway closure during expiration, and redistributes lung water. PEEP redistributes extravascular lung water from alveoli to the perivascular space, where the impact of excess lung water on gas exchange is decreased. Through these mechanisms, PEEP decreases intrapulmonary shunting, increases the functional residual capacity (FRC), improves compliance, decreases the diffusion distance for oxygen, and *improves oxygenation*.

Indications and Relative Contraindications for Use of PEEP

The primary clinical applications of PEEP are to prevent atelectasis both postoperatively and in the bedridden patient and to reverse established atelectasis. In patients whose PaO$_2$ is 60 mm Hg or less (O$_2$ saturation ≤90%) on an FiO$_2$ of 0.5 or greater, PEEP is therapeutically indicated to improve oxygenation. With the addition of PEEP, it is usually possible to provide oxygenation with a lower FiO$_2$, thus reducing the chance of pulmonary oxygen toxicity. Before or simultaneous to the addition of PEEP, therapies designed to treat the underlying condition and improve oxygenation (e.g., diuresis, postural drainage, chest physiotherapy, antibiotics, and body positioning) should be applied. PEEP will not correct underlying disorders such as congestive heart failure, fluid overload, and pneumonia. It only supports oxygenation until the underlying condition is corrected. PEEP may also be used to provide internal stabilization of the chest wall and minimize paradoxical chest wall movement in flail chest. Some caregivers consider a small amount of PEEP, 3 to 5 cm H$_2$O, "physiologic" when it is applied to patients with artificial airways, purporting that it mimics the amount of PEEP usually created by the glottic apparatus, which is interrupted by the artificial airway. This latter point is a controversial one. However, 5 cm H$_2$O PEEP may be applied to preserve a more normal FRC, which is decreased in the supine position, a position that is assumed the majority of the time by the critically ill patient supported by mechanical ventilation.

Relative contraindications to the use of PEEP include unilateral lung disease, because the application of PEEP may result in alveolar overdistention in the healthy lung, which both increases dead space and redistributes perfusion to the bad lung. This redistribution of perfusion to the relatively less ventilated lung results in an increase in intrapulmonary shunt. Under these conditions, independent lung ventilation may be indicated (see Chapter 11). In obstructive lung disease, patients already have an increased FRC because of air trapping. PEEP may not improve oxygenation in these patients while subjecting them to the possibilities of pulmonary barotrauma and decreased cardiac output. Other conditions are relative contraindications because the positive intrathoracic pressure created by PEEP may exacerbate these conditions, which include pneumothorax, bronchopleural fistula, hypovolemia, intracardiac shunt, and increased intracranial pressure. The clinical significance of these relative contraindications is that one needs to be aware of the effect of PEEP on these conditions so that the risk/benefit ratio can be weighed properly and preventive measures, such as volume loading and use of a chest tube, can be readied.

PEEP Versus Continuous Positive Airway Pressure

PEEP and continuous positive airway pressure (CPAP) are identical in their mechanism, but the terms are not interchangeable. The use of one term rather than the other provides a description of the amount of ventilatory support the patient is receiving. Positive pressure applied at the end of expiration may be administered to patients who are either spontaneously breathing or undergoing mechanical ventilation. PEEP is the correct term when patients are receiving positive end-expiratory pressure along with any other mechanical ventilatory assistance, such as pressure support or assist/control ventilation (Fig. 6–10). CPAP is the correct term when positive pressure is being used with the spontaneously breathing patient who is receiving no other ventilatory assistance. CPAP is measured in centimeters of H_2O pressure and may be administered through a ventilator or with a CPAP mask. See Chapter 7 for further information about indications for CPAP use and patient monitoring.

Adverse Effects

It is important to be aware of the adverse effects of PEEP and how they are prevented or managed. Problems related to the use of PEEP lie in the possibly precipitous reduction in cardiac output (CO), and thus in tissue oxygen delivery, that can occur as a result of the increase in intrathoracic pressure. Three primary factors result in a decrease in CO. First, much of the reduction in CO is attributable to a decrease in venous return, which occurs because of an increase in

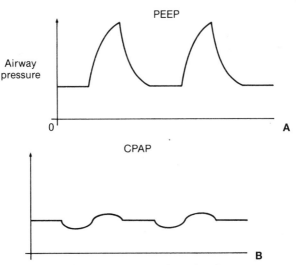

FIGURE 6–10   (A) *Positive end-expiratory pressure* (PEEP) is the correct term when positive end-expiratory pressure is applied with any other form of ventilatory support. (B) CPAP is positive pressure applied to the spontaneously breathing patient (with or without use of the ventilator) who is receiving no other ventilatory assistance. (Modified from Dupuis, YG: *Ventilators: Theory and Clinical Application.* 2nd ed. St. Louis: Mosby–Year Book, 1992.)

right atrial transmural pressure. Second, pulmonary vascular resistance is increased because of referred positive pressure from the alveoli. This increases RV afterload, impairing RV emptying. Third, as RV end-systolic volume increases, the interventricular septum shifts, impairing diastolic filling of the left ventricle and further depressing CO.

Management of the adverse hemodynamic effects of PEEP begin by ensuring that the patient has adequate intravascular volume. After optimal preload has been achieved, inotropic and afterloading agents are added in the appropriate setting. These agents may be necessary to maintain adequate tissue oxygen delivery, the ultimate goal. Use of a pulmonary artery catheter for monitoring CO and calculation of tissue oxygenation should be considered when 10 cm H_2O or more PEEP is applied.

Institution and Withdrawal of PEEP

When PEEP is indicated, the initial setting is generally 5 cm H_2O. PEEP may then be increased in increments of 3 to 5 cm H_2O until satisfactory oxygenation is obtained. The response to each change should be evaluated, either with the use of pulse oximetry or with assessment of arterial blood gas values and the patient's condition. As a general guideline, arterial blood gas values should be obtained 20 minutes after the change in PEEP, but the time frame varies by institution. The goal is to find the "best" PEEP, which is the least amount of PEEP required to obtain an O_2 saturation $\geq 92\%$, PaO_2 ≥ 60 mm Hg, on an FIO_2 ideally <0.6, which does not impair delivery of oxygen to the tissues. If PEEP decreases CO in an uncorrectable fashion, then the preservation of tissue oxygenation will require the PEEP to be lowered and the FIO_2 increased—if necessary, to toxic levels. Excess PEEP will overdistend the alveoli, causing compression of the adjacent pulmonary capillaries and thus creating dead space and its attendant hypercapnia (Fig. 6–11).

Once the FIO_2 is reduced to 0.6 or less, the patient is hemodynamically stable, and active sepsis is controlled, then withdrawal of PEEP may begin. PEEP should be decreased in increments of 5 cm H_2O, with the adequacy of oxygenation evaluated after each change. The patient's condition should be allowed to stabilize

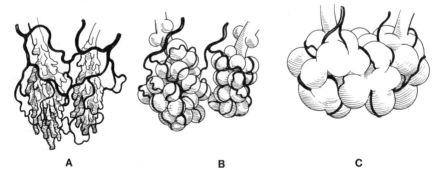

| A | B | C |

Figure 6–11 Effect of the application of PEEP on the alveoli. (A) Atelectatic alveoli before PEEP application. (B) Optimal PEEP application has reinflated alveoli to normal volume. (C) Excessive PEEP application overdistends the alveoli and compresses adjacent pulmonary capillaries, creating dead space with its attendant hypercapnia.

for 6 hours after each 5 cm H_2O decrease in PEEP, or for 6 to 12 hours if the underlying disease process affecting oxygenation has been prolonged. Abrupt withdrawal of PEEP may rapidly result in hypoxemia because of airway closure and the need to reinstate PEEP at possibly higher levels than were previously required. For this reason an in-line suction catheter should be used for patients receiving high levels of PEEP. Furthermore, if the ventilator circuit is disrupted, manual ventilation with a bag-valve-mask device, with an appropriately set PEEP valve, should be instituted.

Interpretation of Vascular Pressures During PEEP

Positive pressure applied to the lungs is referred throughout the thoracic cavity and therefore to the vascular structures. Formulas have been developed to determine the effect of positive pressure applied to the lungs on the vascular pressure readings, specifically the pulmonary capillary wedge pressure (PCWP). These formulas provide the "corrected PCWP" by subtracting a percentage of the PEEP from the PCWP. The use of these calculations is misleading, however, because the compliance of the lungs (which is not a variable in the equation) affects the amount of pressure referred beyond the lungs into the thoracic cavity and vascular structures. Another method used in some clinical settings is to subtract the amount of PEEP being used from the PCWP to obtain a corrected PCWP. This method has no scientific basis, either. Saying that 5 cm H_2O PEEP adds 5 mm Hg pressure to the PCWP is incorrect simply because the units of measure are not equal. Finally, removing the patient from the ventilator to eliminate the effect of PEEP on the vascular pressure is fraught with potential hazards because of the wide fluctuations in oxygenation that could occur. For consistency, vascular pressures should be measured while the patient-ventilator system remains intact.

There is no magic formula for determining the effect of PEEP on the vascular pressures; however, the amount of PEEP (set and auto) must be documented and taken into consideration as the vascular pressures are interpreted. For example, if the patient's vascular pressure readings rise concurrently with an increase in PEEP, then making this connection will assist in ruling out new-onset heart failure or hypervolemia as a cause of the elevation.

Intrinsic PEEP

Intrinsic PEEP (auto-PEEP), by definition, is the spontaneous development of PEEP as a result of insufficient expiratory time. Causes of auto-PEEP formation include rapid respiratory rate, high minute ventilatory demand, airflow obstruction, and inverse I:E ratio ventilation. Expiratory time is inadequate when the lung has not reached its resting expiratory volume before the next inspiration begins. Inadequate expiratory time causes gases to become trapped in the lung. These trapped gases create positive pressure in the thorax. Auto-PEEP will continue to develop until the elastic recoil forces in the lung overcome the tendency to trap further gases, as previously shown in Figure 6–8. Auto-PEEP is also known as pulmonary gas trapping, endogenous PEEP, occult PEEP, intrinsic PEEP, or inadvertent PEEP when it has occurred unwittingly.

Extrinsic PEEP is the amount of PEEP that the clinician sets on the ventilator. It is the PEEP that you know about and can readily read on the pressure manometer on the ventilator display panel at end-expiration. Auto-PEEP (intrinsic PEEP) is the PEEP that you may not know about and cannot readily detect by reading the pressure manometer on the ventilator without performing a special maneuver. When auto-PEEP forms, the end-expiratory pressure is above the ambient level but is not read by the ventilator pressure manometer because the manometer is open to the atmosphere during exhalation and reads only the set PEEP. For measurement of auto-PEEP, the exhalation valve must be occluded just before the next breath would begin (similarly to performing the end-inspiratory hold maneuver when static compliance is being measured). An end-expiratory hold should be performed as quickly as possible to prevent discomfort from interrupting the respiratory cycle and pattern. Occluding the exhalation port for several seconds allows the ventilator pressure manometer to read both the circuit pressure (set-PEEP) and the airway pressure (auto-PEEP) (Fig. 6–12). The airway-pressure manometer reading therefore reflects *total* PEEP. For determination of the auto-PEEP value, the following calculation is then performed:

$$\text{Auto-PEEP} = \text{Total PEEP} - \text{Set-PEEP}$$

The effective PEEP is the total PEEP—that is, both set-PEEP and auto-PEEP function physiologically in the same manner.

The detection and monitoring of auto-PEEP are important because of its physiologic effects. If auto-PEEP is being used therapeutically, then it should be monitored and adjusted like all other ventilator settings. If it is unintentional, then the clinician who is unaware of its presence is unable to manage its poten-

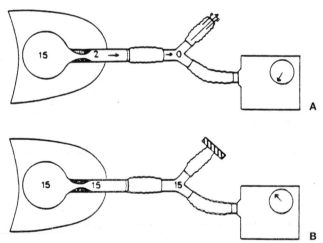

FIGURE 6–12 Measurement of auto-PEEP. *(A)* Auto-PEEP is not constantly read by the ventilator pressure manometer because the manometer is open to atmosphere during exhalation and reads only the set-PEEP. *(B)* For determination of auto-PEEP, the exhalation port is occluded just before the beginning of the subsequent breath. Circuit and airway pressure equilibrate, allowing for the measurement of total PEEP. The following calculation is used to determine auto-PEEP: Auto-PEEP = Total PEEP − Set-PEEP. *Shaded area* represents an area of airway obstruction. For additional causes of formation of auto-PEEP, see the text. (From O'Quin, R, and Marini, JJ: Pulmonary artery occlusion pressure: Clinical physiology, measurement and interpretation. *Am Rev Respir Dis* 1983;128: 319–326.)

tially adverse effects on the patient. Just as with set-PEEP, auto-PEEP places the patient at risk of having barotrauma and hemodynamic compromise. Not being aware of the presence of auto-PEEP may also lead to the misinterpretation of vascular pressures. Auto-PEEP may subject the patient to an increased work of breathing in modes that require the patient to draw back a preset amount of pressure to trigger the inspiratory flow of gases. When auto-PEEP is present, the patient must draw back through both the auto-PEEP and the set sensitivity level (usually -2 cm H_2O) to initiate inspiratory flow. A final problem that may occur when the presence of auto-PEEP is unknown is the miscalculation of compliance. In measurements of both static and dynamic compliance, the total PEEP value must be used or errors will result (see Chapter 2).

Correction of unwanted auto-PEEP requires making ventilator adjustments that provide for a longer expiratory time to allow the lungs to return to their resting volume before the next breath. Such ventilator adjustments include decreasing the RR or VT or increasing the peak inspiratory flow rate so that the desired volume is given in a shorter inspiratory time. Another mechanism is removal of any set-PEEP so that the total PEEP is reduced. Bronchodilators may also be used as a method of reducing obstruction to expiratory flow.

Clues to the presence of auto-PEEP are excessive negative inspiratory effort by the patient to trigger the ventilator, rapid respiratory rates, and high minute ventilation. Auto-PEEP should also be suspected when causes of flow obstruction, such as wheezing, are present, which may indicate high expiratory resistance or a history of COPD.

CORRECTING OXYGENATION AND VENTILATION PROBLEMS

Once the initial ventilator settings have been applied, the analysis of arterial blood gases should be performed, generally 20 minutes later. The arterial blood gas values will allow assessment of the adequacy of oxygenation and ventilation and determination of the correlation between the pulse oximeter SaO_2 value and the laboratory-quantified SaO_2 value. Ventilator adjustments, if necessary, may then be made to correct problems with oxygenation and ventilation (Table 6–5). The adjustment of ventilator settings will be explored further in Chapters 7 and 8.

TABLE 6–5 Correction of Oxygenation and Ventilation Problems Through Adjustment of the Ventilator Settings

Problem	ABG Findings	Ventilator Setting Adjustments
Excessive oxygenation	PaO_2 >100 mm Hg	Decrease FIO_2
	SaO_2 100%	Decrease PEEP
Inadequate oxygenation	PaO_2 <60 mm Hg	Increase FIO_2
	SaO_2 <90%	Increase PEEP
Respiratory acidosis	$PaCO_2$ >45 mm Hg	Increase VT
	pH ≤7.35	Increase RR
Respiratory alkalosis	$PaCO_2$ <35 mm Hg	Decrease VT
	pH ≥7.45	Decrease RR

ABG = Arterial blood gas.

RECOMMENDED READINGS

Aldrich, T.K., and Prevant, D.J. (1994). Indications of mechanical ventilation. In M.J. Tobin (Ed.). *Principles and Practice of Mechanical Ventilation* (pp. 155–189). New York: McGraw-Hill.

American Association for Respiratory Care (1992). Consensus Statement on the Essentials of Mechanical Ventilators. *Respir Care* 37(9), 1000–1008.

Banner, M.J., Blanch, P.B., and Kirby, R.R. (1993). Imposed work of breathing and methods of triggering a demand-flow, continuous positive airway pressure system. *Crit Care Med* 21(2), 183–190.

Benson, M.S., and Pierson, D.J. (1988). Auto-PEEP during mechanical ventilation in adults. *Respir Care* 33(7), 557–568.

Bone, R.C. (1993). Acute respiratory failure: Definition and overview. In R.C. Bone (Ed.). *Pulmonary and Critical Care Medicine* (pp. 1–7). St. Louis: Mosby–Year Book.

Branson, R.D. (1991). Enhanced capabilities of current ICU ventilators: Do they really benefit patients? *Respir Care* 36(5), 362–376.

Branson, R.D. (1994). Flow-triggering systems. *Respir Care* 39(2):138–144.

Chatburn, R.L. (1992). Classification of mechanical ventilators. *Respir Care* 37(9), 1009–1025.

Dettenmeier, P.A., and Johnson, T.M. (1991). The art and science of mechanical ventilator adjustments. *Crit Care Nurs Clin North Am* 3(4), 575–583.

Dupuis, Y. (1992). Flow-by. In Y. Dupuis (Ed.). *Ventilators: Theory and Clinical Application* (pp. 230–235). St. Louis: Mosby–Year Book.

Gurevitch, M.J. (1988). Selection of the inspiratory:expiratory ratio. In R.M. Kacmarek, and J.K. Stoller (Eds.). *Current Respiratory Care* (pp. 148–152). Toronto: B.C. Decker.

Hyzy, R.C., and Popovich, J. (1993). Mechanical ventilation and weaning. In R.W. Carlson and M.A. Geheb (Eds.). *Principles and Practice of Medical Intensive Care* (pp. 924–943). Philadelphia: W.B. Saunders.

Kreit, J.W., and Eschenbacher, W.L. (1988). The physiology of spontaneous and mechanical ventilation. *Clin Chest Med* 9(1), 11–21.

Lanken, P.N. (1993). Respiratory failure: An overview. In R.W. Carlson and M.A. Geheb (Eds.). *Principles and Practice of Medical Intensive Care* (pp. 754–763). Philadelphia: W.B. Saunders.

Marcy, T.W., and Marini, J.J. (1991). Inverse ratio ventilation in ARDS: Rationale and implementation. *Chest* 100(2), 494–504.

Rau, J.L., and Shelledy, D.C. (1991). The effect of varying inspiratory flow waveforms on peak and mean airway pressures with a time-cycled volume ventilator: A bench study. *Respir Care* 36(5), 347–356.

Rossi, A., and Ranieri, M.V. (1994). Positive end-expiratory pressure. In M.J. Tobin (Ed.). *Principles and Practice of Mechanical Ventilation* (pp. 259–303). New York: McGraw-Hill.

Sassoon, C.S.H. (1992). Mechanical ventilator design and function: The trigger variable. *Respir Care* 37(9), 1056–1069.

Sassoon, C.S.H., et al. (1989). Inspiratory work of breathing on flow-by and demand-flow continuous positive airway pressure. *Crit Care Med* 17(11), 1108–1114.

Stoller, J.K. (1988). Respiratory effects of positive end-expiratory pressure. *Respir Care* 33(6), 454–463.

Modes of Mechanical Ventilation

There are many methods by which the patient and ventilator interact to perform the ventilatory cycle. These variable techniques are called *modes* of mechanical ventilation. The number of modes continues to increase in the effort to improve the efficiency of mechanical ventilation. As each new mode emerges, so do pro and con arguments about its use and about its advantages and disadvantages over previously described modes. There is no one best mode for management of the patient in need of ventilatory support, just as there is no exact science to the application of the various modes. Experience and skill probably rank very high in the success of a mode's application. That there are so many modes should be viewed as advantageous in the approach to the complex indications for mechanical ventilation. Confusion about differing modes is compounded by the fact that the various authors and manufacturers use different terms to describe the same mode.

This chapter will describe the modes of mechanical ventilation, their indications, their advantages and disadvantages, and the focus areas of patient monitoring. The focus areas of patient monitoring are key areas of total assessment that may have greater variability when the mode being discussed is used and that therefore need to be monitored closely. It is assumed that a complete assessment will always be performed on each patient and will include physical examination, laboratory and x-ray findings, ventilator settings, and patient data such as the peak inspiratory pressure (PIP), exhaled tidal volume (EVT) and minute ventilation ($\dot{V}E$).

Modes of ventilation are classified by the mechanism that begins inspiration. Thus there are two basic categories of modes: controlled and assisted. In controlled ventilation, the ventilator initiates the breath and performs all the work of breathing. In assisted ventilation, the patient initiates and terminates all or some of the breaths, with the ventilator giving variable amounts of support throughout the respiratory cycle. Hence the modes of ventilation vary in degree of patient versus ventilator effort. The mode chosen for a particular patient will depend on how much of the work of breathing the patient can perform—that is, on how much work it is desirable for the patient to perform, considering the patient's pathologic condition.

There are four different breath types that a patient using a ventilator may demonstrate clinically (Table 7–1). Breath types are classified by whether the patient or the ventilator triggers the breath and how the patient and ventilator interact to perform the work of breathing. Machine-cycled breaths may be manda-

TABLE 7-1 Mechanical Ventilation Breath Types

Breath Type	Description
Machine-cycled mandatory breath	A breath that is triggered by the ventilator, and then the ventilator performs all of the work of breathing throughout the phases of ventilation
Machine-cycled assisted breath	A breath that is triggered by the patient, but the ventilator performs the rest of the ventilatory work
Patient-cycled supported breath	A breath that is triggered by the patient, but the patient and ventilator interact to perform the work of ventilation throughout the remaining phases of ventilation
Patient-cycled spontaneous breath	A breath that is triggered by the patient, and the patient then performs all of the work of ventilation

tory or assisted, and patient-cycled breaths may be supported or spontaneous. Recall from Chapter 6 that "cycling" is the changeover from the inspiratory to the expiratory phase.

Throughout this chapter, pressure and/or flow waveforms will be used to depict the typical ventilation pattern resulting from the use of a mode. Figure 7-1, a graph of spontaneous ventilation, serves as an example of these waveforms.

FULL VERSUS PARTIAL VENTILATORY SUPPORT

The question of which mode is the "right" mode of ventilation for respiratory failure of a particular cause has no simple answer. It continues to generate stimulating academic discussion because there are many therapeutic options. Ventilatory support can be classified according to two general approaches: full ventilatory support (FVS) and partial ventilatory support (PVS). FVS constitutes mechanical ventilation in which the ventilator performs essentially all of the work of breathing (WOB) and must be adjusted to completely maintain CO_2 homeo-

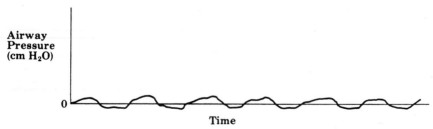

FIGURE 7-1 Spontaneous ventilation. Pressure, in centimeters of H_2O, is graphed on vertical axis against time on horizontal axis. Negative deflections represent patient inspiratory effort. (From Pilbeam, SP: *Mechanical Ventilation: Physiological and Clinical Applications*. St. Louis: Mosby–Year Book, 1992.)

stasis without any contribution from the patient. PVS occurs when both the ventilator and the patient contribute toward the WOB and in maintaining CO_2 homeostasis.

Normally FVS is the initial application of mechanical ventilation required by patients with acute respiratory failure. FVS may be necessary for the first 24 to 72 hours to relieve the patient of the WOB, allow the diaphragm and ventilatory muscles to recuperate from fatigue, and allow time for the underlying pulmonary abnormality to begin to resolve. FVS is also indicated in patients with apnea; patients who are heavily sedated or paralyzed; patients with depressed neurologic status, such as those with head trauma (particularly when controlled hyperventilation is being employed), drug overdose, or cerebrovascular accident; and when negative respiratory effort is contraindicated, such as in severe flail chest. Almost all modes of ventilation, if properly adjusted, can provide FVS. The term FVS should not be construed to mean that the ventilator has complete control of ventilatory processes; instead, it means that the ventilator provides all of the patient's ventilatory needs.

The advantages of PVS include allowing the patient to respond to increases in CO_2 by increasing $\dot{V}E$ and promoting use of the respiratory muscles, thereby preventing disuse atrophy. PVS can be provided by all the modes described below by titrating the amount of support offered. Exceptions are those modes that control ventilation—controlled mechanical ventilation (CMV) and pure pressure-control (PC) ventilation.

When PVS is used as the patient becomes better able to generate more of the WOB, the amount of machine assistance should be reduced commensurately. The workload must be balanced between the patient and the ventilator in a way that prevents ventilatory muscle atrophy or fatigue. To objectively apply this principle, one must appreciate all the components of the patient's WOB: normal physiologic WOB, the WOB imposed by the airway and ventilator circuitry, and the physiologic WOB imposed by the disease process. Thorough assessment of the patient's condition and an understanding of how each mode interacts with the patient to perform the WOB are essential. No formulas or exact parameters can be given to guide PVS. In titrating ventilatory support, clinical judgment plays a key role in preventing disuse atrophy and respiratory muscle fatigue, as well as in maintaining oxygenation, ventilation, and acid-base homeostasis.

MODES

Controlled Mechanical Ventilation

DEFINITION AND DESCRIPTION

With CMV the patient receives a preset number of breaths per minute, of a preset tidal volume (VT). Patient effort will not trigger a mechanical breath. The ventilator performs all the WOB (Fig. 7–2). On many ventilators the CMV mode differs from the assist/control (A/C) mode only when the sensitivity is set so that the ventilator will not respond to the patient's inspiratory efforts. Some manufacturers use the term CMV to refer to the A/C mode, which leads to confusion between these two modes. The rationale for their use of the term CMV involves redefining CMV to mean controlled *mandatory* ventilation, in which every breath is of a mandatory VT.

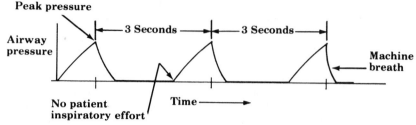

Figure 7-2 Controlled mechanical ventilation (CMV). Patient receives a preset number of breaths of a preset tidal volume, delivered at equal time intervals. Patient effort will not trigger either a spontaneous or mechanical breath. (From Pilbeam, SP: *Mechanical Ventilation: Physiological and Clinical Applications*. St. Louis: Mosby–Year Book, 1992.)

Indications

1. Patients with minimal or no respiratory effort because of dysfunction of the central nervous system (e.g., Guillain-Barré syndrome, high-level spinal cord lesions, or drug overdose). Respiratory suppression may also be intentional, such as when heavy sedation and neuromuscular blockage are used.
2. When negative inspiratory effort is contraindicated, as in some cases of severe flail chest.
3. To provide a fail-safe method of ventilating the patient's lungs under conditions such as anesthesia or as a backup to assisted ventilation.

Advantages and Disadvantages

CMV was used widely before the advent of A/C ventilation. Because the patient cannot achieve a spontaneous breath, if he is awake and attempts to breathe, CMV will lock him out. This can lead to sensations of air hunger and significantly increase the WOB. This disadvantage has relegated the use of CMV to the indications previously listed.

This mode is inefficient if the patient attempts to breathe, because breathing may cause patient-ventilator asynchrony. Evidence that the patient is attempting to initiate a breath may include contractions of the accessory muscles of inspiration and sternal retractions. Accordingly, patients who can generate spontaneous respiratory efforts must be heavily sedated and/or paralyzed to improve patient comfort and ventilating efficiency. The use of such sedation and/or paralysis is not without its own potential complications; therefore, if patient-initiated breaths are not contraindicated, another mode of ventilation should be chosen. If the patient splints the chest wall or exhales during inspiration, then the peak airway pressure limit set on the ventilator may be reached. This causes the remainder of the inspiratory volume to be dumped from the ventilator into the atmosphere. This is commonly called "bucking the ventilator."

With CMV, alveolar ventilation and the respiratory contribution to acid-base balance are completely controlled by the clinician. Acid-base balance must be closely monitored and ventilator settings adjusted with changing physiologic scenarios, such as fever, change in nutritional intake, and stress.

Respiratory muscle weakness and atrophy may result from disuse if CMV is used for an extended period, making it harder to wean the patient from the ventilator. Adverse hemodynamic effects may occur with use of this mode because every breath is delivered under positive pressure.

FOCUS AREAS OF PATIENT MONITORING

1. Peak inspiratory pressure (PIP) because it is variable in this volume-cycled mode of ventilation and will increase with changes in compliance and resistance.
2. Exhaled tidal volumes (EVT) because even though VT is preset on the ventilator control panel, delivery is not guaranteed. If EVT deviates from the set VT by 100 cc or greater in adults, look for a source of the loss of VT (see Chapter 8).
3. Acid-base balance because the respiratory component is controlled by the operator.
4. Patient-ventilator asynchrony that may be due to flow rate or respiratory rate settings that are inadequate to meet the patient's ventilatory needs.
5. Adequate sedation of the patient with ability to initiate spontaneous respirations.

Assist/Control Mode

DEFINITION AND DESCRIPTION

The A/C mode is a method of ventilation in which the ventilator delivers a preset number of breaths of a preset VT. Between these machine-initiated breaths, the patient may trigger spontaneous breaths. When the ventilator senses the patient's spontaneous respiratory effort, it delivers a breath of the preset VT. The patient cannot vary the volume of spontaneously initiated breaths (Fig. 7–3). The only work that the patient must perform is the negative inspiratory effort required to trigger the vent on the patient-initiated breaths. The ventilator performs the rest of the work. The difference between A/C and CMV is that with the A/C mode the ventilator is sensitive and responds to the patient's spontaneous respiratory efforts. Some manufacturers use the term CMV to mean A/C. Their rationale involves redefining CMV to mean controlled *mandatory* ventilation, in which every breath is of a mandatory VT.

INDICATIONS

1. Normal respiratory drive, but respiratory muscles are too weak to perform the WOB (e.g., when a patient is emerging from anesthesia).

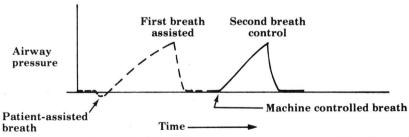

FIGURE 7–3   Assist/control (A/C) ventilation pressure curve. Patient receives a preset number of control breaths of a preset tidal volume. The patient may trigger additional breaths. These machine-assisted breaths will be of the preset tidal volume. An assisted breath is evident by the negative pressure deflection created by the patient when triggering the ventilator. A control breath shows no negative deflection. (From Pilbeam, SP: *Mechanical Ventilation: Physiological and Clinical Applications*. St. Louis: Mosby–Year Book, 1992.)

2. Normal respiratory drive, but respiratory muscles are unable to perform the WOB because it is increased, as in pulmonary abnormalities in which lung compliance is decreased.
3. When it is desirable to allow patients to set their own rate and thereby assist in maintaining a normal $PaCO_2$.

ADVANTAGES AND DISADVANTAGES

The A/C mode allows the patient to control the rate of breathing, and yet it guarantees the delivery of a minimal preset rate and volume. The A/C mode also allows some work to be performed by the respiratory muscles, though it is minimal if the flow rate and sensitivity are set appropriately. It is indicated when it is desirable for the ventilator to perform the bulk of the ventilatory work. Under these conditions the WOB with the A/C mode is less than that of intermittent mandatory ventilation (IMV) at the same settings.

Disadvantages include patients' tendency to hyperventilate because of anxiety, pain, or neurologic factors, because respiratory alkalosis will ensue. Significant alkalosis suppresses the ventilatory drive and is detrimental to many metabolic functions. Hyperventilation may also lead to the formation of intrinsic positive end-expiratory pressure, also known as auto-PEEP, because of a shortened expiratory time. Variability in the patient's hemodynamic status may occur with the A/C mode because every breath is delivered under positive pressure.

FOCUS AREAS OF PATIENT MONITORING

1. Peak inspiratory pressure (PIP) because it is variable in this volume-cycled mode of ventilation and will increase with changes in compliance and resistance.
2. Exhaled tidal volume (EVT) because, even though VT is preset on the ventilator control panel, delivery is not guaranteed. If EVT deviates from set VT by 100 cc or greater in adults, look for a source of the loss of VT (see Chapter 8).
3. Evaluation of patient's subjective sense of comfort. Monitor airway pressure manometer during patient's spontaneous respiratory effort and adjust sensitivity to allow for minimal triggering effort. Adjust flow rate to meet patient's inspiratory demands. The trigger sensitivity and the flow rate are the chief variables affecting the patient's WOB when the A/C mode is used.
4. Close monitoring of acid-base status. If the patient is hyperventilating, consider sedation or changing to a mode in which the patient has greater control (i.e., IMV, synchronized IMV, or pressure support ventilation).

Intermittent Mandatory Ventilation

DEFINITION AND DESCRIPTION

Intermittent mandatory ventilation (IMV) is a mode of ventilation in which the patient receives a preset number of breaths of a preset VT. Between these mandatory breaths, the patient may initiate spontaneous breaths. The volume of the spontaneous breaths is dependent on the muscular respiratory effort that the patient is able to generate (Fig. 7–4A). The main difference between the IMV and A/C modes is the volume of the patient-initiated breaths. In the A/C mode the VT is guaranteed, whereas in IMV it is variable. IMV was originally developed in an effort to create a mode in which the patient could interact with the

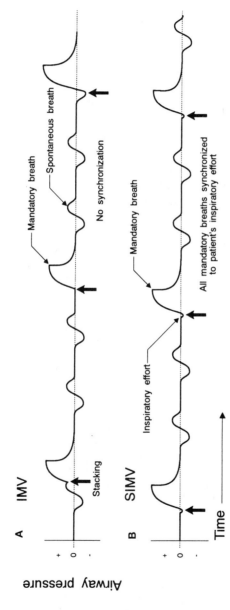

Figure 7-4 Intermittent mandatory ventilation (IMV) and synchronized intermittent mandatory ventilation (SIMV). Pressure waveform shows essential differences between IMV and SIMV. Mandatory breaths are marked with vertical arrows. In IMV (A), mandatory breaths are given at equal time intervals regardless of where the patient is in the ventilatory cycle. This can result in breath stacking. In SIMV (B), mandatory breaths are delivered in synchrony with the patient's negative inspiratory effort. (From Dupuis, YG: *Ventilators: Theory and Clinical Application*. 2nd ed. St Louis: Mosby–Year Book, 1992.)

ventilator, using the respiratory muscles; it would thus be useful for weaning patients from ventilatory support. The lower the IMV rate, the more spontaneous breaths the patient will initiate, therefore assuming a greater portion of the ventilatory work. As the patient demonstrates the ability to generate more work, the mandatory breath rate is decreased accordingly.

INDICATIONS
1. Normal respiratory drive but respiratory muscles unable to perform all WOB.
2. In situations where it is desirable to allow patients to set their own respiratory rate and thus assist in maintaining a normal $PaCO_2$.
3. Need to wean patient from mechanical ventilation.

ADVANTAGES AND DISADVANTAGES
Hyperventilation is less of a problem in this mode than in the A/C mode because the patient can modify rate and volume of ventilation on the spontaneous breaths and therefore maintain normal CO_2 levels. Less atrophy of the respiratory muscles will occur because the patient participates more in ventilation, using the ventilatory muscles to a greater degree than when CMV or A/C is used. The hemodynamic effects of positive-pressure ventilation may be less with IMV than CMV or A/C because ventilation will occur at a lower mean airway pressure when spontaneous breaths are taken; therefore the average mean airway pressure over time will be less.

IMV fails to monitor the patient's spontaneous respiratory efforts and may deliver a mandatory breath during the patient's own ventilatory cycle. This may lead to breath stacking, in which a mechanical breath falls during or at the end of the patient's breath. This creates patient-ventilator dyssynchrony, discomfort, inadequate ventilation, and potentially barotrauma. If breath stacking leads to pressure limiting on inspiration, then the ventilator will vent the rest of the V_T to the atmosphere.

FOCUS AREAS OF PATIENT MONITORING
1. The patient's respiratory rate (RR). If the RR increases, then the V_T of the spontaneous breaths should be reassessed. The V_T of the spontaneous breaths should be 5 to 8 cc/kg. If the patient is beginning to fatigue, a more shallow and rapid respiratory pattern may develop. This ventilatory pattern will lead to atelectasis, a reduction in compliance, further increase in the WOB, and the need for greater ventilatory support.
2. Peak inspiratory pressure (PIP) because it is variable in this volume-cycled mode of ventilation and will increase with changes in compliance and resistance.
3. Exhaled tidal volumes (EV_T) of mandatory breaths because even though a preset V_T is set on the ventilator control panel, delivery is not guaranteed. If EV_T deviates from set V_T by 100 cc or greater in adults, look for a source of the loss of V_T (see Chapter 8).
4. EV_T of spontaneous breaths. Volume should be 5 to 8 cc/kg. Volumes <5 cc/kg promote the development of atelectasis and indicate that the patient does not have sufficient respiratory muscle strength to generate an adequate V_T.
5. Patient comfort and patient-ventilator synchrony. If the patient complains of feeling unable to get enough air, ensure that the sensitivity and flow

rates are adjusted appropriately. If patient-ventilator dyssynchrony is a problem, especially during weaning trials, talk with the patient calmly and reassuringly, coaching him or her to work with the ventilator, that is, to relax and allow the ventilator to deliver the mandatory breaths. Provide sedation and anxiolytic medications as necessary in doses that will not suppress the respiratory drive. If patient discomfort remains a problem and weaning is the goal, T-piece trials alternating with use of the A/C mode may be another option. Also consider a mode that allows the patient more control, such as synchronized IMV or pressure-support (PS) ventilation.

Synchronized Intermittent Mandatory Ventilation

DEFINITION AND DESCRIPTION

Synchronized intermittent mandatory ventilation (SIMV) is a mode in which the patient is guaranteed a preset number of breaths of a preset VT. Between these mandatory breaths the patient may initiate spontaneous breaths. The volume of the spontaneous breaths is dependent on the muscular respiratory effort that the patient is able to generate. SIMV differs from IMV in that instead of delivering the mandatory ventilator breath at a precise time, regardless of where the patient is in the ventilatory cycle, the ventilator delivers the mandatory breath simultaneously as it senses the patient's negative inspiratory effort (Fig. 7–4B). This is achieved in SIMV by the ventilator's monitoring for the patient's spontaneous, negative inspiratory effort within a window of time and then delivering the mandatory breath in synchrony with the patient's inspiratory effort within this timing window. If the patient does not make a negative inspiratory effort within the timing window, the mandatory breath is delivered at the scheduled time. The ventilator then resets to respond to the next spontaneous inspiratory effort.

The A/C mode differs from SIMV in regard to the VT of the *patient-initiated* breaths. Patient-initiated breaths in the A/C mode result in the patient's receiving a guaranteed VT, whereas in SIMV the VT is variable because it is dependent on patient effort and lung characteristics. The difference between IMV and SIMV is that, in the latter, the mandatory breaths are synchronized to the patient's spontaneous respiratory efforts.

INDICATIONS

1. Normal respiratory drive but respiratory muscles unable to perform all the WOB.
2. Situations in which it is desirable to allow patients to set their own rate, thus assisting in maintaining a normal $PaCO_2$.
3. Need to wean the patient from mechanical ventilation.

ADVANTAGES AND DISADVANTAGES

Synchronizing the mandatory breaths with the patient's readiness to breathe improves patient comfort, reduces competition between ventilator and patient, and prevents breath stacking and its potential problems, such as barotrauma and loss of VT as a result of pressure limiting. Hyperventilation is less of a problem in this mode than in the A/C mode because the patient can modify the rate and volume of ventilation of the spontaneous breaths to maintain normal CO_2 levels. Less atrophy of the respiratory muscles occurs because the patient uses the ventilatory muscles to a greater degree than with CMV or A/C. The hemodynamic effects of positive-pressure ventilation are less with SIMV than with CMV or A/C because the patient will ventilate at a lower mean airway pressure (Paw) on the spontaneous breaths, so the average Paw over time is less.

A disadvantage of SIMV is that the spontaneous breaths in a SIMV system are provided through a patient-triggered, demand flow system. In most ventilators the opening of the demand valve occurs in response to a drop in circuit pressure. When this drop in pressure is sensed, the flow of fresh gas is initiated to meet the patient's respiratory needs. Demand flow systems vary considerably in circuit resistance and the amount of negative effort the patient must generate to initiate the flow of gases. The WOB associated with the demand valve system comes from several sources: from the amount of work required to open the valve, from the ongoing ventilatory muscle work performed during the lag time which begins at the onset of the flow of gases and ends when the patient actually receives the gas, and from flow rates that are insufficient to meet the patient's ventilatory demand. In some systems the WOB associated with the demand valve may be considerable.

Initially IMV was achieved by the use of a separate continuous flow (CF) circuit attached through a side-arm or one-way valve. One circuit provided the flow necessary for the mandatory breaths, and the other for the spontaneous breaths. The supply of gas to the patient is continuous in such a circuit and does not utilize a demand valve (Fig. 7–5). The WOB is reduced in a CF circuit by the operator's ensuring that the flow rate is set adequately to meet the patient's inspiratory demands. Some problems noted with the CF circuit, which prompted the development of SIMV and the patient-triggered system, include the cost of extra tubing, the potential for incorrect setup, wasted gas flow, and the risk of assembly disconnection. The use of demand flow systems proliferated before their limitations were assessed and reduced.

The realization that the WOB associated with demand valve systems may be considerable has led to the development, in some of the newer ventilators, of demand flow systems that require less work to activate them. A new method of triggering the ventilator, flow-triggering, or the flow-by system, has also been developed; it is designed to provide continuous flow and eliminate the lag time from onset of breath to delivery of gas (see Chapter 6). Finally, the WOB imposed by the ventilator circuit and the artificial airway may be eliminated with the use of pressure support ventilation, which provides inspiratory ventilatory assistance.

Focus Areas of Patient Monitoring

1. The patient's respiratory rate (RR). If the RR increases, then the V_T of the spontaneous breaths should be reassessed. The V_T of the spontaneous breaths should be 5 to 8 cc/kg. If the patient is becoming fatigued, a more shallow and rapid respiratory pattern may develop. This ventilatory pattern will lead to atelectasis, a reduction in compliance, further increase in the WOB, and the need for greater ventilatory support.
2. PIP because it is variable in this volume-cycled mode of ventilation and will increase with changes in compliance and resistance.
3. EV_T of mandatory breaths because, even though a preset V_T is set on the ventilator control panel, delivery is not guaranteed. If EV_T deviates from set V_T by 100 cc or greater in an adult, look for a source of the loss of V_T (see Chapter 8).

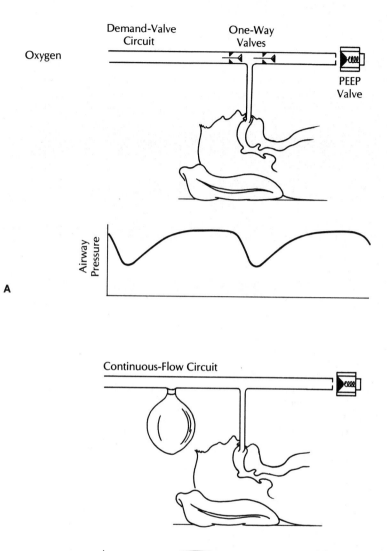

FIGURE 7-5 Demand valve (A) versus continuous-flow (B) circuit. Considerable drop in inspiratory airway pressure (triggering effort) is required to open the demand valve in some ventilators. This effort increases the work of breathing. (Reproduced with permission from Tobin, MJ: Update on strategies in mechanical ventilation. *Hosp Pract* 1986;21(6):80. Illustrations by Alan D. Iselin.)

4. EVT of spontaneous breaths. Volume should be 5 to 8 cc/kg. Volumes <5 cc/kg promote the development of atelectasis and indicate that the patient does not have sufficient respiratory muscle strength to generate an adequate VT. The patient may be given additional assistance with his or her spontaneous breaths by means of PS.

5. Patient comfort. If the patient complains of a feeling of not being able to get enough air, ensure that the sensitivity and flow rates are adjusted appropriately. If the patient is uncomfortable or anxious, especially during weaning trials, talk with the patient in a calm and reassuring manner, coaching him or her to work with the ventilator, that is, to relax and allow the ventilator to deliver the mandatory breaths. Provide sedation and anxiolytic medications as necessary in doses that will not suppress the respiratory drive. If patient discomfort remains a problem and weaning is the goal, T-piece trials alternating with the A/C mode may be another option. Also consider a mode that allows the patient even more control, such as PS ventilation. If patient discomfort during SIMV remains a problem and weaning is the goal, T-piece trials alternating with the A/C or PS mode may be better tolerated.

Continuous Positive Airway Pressure
Definition and Description
Continuous positive airway pressure (CPAP) is positive pressure applied throughout the respiratory cycle to the spontaneously breathing patient (Fig. 7–6). The patient must have a reliable ventilatory drive and an adequate VT, because no mandatory breaths or other ventilatory assistance is given the patient. Furthermore, the patient performs all the WOB.

CPAP provides positive pressure at end-exhalation, thus preventing alveolar collapse, improving the functional residual capacity (FRC), and enhancing oxygenation. As discussed previously (Chapter 6), CPAP is identical to PEEP in its physiologic effects. CPAP is the correct term when the baseline pressure is elevated in the *spontaneously* breathing patient both when the ventilator is used and when it is not. *PEEP* is the term used when the baseline pressure is elevated and

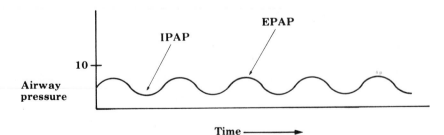

Figure 7–6 Continuous positive airway pressure (CPAP). Patient is breathing spontaneously, with positive pressure applied throughout ventilatory cycle. Therefore both inspiratory positive airway pressure (IPAP) and expiratory positive airway pressure (EPAP) are present. The baseline is always positive, never returning to ambient pressure. (From Pilbeam, SP: *Mechanical Ventilation: Physiological and Clinical Applications.* St. Louis: Mosby–Year Book, 1992.)

the patient is receiving some form of additional respiratory support (e.g., A/C, SIMV, PS).

INDICATIONS
1. Adequate ventilation but incompetent oxygenation because of conditions that decrease the FRC, such as atelectasis or secretion retention.
2. Adequate ventilation but need to maintain artificial airway because of airway edema or obstruction or for pulmonary toilet.
3. Need to wean the patient from mechanical ventilation. During weaning, CPAP is used to promote alveolar stability and improve the FRC, in comparison with breathing on T-piece without CPAP.

ADVANTAGES AND DISADVANTAGES
The primary advantage of CPAP is that it reduces atelectasis. CPAP also maintains and promotes respiratory muscle strength because the patient is given no other ventilatory assistance and therefore performs all the WOB. CPAP is often incorporated into a weaning plan as a mechanism to build respiratory muscle strength. For example, CPAP periods may be alternated with periods of SIMV breathing. The time spent in the CPAP trial should be increased as the patient's respiratory muscle function improves.

Because the patient is still connected to the ventilator, when using CPAP as a weaning mode the practitioner benefits from low EVT and apnea alarms and the delivery of mandatory breaths as a backup in the event of apnea. None of these options are present when weaning is accomplished with a T-piece. Furthermore, the adequacy of the VT can be readily monitored on the display panel of the ventilator. For further information on the use of CPAP as a weaning mode, see Chapter 10: Weaning From Mechanical Ventilation.

The application of positive pressure may cause decreased cardiac output, increased intracranial pressure, and pulmonary barotrauma. Levels of positive pressure generally used with CPAP are 5 to 10 cm H_2O. These levels are unlikely to cause serious adverse effects unless significant hypovolemia or cardiac dysfunction is present. If the latter is present, then a mode that requires the patient to perform less of the WOB is indicated.

FOCUS AREAS OF PATIENT MONITORING
1. The patient's RR. RR should remain less than 25 breaths/min. If the RR increases, then the EVT should be assessed. If the patient is becoming fatigued, a more shallow and rapid respiratory pattern may develop. This pattern will lead to atelectasis and a reduction in compliance, further increasing the WOB and the need for greater ventilatory assistance.
2. The EVT, which should be 5 to 8 cc/kg. Volumes <5 cc/kg promote the development of atelectasis and indicate that the patient does not have sufficient respiratory muscle strength to generate an adequate VT. The mode of ventilation may need to be switched to one that provides additional assistance, such as PS, SIMV, or A/C. If the patient is in a weaning trial and the RR is increasing and VT decreasing, these are signs of fatigue and the chosen resting mode should be reinstated.
3. Patient comfort. If the patient complains of feeling unable to get enough air, ensure that the flow rate is adjusted appropriately. If the patient is anxious, especially during weaning trials, talk with the patient in a calm and

reassuring manner and stay until both you and the patient are confident that ventilation is adequate. Provide sedation and/or anxiolytic medications as necessary in doses that will not suppress respiration.

Pressure Support

Definition and Description

Pressure support (PS) is a mode of ventilation in which the patient's spontaneous respiratory activity is augmented by the delivery of a preset amount of inspiratory positive pressure. When the patient triggers the onset of inspiration, the preselected amount of PS is delivered and then held constant throughout inspiration, thereby promoting the flow of gas into the lungs (Fig. 7–7). With PS there is no set V_T. The V_T is variable, being determined by patient effort, the amount of applied PS, and the compliance and resistance of the system (patient and ventilator). Gas flow is delivered with the decelerating flow-wave pattern, in which the flow rate naturally decays as the patient's lungs fill with air on inspiration. Inspiration ends when the peak inspiratory flow rate decreases to a minimal level, either one fourth of the peak flow or 5 L/min, depending on ventilator model (Fig. 7–8). PS is therefore a flow-cycled mode of ventilation. Because inspiration ends on the basis of a flow criterion (not pressure, time, or volume), the patient retains control over respiratory pattern and volume.

The PS mode may be used alone or in conjunction with SIMV (Fig. 7–9). Straight PS should only be used in patients who display a reliable respiratory drive, because all breaths are patient initiated. When PS is used with SIMV, only the spontaneous breaths are pressure supported. One advantage of using SIMV and PS concurrently is that in the event of apnea the patient will be assured of a preselected, backup number of mandatory breaths.

PS may be delivered at either a high level or a low level. In high-level PS (PSV_{max}), the amount of PS is increased until the patient achieves the V_T tradi-

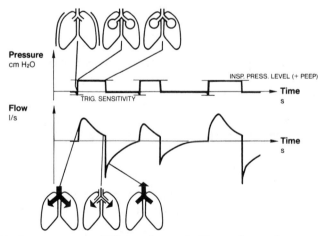

Figure 7–7 Pressure support (PS) ventilation. In PS ventilation the patient's spontaneous respiratory effort is provided inspiratory pressure augmentation to promote the flow of gas into the lungs. The applied PS level is held constant throughout the inspiratory phase. (Courtesy of Siemens Medical Systems, Electromedical Group, Danvers, Mass.)

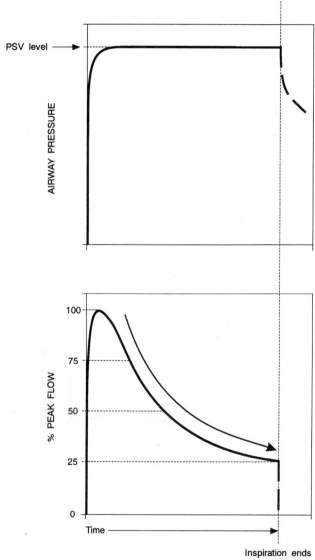

FIGURE 7-8 Decelerating flow pattern used with pressure support ventilation. Airway pressure remains constant throughout inspiration. The changeover from inspiration to expiration occurs when flow decelerates to 25% of peak flow or to some other defined minimal level. (From Dupuis, YG: *Ventilators: Theory and Clinical Application.* 2nd ed. St. Louis: Mosby–Year Book, 1992.)

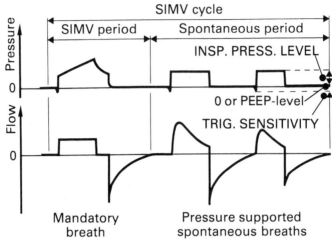

Figure 7-9 Synchronized intermittent mandatory ventilation (SIMV) with pressure support (PS) ventilation. In SIMV and PS, mandatory breaths of a preset tidal volume are administered in the fashion of SIMV. Only spontaneous breaths are pressure supported, not the mandatory breaths. (Courtesy of Siemens Medical Systems, Electromedical Group, Danvers, Mass.)

tionally used in full ventilatory support: 10 to 15 cc/kg. When PS is used in this manner, no additional volume-cycled breaths are required as long as the patient has a consistent respiratory drive. In low-level PS, the amount of support is adjusted until the patient achieves a V_T that is acceptable for spontaneous breathing: 5 to 8 cc/kg. Low-level PS may be used alone; however, it is often used with an SIMV backup rate to ensure minimal alveolar ventilation. With either high- or low-level PS, the amount of support given to the patient is decreased as respiratory muscle strength increases and as the respiratory system mechanics improve, as evidenced by an improving V_T.

When PS is used with PEEP, the peak inspiratory pressure (PIP) is equal to the PS level plus the amount of applied PEEP. On a breath-to-breath basis, the PIP remains constant at this level. The correct terminology, which will also help you to remember what the expected PIP is, is to say that the patient is on both PS and PEEP. For example, one may say, "PS of 8 cm H_2O above 5 cm H_2O PEEP," indicating that the PIP is 13 cm H_2O. It is incorrect to say the patient is on PS and CPAP, because CPAP is a mode in and of itself. Confusion arises about this latter point because of the terms used by ventilator manufacturers. If the PIP increases as a result of such events as splinting, coughing, or kinking of the ventilator circuit or airway, then the high-pressure-limit alarm parameter set by the operator will be reached, causing the ventilator to cycle into expiration. Recall that in PS the pressure limit is not the mechanism that routinely causes the ventilator to cycle from inspiration to expiration. PS is a flow-cycled, pressure-limited mode of ventilation.

Indications
1. Need to wean patient from mechanical ventilation. The quality and quantity of work applied to the respiratory muscles can be tightly controlled by varying the level of PS. PS is primarily used as a mode of weaning.

2. Long-term mechanical ventilation. PS, by augmenting inspiratory flow, reduces the WOB associated with the artificial airway and the ventilator circuitry. Respiratory muscle wasting is reduced because the patient will use the ventilatory muscles throughout inspiration.

ADVANTAGES AND DISADVANTAGES

PS may be used to overcome the resistance work associated with moving inspiratory flow through an artificial airway and the ventilatory circuitry. If the WOB is decreased, so is the oxygen consumption in relation to ventilation. Decreasing the WOB also increases the likelihood that the patient will better tolerate weaning. PS improves patient-ventilator synchrony and patient comfort because the patient has control over the process of ventilation. The patient determines when to initiate a breath, the timing of inspiration and expiration, and the ventilatory pattern. Therefore the patient also maintains greater control over the $PaCO_2$ and acid-base balance.

PS allows the operator to augment inadequate spontaneous VT to any desired degree and to set the PIP. The amount of assistance afforded the patient and the quality and quantity of work applied to respiratory muscles for reconditioning are more "titratable" than with the volume-cycled modes of ventilation. With PS, every spontaneous breath is assisted and the amount of assistance can be reduced in increments as small as 2 cm H_2O, thereby gradually titrating the amount of work being relinquished to the patient. In comparison, when the number of mandatory breaths is reduced in SIMV, all WOB previously done by the ventilator to achieve those breaths is handed over to the patient. The kind of work (high volume/low pressure) performed by the respiratory muscles during PS promotes endurance, as opposed to strength (see Chapter 10: Weaning From Mechanical Ventilation). Finally, a lower mean airway pressure is achieved because PIPs are generally lower than with volume-cycled ventilation.

The main disadvantage of PS is that the VT is variable and therefore the alveolar ventilation is not guaranteed. If compliance decreases or resistance increases, because of either patient or ventilator circuitry factors, then VT decreases. PS should be used with great caution in patients who exhibit an extremely variable respiratory system impedance, such as those with bronchospasm or significant secretions.

The ventilator may fail to cycle to expiration if an extensive air leak occurs, either around the airway or elsewhere in the system, because the flow rate that terminates inspiratory pressure support will not be reached. This will result in the application of positive pressure throughout the respiratory cycle, much as in CPAP. Finally, the use of in-line nebulizers should be limited with PS ventilation because the increased flow created by the nebulizer may be erroneously sensed by the ventilator as the patient's minute ventilation. This may result in failure to detect apnea. Medications should be administered with metered dose inhalers to avoid this potential complication.

FOCUS AREAS OF PATIENT MONITORING

1. Exhaled VT. When PS is used for full ventilatory assistance, the VT should be 10 to 15 cc/kg. Partial ventilatory assistance VTs should be 5 to 8 cc/kg. The cause of low EVT needs to be rapidly investigated because volumes less than the goal for the patient promote the development of atelectasis. Systematically assesss the patient-related versus ventilator circuitry–related causes of decreased exhaled VT (Table 7–2). VT is increased by increasing

TABLE 7–2   Troubleshooting Potential Causes of Low Exhaled Tidal Volume (EVT) With a Pressure Mode of Ventilation

Patient Related

Reduction in compliance: for example, pleural space disease, infiltrative process
Increase in resistance: airway narrowing, as in bronchospasm, secretions in airway
Insufficient respiratory muscle strength to meet ventilatory demands
Loss of tidal volume through pleural air leak

Ventilator Circuit Related

Increase in resistance to gas flow: kinking of endotracheal tube, patient biting on airway, circuit tubing compressed between bed rail and mattress or patient lying on it, water in tubing
Loose connection in exhaled gas limb of circuitry, allowing gases to escape
Loss of tidal volume from around artificial airway cuff

the amount of PS. If the patient is in a weaning trial and the RR is increasing and EVT is decreasing, these are signs of fatigue. The patient should be provided more ventilatory support: increase the PS level, increase the number of mandatory breaths, or return the patient to the chosen resting mode.

2. Airway cuff leaks because the ventilator will not reach the PS level and may persist in the inspiratory phase of respiratory cycle.

3. The patient's RR, which should remain at less than 25 breaths/min. If the RR increases, then the VT should be assessed. If the patient is becoming fatigued, a shallower and more rapid respiratory pattern may develop. This ventilatory pattern will lead to atelectasis, a reduction in compliance, further increase in the WOB, and the need for greater ventilatory assistance.

4. Hemodynamic effects of positive-pressure ventilation when PS_{max} is being used.

Noninvasive Pressure Support Ventilation

DEFINITION AND DESCRIPTION

Noninvasive PS ventilation (NIPSV), also known as bi-level positive airway pressure ventilation, is a noninvasive mode of ventilation in which there is both a set level of inspiratory positive airway pressure (IPAP) and a set level of expiratory positive airway pressure (EPAP) (Fig. 7–10). In comparison with conventional ventilation, IPAP is equivalent to PS, and EPAP is equivalent to PEEP.

This mode is essentially the same as PS ventilation, the differences being that NIPSV is a flow-triggered system and is applied through a nasal mask; therefore an artificial airway is not needed. Tidal volume, flow rate, and inspiratory time vary with patient effort, the set pressure differential, and changes in compliance and resistance. Various names for this mode of ventilation can be found in the literature, including nasal intermittent positive-pressure ventilation (NIPPV) and bi-level positive airway pressure (BiPAP). A device for delivering this method of ventilation, the BiPAP pressure support ventilator, is made by Respironics (Fig. 7–11). Possibly as an extension of this trade name, some authors erroneously refer to the mode as BiPAP. NIPSV is a very new mode of ven-

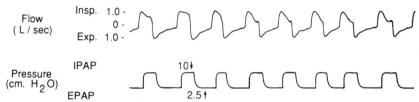

FIGURE 7-10 Noninvasive pressure support ventilation (NIPSV). Tracings of mask pressure and patient airflow during administration of 10 cm H_2O inspiratory positive airway pressure (IPAP) and 2.5 cm H_2O expiratory positive airway pressure (EPAP). This mode is essentially the same as PS applied with PEEP (see text for further discussion). (Modified from Sanders, MH, et al.: Nocturnal ventilatory assistance with bi-level positive airway pressure. *Operative Techniques in Otolaryngology–Head and Neck Surgery* 1991;2:57.)

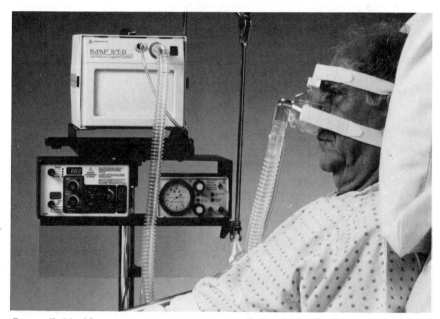

FIGURE 7-11 Noninvasive pressure support ventilation (NIPSV), also known as bi-level positive airway pressure, may be administered through a nasal mask with the BiPAP ventilatory support system (BiPAP; Respironics, Murrysville, Pa.). This system is capable of operating in four "modes." In the spontaneous (S) mode, the unit synchronizes with the patient's respiratory pattern, cycling from inspiratory to expiratory positive airway pressure (IPAP to EPAP). In the spontaneous/timed (S/T) mode, the unit cycles as in the spontaneous mode, but in the event of apnea, assisted breaths are given on the basis of a clinician set breaths-per-minute setting. In the timed (T) mode, the unit cycles between IPAP and EPAP levels according to set RR and percent IPAP time controls. The continuous positive airway pressure (CPAP) mode allows the BiPAP system to be used for the delivery of CPAP. (Photo courtesy of Respironics, Murrysville, Pa.)

tilation, and further research is needed to define its applications and discern its benefits and the precautions needed during use.

INDICATIONS
1. Chronic ventilatory failure superimposed by an acute process.
2. Nocturnal ventilatory support in patients with chronic ventilatory failure and limited functional capacity of the respiratory muscles. These conditions may be due to chest wall disorders, neuromuscular disease, or chronic obstructive pulmonary disease.
3. Nocturnal ventilatory support in patients with obstructive sleep apnea.
4. As a transitional method of variable ventilatory assistance after extubation and before purely spontaneous breathing begins.
5. As a method of providing ventilatory assistance while avoiding intubation.

ADVANTAGES AND DISADVANTAGES
NIPSV was originally developed for the relief of obstructive sleep apnea, the IPAP creating an adequate VT and EPAP stenting the airway. As NIPSV gained in popularity, it gradually moved into the inpatient setting. The main advantage of NIPSV is the ability to provide ventilatory assistance without intubation. This eradicates intubation-related complications, enables patients to eat and speak normally, and eliminates discomfort from an artificial airway. Because NIPSV is easy to apply, it is useful in general care settings, postanesthesia care units, and emergency departments, as well as intensive care units. If the patient requires home ventilation, the same system can be used in the home setting, smoothing the transition from the hospital setting into the home.

The theoretical advantage of NIPSV over negative-pressure ventilation is that in the latter a fixed rate of ventilation is required and upper airway obstruction can be exacerbated. In comparison with nasal CPAP, a theoretical advantage of NIPSV is that it provides inspiratory assistance to augment VT and offload weak respiratory muscles, whereas CPAP provides no inspiratory assistance and may actually impose an increase in the WOB. Controlled clinical trials comparing these modes and studying the indications for NIPSV are needed.

It may be difficult to create a perfect seal; therefore a system that detects leaks around the mask and compensates for them by increasing flow is ideal. The Bi-PAP system operates under such a principle and does so without affecting the sensitivity of the flow-triggering mechanism. Because flow-triggering is utilized, as opposed to pressure-triggering, the WOB associated with triggering the ventilator is eliminated.

Disadvantages include the limitation in the amount of support that the ventilator can offer to the patient. The intent, however, of the portable NIPSV machine is to assist the patient's respiratory efforts not to override them. When resources for ventilator purchases are limited, the purchase of a separate system for the delivery of NIPSV may be prohibitive. These costs must be weighed against potential savings from moving patients out of the intensive care setting and from eliminating morbidity caused by use of the artificial airway. Use of a noninvasive system, however, results in less control of the airway. Patients must therefore be able to clear their own secretions.

FOCUS AREAS OF PATIENT MONITORING
1. Exhaled VT (EVT), which will be variable in this pressure mode of ventilation. The EVT should be at least 5 to 8 cc/kg. Prevent all factors that will

increase resistance to ventilation and decrease VT; for example, drain water from the tubing. If the EVT is less than the goal, atelectasis may develop, resulting in the need for increased ventilatory assistance.

2. The PIP. Determine whether altering the EPAP level also changes the IPAP level in the system being used to deliver NIPSV.

3. Mouth breathing. Consider the use of a chin strap if the patient tends to breathe through the mouth.

4. Pressure areas, particularly over the bridge of the nose, caused by the mask. Comfort between the interface of patient's skin and the mask is probably one of the most important areas of patient compliance. At the first sign of pressure, the application of a patch of wound care dressing may prevent further problems.

5. Monitor for gastric distention and place a nasogastric (NG) tube as necessary. The nasal mask can be fitted around the NG tube.

6. Monitor patient's nasal passages and upper airways for excessive drying. The addition of a humidification system is optional (nonheated, passover) and should be added on the basis of patient comfort and assessment of the secretions and upper airways.

Pressure Control

DEFINITION AND DESCRIPTION

Pressure control (PC) is a mode of ventilation in which there is a preset RR and every breath is augmented by a preset amount of inspiratory pressure (Fig. 7–12). In pure PC, each breath is time triggered and the patient is unable to trigger the ventilator to take additional breaths above the preset rate. This is achieved by setting the sensitivity so that it will not respond to the patient. Thus, with pure PC, each breath is a machine-cycled mandatory breath.

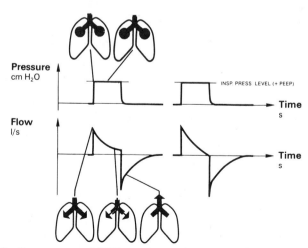

FIGURE 7–12   Pressure control (PC) ventilation. A preset number of breaths per minute are delivered, every breath being augmented by a preset amount of inspiratory pressure. Flow is delivered with the use of the decelerating flow-wave curve. Tidal volume is variable. Inspiratory/expiratory changeover is time-cycled. (Courtesy of Siemens Medical Systems, Electromedical Group, Danvers, Mass.)

However, PC may also be applied with a sensitivity setting that will respond to the patient, allowing additional breaths to be triggered. These additional patient-triggered breaths, called machine-cycled assisted breaths, are also augmented by the preset amount of pressure. Some authors refer to this latter application of PC as the pressure assist/control mode. With PC there is no set Vt. The Vt that the patient will receive with each breath is variable and is determined by the set inspiratory pressure, the RR, the inspiratory time, pulmonary compliance, and airway and circuit resistance.

The onset of inspiration is determined primarily by the timing mechanism. Once triggered, the inspiratory flow of gas is augmented by the preselected amount of pressure, that is, the PC level. This amount of pressure is held constant throughout inspiration. Flow is delivered with the decelerating flow-wave pattern, as opposed to the square or sinusoidal-wave patterns primarily used with volume-cycled modes of ventilation. With the decelerating flow-wave pattern, flow rate naturally decays as the patient's lungs fill with air on inspiration. Unlike pressure support, which is a flow-cycled mode of ventilation that gives the patient control over the ventilatory pattern, PC is time-cycled to end inspiration and begin expiration. The patient has no control over the ventilatory pattern.

INDICATIONS

PC may be used as a method of providing full ventilatory support in patients with noncompliant lungs who exhibit high airway pressures and poor oxygenation while supported by volume-cycled ventilation. PC can be utilized to get the airway pressure under the control of the clinician, who uses only the amount of inspiratory pressure necessary to achieve the desired Vt. In comparison with volume ventilation, in the same noncompliant lung conditions, the PIP may be reduced, thereby reducing the potential for pulmonary barotrauma. Concurrently, the mean airway pressure is increased, which improves oxygenation.

ADVANTAGES AND DISADVANTAGES

PC ventilation is useful as a therapeutic option for patients with adult respiratory distress syndrome (ARDS). Despite the use of volume modes of ventilation to support the respiratory system in ARDS, the mortality rate remains 40% to 70%. ARDS is a syndrome characterized by interstitial and, progressively, alveolar edema caused by increased permeability of the pulmonary capillaries. On the chest radiograph, the abnormality is evident as a diffuse alveolar pattern. The patient also presents with reduced pulmonary compliance, increased intrapulmonary shunt, and persistent hypoxemia despite increasing FIO_2 and levels of PEEP. Physiologic dead space increases because of extensive capillary leak and intravascular coagulation and eventually leads to a rise in the $PaCO_2$. Because of the nonhomogeneous distribution of the disease process, airways and alveoli with differing resistances and compliances (time constants) exist in adjacent areas of the lung.

Under the conditions described above, in which the lungs are very noncompliant and the disease process is diffuse, the delivery of volume-cycled ventilation with a square wave pattern may result in a high PIP and maldistribution of gases. The high PIP that is generated is associated with pulmonary barotrauma. That is not to say that the higher the PIP, the more barotrauma. Pulmonary barotrauma occurs when the PIP is high and there is uneven expansion of the lung and uneven pressure gradients between the alveoli. These conditions, which exist in nonuniform disease processes such as ARDS, lead to shear forces and injury in the lung. Reducing the PIP may reduce pulmonary barotrauma.

PC ventilation is postulated to reduce pulmonary barotrauma associated with high ventilating pressures and uneven gas distribution. Reduced airway pressures are promoted by limiting the application of inspiratory pressure to that which achieves the desired VT. This pressure is typically much lower than that which is generated with volume-cycled ventilation and a square flow-wave pattern. When the lungs are stiff and gases are delivered with "bulk flow," as with a square wave pattern, flow in the lung is turbulent, causing increases in lateral pressure and airway trauma. The decelerating flow-wave pattern used with PC ventilation changes the nature of the flow patten in the lung and promotes laminar flow, which is more ideal because it leads to a more even distribution of gas (Fig. 7–13). Laminar flow waves wedge their way into airways and alveoli, creating less airway trauma and a more uniform gas distribution. The decelerating flow-wave pattern has been associated with a significant reduction in total resistance, improved pulmonary compliance, a decrease in dead space ventilation, and an increase in oxygenation.

PC ventilation is more proficient than other modes in maintaining open airways and improving gas distribution. Greater proportions of average flow, pressure, and volume are delivered earlier in inspiration than when volume ventilation with a square wave pattern is used. The rapid initial pressure possibly assists in opening collapsed alveoli at the beginning of inspiration. Pressure is then sustained throughout the inspiratory phase, splinting the airways and allowing for improved gas distribution. In volume-cycled ventilation, flow is constant while airway pressure gradually rises to a maximum, possibly reaching the critical opening pressure of noncompliant alveoli at the peak of inspiration. However, at that point the flow stops and expiration begins, preventing noncompliant lung units from filling adequately.

When a pressure mode of ventilation is used, the mean airway pressure, which is the mean pressure in the airway throughout the ventilatory cycle, increases.

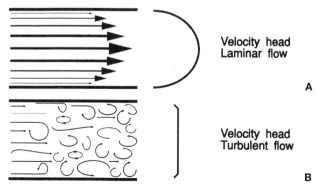

Velocity head
Laminar flow

A

Velocity head
Turbulent flow

B

FIGURE 7–13   Velocity profile of gas particles moving along the airways during (A) laminar flow and (B) turbulent flow. The decelerating flow-wave pattern used with pressure support (PS) and pressure control (PC) ventilation promotes laminar flow. Laminar flow creates less airway trauma and promotes a more even distribution of gas. (From Dupuis, YG: *Ventilators: Theory and Clinical Application.* 2nd ed. St. Louis: Mosby–Year Book, 1992.)

Mean airway pressure increases in pressure ventilation because airway pressure rapidly rises and is sustained at the PIP throughout inspiration. Mean airway pressure is a key determinant of lung volume and therefore oxygenation, both of which are sources of problems in ARDS. Manipulation of the mean airway pressure contributes to achieving the goal of restoring lung volume through the recruitment of collapsed alveoli and the redistribution of lung water, thereby improving oxygenation. Increases in mean airway pressure may be unfavorable in that they are also associated with reductions in cardiac output because of lung distention, which reduces preload and increases right ventricular afterload. Appropriate monitoring should be implemented when a pressure mode of ventilation is applied, so that a reduction in cardiac output can be detected rapidly and managed as necessary with preload augmentation and inotropic agents. The patient will not benefit from an improved PaO$_2$ if overall tissue oxygen delivery is compromised.

FOCUS AREAS OF PATIENT MONITORING

1. Be thoroughly familiar with all ventilator settings, including the inspiratory pressure level—for example, PC of 40 cm H$_2$O, respiratory rate of 20 breaths/min, 15 cm H$_2$O PEEP, and FIO$_2$ 0.6. In this example, PC of 40 cm H$_2$O refers to an inspiratory pressure level of 40, not 40 breaths/min. A common error is to believe that the PC level is the set RR. The likely reason is that an A/C or SIMV of 8 means 8 breaths/min.
2. With the pressure A/C mode, rapid RRs may result in respiratory alkalosis, air trapping, the formation of auto-PEEP, and hemodynamic compromise. Sedate the patient as necessary.
3. Monitor exhaled VT and minute ventilation closely, because any factor that reduces compliance or increases airway resistance will adversely affect VT. Conversely, if the PC level is not decreased commensurately with improvement in the patient's lung characteristics, the increase in VT may result in overdistention and excessive ventilation.
4. Monitor PIP, which should equal the PC level plus any level of applied PEEP.
5. Monitor hemodynamics closely, anticipating possible compromise as a result of increases in mean airway pressure.
6. Monitor and prevent airway cuff leaks, because the ventilator may not reach PC level and may persist in the inspiratory phase of the respiratory cycle.
7. See the discussion of PC inverse inspiratory-to-expiratory ratio ventilation, below, to learn how to make ventilator setting changes for optimal gas exchange.

Pressure Control With Inverse Inspiratory-to-Expiratory Ratio Ventilation

DEFINITION AND DESCRIPTION

Pressure control (PC), as previously discussed, is a mode of ventilation in which there is a preset RR and every breath is augmented by a preset amount of inspiratory pressure. Inversion of the inspiratory-to-expiratory (I:E) ratio is an additional strategy used with this mode of ventilation when further efforts to improve oxygenation are needed. The I:E ratio is inverted, 1:1, 2:1, 3:1, 4:1, in such a way that inspiratory time equals or exceeds expiratory time. This is done to improve gas distribution in the lung and increase the mean airway pressure for improvement of oxygenation. In addition to changing the inspiratory and expiratory times, the RR must be set rapidly enough so that the patient does not exhale completely before the initiation of the next breath. A shortened expiratory time results in gas trapping in the lung (auto-PEEP), which keeps the critical closing volume above the point of alveolar collapse (Fig. 7–14). Utilization of a terminal flow curve, if available, assists in the appropriate rate selection. Continuous monitoring of the flow curve can be performed by feeding this information from the ventilator into either the bedside cardiac monitor or a separate computer monitor. Because the ventilatory pattern is altered, sedation and medical paralysis are usually necessary to maintain patient-ventilator synchrony. Inversion of the I:E ratio, use of a sufficient inspiratory pressure to overcome the opening pressure of the lung, and use of a critical rate to promote the formation of auto-PEEP are strategies to improve oxygenation that build on the previously described benefits of PC ventilation. The section on PC ventilation, above, should be read as a foundation for understanding PC with inverse I:E ratio ventilation. In addition, please see the sections in Chapter 6 on inverse I:E ratios and auto-PEEP for a thorough discussion of these critical topics.

Indications

PC inverse I:E ratio ventilation may be used as a means of providing full ventilatory support in patients with noncompliant lungs who exhibit high airway pressures and poor oxygenation when volume-cycled ventilation is used. PC ventilation can be used to get the airway pressure under the control of the clinician, with only the necessary amount of inspiratory pressure used to achieve the desired VT. In comparison with volume ventilation, in the same noncompliant lung conditions, the PIP may be reduced, thereby reducing the potential for pulmonary barotrauma. Concurrently, the mean airway pressure is increased, which improves oxygenation. Inversion of the I:E ratio further increases mean airway pressure and promotes optimal gas distribution in the lung.

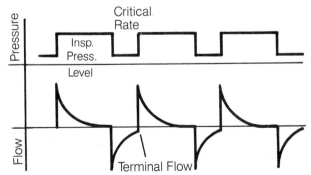

Figure 7–14 Pressure control (PC) with inverse inspiratory-to-expiratory (I:E) ratio ventilation. A critical pressure achieves the desired tidal volume and splints the alveoli throughout inspiration. The critical rate is determined by setting each new breath to begin just before terminal flow of the previous breath returns to zero. Appropriate rate and I:E ratio settings result in the desired formation of auto-PEEP. (Courtesy of Siemens Medical Systems, Electromedical Group, Danvers, Mass.)

Advantages and Disadvantages

In surfactant deficient lung disease such as ARDS, the pattern of pulmonary abnormality is diffuse and nonuniform throughout the lung. Lung units with varying resistances and compliances exist in adjacent areas of the lung. Alveoli with relatively more disease have longer time constants and require more time to fill. In conventional ratio ventilation, alveoli with long time constants may not have adequate time to fill and may remain in a collapsed state, resulting in persistent intrapulmonary shunt and hypoxemia. Inverting the I:E ratio increases the inspiratory time and thereby allows the alveoli with long time constants adequate time to fill, which improves overall gas distribution in the lung. Inspiratory time is prolonged to the point where it encroaches on expiratory time. On exhalation, the alveoli then do not have time to empty to their resting volume, and gas is trapped in the lung (dynamic hyperinflation). This trapped gas creates pressure in the lung known as auto-PEEP. Auto-PEEP splints the unstable alveoli at end-expiration. After this shortened expiratory phase, the lungs are rapidly reinflated before the alveoli reach their closing volume; therefore, fewer lung units collapse.

PC with inverse I:E ratio ventilation results in an increase in the functional residual capacity, a reduction in intrapulmonary shunt, improved oxygenation, and a reduction in dead space ventilation. The primary disadvantage of this mode of ventilation is that hemodynamic embarrassment may occur as a result of increases in both the mean airway pressure and the level of total PEEP.

Institution of PC With Inverse I:E Ratio Ventilation

The typical patient for whom inverse I:E ratio ventilation should be considered has progressively worsening radiographic infiltrates, increasing PIP, worsening oxygenation despite a high FIO_2 and a high level of PEEP, and a high minute ventilation. Table 7–3 outlines guidelines for initial ventilator settings.

The following important patient management and monitoring principles apply to the patient who is to receive support with PC inverse I:E ratio ventilation:

- Before implementing PC with inverse I:E ratio ventilation, ensure that appropriate patient monitoring has been implemented. Monitoring equip-

TABLE 7–3 Pressure Control With Inverse I:E Ratio Ventilation: Guidelines for Initial Ventilator Setting

Parameter	Initial Setting
FIO_2	1.0
I:E ratio	1:1
Inspiratory pressure (pressure control level)	Adjust to achieve VT of 10 to 12 cc/kg, usually accomplished at one half to one third of the PIP on volume ventilation; use lowest pressure that achieves best VT, minute ventilation, and $PaCO_2$ (in disease processes resulting in severely noncompliant lungs, smaller VTs may be desirable)
Respiratory rate	Adjust at sufficiently rapid rate so that before exhalation is completed, subsequent breath begins—usually around 20 to 25 breaths per minute; use terminal flow curve if available
Set-PEEP	Around 5 cm H_2O; remember that auto-PEEP will form because of inversion of I:E ratio

ment should include a pulse oximeter, electrocardiograph, pulmonary artery catheter, arterial line, and, ideally, an end-tidal CO_2 monitor. The clinician should be prepared to stay with the patient on implementation of this mode, to monitor cardiac and pulmonary response, and to manage hemodynamic alterations. All supplies should be in the room, including intravenous fluid for volume resuscitation and an inotropic agent, to be initiated and titrated especially if the patient has questionable cardiac reserve. All components of oxygen delivery should be optimized.

- The patient must be sedated and paralyzed. This will ensure patient comfort and prevent the patient from breathing out of phase with the ventilator. Patient interruption of the I:E ratio will result in a loss of PEEP, a reduction in the functional residual capacity (FRC), and hypoxemia.
- If available, a closed system should be utilized for suctioning the patient. This type of system eliminates the need to break the patient-ventilator circuit, with a resultant loss of PEEP. Suction as indicated by chest assessment and provide hyperoxygenation before each pass of the suction catheter.

VENTILATOR SETTING ADJUSTMENTS

As pulse oximetry and end-tidal CO_2 monitoring are performed and arterial blood gas values are obtained, the ventilator must be adjusted appropriately to achieve optimal gas exchange. It is important to introduce a key concept before oxygenation and ventilation are discussed as separate issues. When the PEEP is changed, an appreciation must exist that *any increase in the baseline pressure will decrease the VT* because the change in pressure from baseline to PIP is a primary determinant of inspired volume (Fig. 7–15). Consequently, when adjustments are being made in the PEEP to affect oxygenation, ventilation may also be

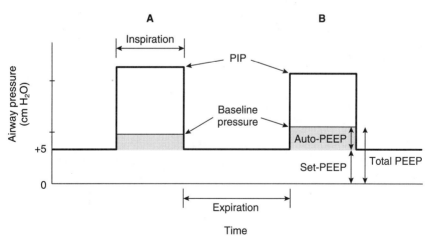

FIGURE 7–15 Pressure control (PC) and PC inverse inspiratory-to-expiratory (I:E) ratio ventilation. Any change in the baseline pressure that is not associated with a concurrent change in the applied inspiratory pressure will affect VT. The important concept here is that the change in pressure from baseline (total PEEP) to peak inspiratory pressure (PIP) is a key determinant of VT. In this example, both breaths A and B have 5 cm H_2O set-PEEP applied to them. Hashed area represents auto-PEEP, which is greater in breath B. Breath A will therefore have a larger change in pressure from baseline (total PEEP) to PIP than breath B and consequently a larger VT.

affected. The clinician must develop an understanding of this concept, which requires new thought processes regarding how to make ventilator setting changes and differs from the effect these parameters have on each other during use of volume-cycled modes.

Strategies to Improve Oxygenation (PaO₂)

- Increase the FIO_2, trying to keep it in a nontoxic range (<0.6).
- Increase the auto-PEEP by adjusting either the RR or the I:E ratio. Increasing the respiratory frequency shortens the duty cycle, shortening expiratory time, and promoting gas trapping and auto-PEEP formation. The RR should be increased in increments of 3 to 5 breaths/min. Utilization of a terminal flow curve provides visual guidance for the changes. Progressively altering the I:E ratio from $1:1 \rightarrow 2:1 \rightarrow 3:1$ will also increase auto-PEEP formation as expiratory time is shortened. The clinician must be prepared because this setting is the most difficult to change because of hemodynamic instability. Adjustment of the I:E ratio beyond $2:1$ should be done after the above-mentioned maneuvers have been used to their fullest extent.

Strategies to Improve Ventilation (PaCO₂)

- If the patient has respiratory acidosis, then the suitable response is to increase the minute ventilation. This may be achieved by increasing the inspiratory pressure level or increasing the RR.
- Increases in the inspiratory pressure level should be made in increments of 3 to 5 cm H_2O while EVT is monitored to assess patient response. An increase in the EVT is the desired response. If there is no change in the EVT and the PaCO₂ is worsening, then the pressure is exceeding the distensibility of the pulmonary tissue. Go back to the prior inspiratory pressure level and tolerate an elevated PaCO₂ (permissive hypercapnia; see Chapter 11).
- Increase the RR. After reaching a rate at which subsequent breaths encroach on the prior breath, further rate increases may raise the auto-PEEP, worsening the VT and CO_2 excretion. Be cautious regarding hemodynamic instability resulting from increased auto-PEEP.
- Conversely, if the patient presents with a respiratory alkalosis the minute ventilation should be decreased by decreasing either the RR or the inspiratory pressure level. When the RR is decreased, auto-PEEP may decrease, affecting oxygenation.

WEANING FROM PC WITH INVERSE I:E RATIO VENTILATION

When the patient is weaned from PC, the mean airway pressure should be maintained with the PC level and the total PEEP until the FIO_2 can be reduced to 0.5 or less while an O_2 saturation $\geq 90\%$ is maintained. When the patient demonstrates stability, the I:E ratio is the next setting to change. The inspiratory time is decreased cautiously because the response can be unpredictable. The mean airway pressure may drop significantly, especially on the initial change, allowing alveolar units to collapse, reducing the FRC, and leading to a deterioration in oxygenation. No less than a 6-hour period of stability should elapse before another change is made. Once the I:E ratio is at $1:2$, and if a set-PEEP greater than 10 cm H_2O has been utilized, the PEEP should be reduced before further weaning from ventilatory support.

FOCUS AREAS OF PATIENT MONITORING

1. Be familiar with all the ventilator settings and where to find both ventilator settings and patient data on the ventilator's control and display panels.

2. Monitor exhaled tidal volumes (EVт) because any factor that reduces pulmonary compliance or increases airway and circuit resistance will decrease the EVт.
3. Monitor the level of auto-PEEP by performing an end-expiratory pause maneuver for 2 to 4 seconds (see Chapter 6). The reading on the pressure manometer will be total PEEP:

$$\text{Auto-PEEP} = \text{Total PEEP} - \text{Set-PEEP.}$$

4. Monitor the PIP, which should equal the inspiratory pressure level plus the level of *set* PEEP.
5. Document data clearly and completely, ensuring that all caregivers are utilizing the same terminology, particularly when referring to the various forms of PEEP.
6. Monitor the patient's hemodynamic status closely because the hemodynamic effects of this mode of ventilation can be profound. Optimize all aspects of tissue oxygen delivery.
7. Ensure sedation to a level that suppresses the patient's respiratory drive. Institute paralysis as necessary. See Box 7–1 for PC inverse I:E ventilation case study.

Box 7–1 Pressure Control Inverse I:E Ventilation: Case Study

Male, 52 years old, who suffered multiple-system trauma including bilateral hemopneumothoraces. The patient had multiple hypotensive episodes that necessitated massive volume resuscitation. Two days after injury:

1. *Ventilator settings:* A/C 32, patient's rate 32, FIO_2 1.0, Vт 800, PEEP 18 cm H_2O, PIP 108 cm H_2O
2. *ABG values:* pH 7.29; PaO_2 45.5; $PaCO_2$ 47.5; HCO_3^- 22.9; BE −3.7/87% saturation

PC inverse I:E ratio ventilation was initiated:

Ventilator Settings	Patient Data	ABG
PC 40	PIP 50 cm H_2O	PaO_2 43
RR 28	EVт 630	$PaCO_2$ 55
FIO_2 1.0	$\dot{V}E$ 18	pH 7.25
PEEP (set/total) 8/22		Saturation 83%
I:E ratio 2:1		HCO_3^-/BE 24.5/−3.0

For correction of the respiratory acidosis, minute ventilation was increased by increasing the inspiratory pressure level. Oxygenation was improved by increasing the RR to increase the auto-PEEP formation. This made it possible to reduce the FIO_2. Recall that any increase in the baseline pressure will decrease the EVт if there is not an associated increase in the PC level. In this example, despite the increase in the PC level, the EVт decreased with the increase in total PEEP. This is likely explained

---

ABG = Arterial blood gas; *BE,* = base excess.   *Continued on following page.*

Box 7-1   Pressure Control Inverse I:E Ventilation: Case Study *Continued*

by the concurrent markedly shortened expiratory time. These ventilator changes were guided by pulse oximetry and end-tidal CO_2 monitoring and validated with arterial blood gas determinations.

Ventilator Settings	Patient Data	ABG
PC 50 ↑	PIP 58 cm H_2O	Pao_2 110
RR 44 ↑	EVT 500	$Paco_2$ 32
Fio_2 0.5 ↓	$\dot{V}E$ 22.4	pH 7.47
PEEP (set/total) 8/32 ↑		Saturation 96%
I:E ratio 2:1		HCO_3^-/BE 23.4/+1.5

Three hours later:

Ventilator Settings	Patient Data	ABG
PC 50	PIP 58 cm H_2O	Pao_2 173 ↑
RR 44	EVT 500	$Paco_2$ 25 ↓
Fio_2 0.5	$\dot{V}E$ 22.3	pH 7.50 ↑
PEEP (set/total) 8/34		Saturation 97%
I:E ratio 2:1		HCO_3^-/BE 20/0.0

The PC level was decreased to reduce the minute ventilation and correct the respiratory alkalosis:

Ventilator Settings	Patient Data	ABG
PC 42 ↓	PIP 50 cm H_2O	Pao_2 152
RR 44	EVT 460	$Paco_2$ 30 ↑
Fio_2 0.5	$\dot{V}E$ 20.4	pH 7.46
PEEP (set/total) 8/30 ↓		Saturation 97%
I:E ratio 2:1		HCO_3^-/BE 21/-0.3

SUMMARY

The various modes of ventilation give the clinician the opportunity to change the therapeutic option when the patient's condition changes. A thorough understanding of what is known to date about each mode's "mechanism of action" will contribute to sound clinical judgment regarding their use. Much is still to be learned about the appropriate choice of ventilator mode for the various conditions for which mechanical ventilation may be required. New knowledge continues to bring about change in the way we perceive and use the current modes. What remains the same is the clinical outcome goal: the provision of adequate oxygenation and alveolar ventilation, without compromise of pulmonary or systemic perfusion, while complications of applied therapy are prevented.

RECOMMENDED READINGS

Abraham, E., and Yoshihara, G. (1990). Cardiorespiratory effects of pressure controlled ventilation in severe respiratory failure. *Chest* 98(6), 1445–1449.

Al-Saady, N., and Bennett, E.D. (1985). Decelerating inspiratory flow waveform improves lung mechanics and gas exchange in patients on intermittent positive-pressure ventilation. *Intensive Care Med* 11, 68–75.

Branson, R.D., and Chatburn, R.L. (1992). Technical description and classification of modes of ventilator operation. *Respir Care* 37(9), 1026–1044.

Brathwaite, C.E.M., and Borg, U. (1990). Ventilatory support: Use of pressure modes in critically ill patients. *Critical Care Report* 1(3), 300–307.

Brochard, L. (1994). Pressure support ventilation. In M.J. Tobin (Ed.). *Principles and Practice of Mechanical Ventilation* (pp. 239–257). New York: McGraw-Hill.

Civetta, J.M. (1993). Nosocomial respiratory failure or iatrogenic ventilator dependency [Editorial]. *Crit Care Med* 21(2), 171–173.

Dupuis, Y. (1992). Pressure support ventilation. In Y. Dupuis (Ed.). *Ventilators: Theory and Clinical Application* (pp. 224–229). St. Louis: Mosby–Year Book.

Gurevitch, M.J. (1988). Selection of the inspiratory:expiratory ratio (pp. 148–152). In R.M. Kacmarek and J.K. Stoller (Eds.). *Current Respiratory Care*. Toronto: B.C. Decker.

Kacmarek, R.M. (1992). Methods of providing mechanical ventilatory support. In D.J. Pierson and R.M. Kacmarek (Eds.). *Foundations of Respiratory Care* (pp. 953–971). New York: Churchill Livingstone.

Luce, J.M. (1991). What to consider when choosing a positive-pressure ventilation mode. *Journal of Critical Illness* 6(4), 339–347.

Marcy, T.W., and Marini, J.J. (1991). Inverse ratio ventilation in ARDS: Rationale and implementation. *Chest* 100(2), 494–504.

Marini, J.J. (1994). Mechanical ventilation and newer ventilatory techniques. In. R.C. Bone (Ed.). *Pulmonary and Critical Care Medicine* (pp. 1–26). St. Louis: Mosby–Year Book.

Marini, J.J., and Ravenscraft, S.A. (1992). Mean airway pressure: physiologic determinants and clinical importance. Part 2. Clinical implications. *Crit Care Med* 20(11), 1604–1616.

Papadakos, P.J., et al. (1991). The use of pressure-controlled inverse ratio ventilation in the surgical intensive care unit. *J Trauma* 31(9), 1211–1215.

Pennock, B.E., et al. (1991). Pressure support ventilation with a simplified ventilatory support system administered with a nasal mask in patients with respiratory failure. *Chest* 100(5), 1371–1376.

Pilbeam, S.P. (1992). *Mechanical Ventilation: Physiological and Clinical Applications*. St. Louis: C.V. Mosby.

Poelaert, J.I., Vogelaers, D.P., and Colardyn, F.A. (1991). Evaluation of the hemodynamic and respiratory effects of inverse ratio ventilation with a right ventricular ejection fraction catheter. *Chest* 99(6), 1444–1450.

Sanders, M.H., et al. (1991). Nocturnal ventilatory assistance with bi-level positive airway pressure. *Operative Techniques in Otolaryngology–Head and Neck Surgery* 2(2), 56–62.

Sassoon, C.S.H. (1991). Positive pressure ventilation: Alternate modes. *Chest* 100(5), 1421–1429.

Sassoon, C.S.H., Mahutte, C.K., and Light, R.W. (1990). Ventilator modes: Old and new. *Crit Care Clin* 6(3), 605–634.

Tharratt, R.S., Allen, R.P., and Albertson, T.E. (1988). Pressure controlled inverse ratio ventilation in severe adult respiratory failure. *Chest* 94(4), 755–762.

Toben, B.P., and Lewandowski, V. (1988). Nontraditional and new ventilatory techniques. *Crit Care Nurse Q* 11(3), 12–28.

Tobin, M.J. (1986). Update on strategies in mechanical ventilation. *Hosp Pract* 21(6), 69–84.

Udwadia, Z.F., Santis, G.K., and Simonds, A.K. (1992). Nasal ventilation to facilitate weaning in patients with chronic respiratory insufficiency. *Thorax* 47, 715–718.

Wysocki, M., et al. (1993). Noninvasive pressure support ventilation in patients with acute respiratory failure. *Chest* 103(3), 907–913.

Complications of Mechanical Ventilation and Troubleshooting the Patient-Ventilator System

It is indisputable that in many circumstances mechanical ventilation is a life-saving therapy. However, the introduction of a machine to any clinical setting presents the need for the mastery of skills associated with a highly technical therapy and its potential complications. It is imperative that the clinician appreciate the problems associated with the use of mechanical ventilators, understand how to perform a respiratory assessment of the ventilated patient, and understand the proper function and troubleshooting of the patient-ventilator system.

COMPLICATIONS OF MECHANICAL VENTILATION

When mechanically ventilated, the lungs fill with gas through the application of positive pressure. Though positive-pressure ventilation (PPV) provides the benefit of adequate ventilation to the patient, it is also associated with complications. These complications are related to increases in thoracic pressure in general and, more specifically, to increases in mean and peak airway pressures.

Problems Related to Positive Pressure

BAROTRAUMA

In barotrauma, alveolar injury or rupture has occurred as a result of excessive pressure, excessive peak inflating volume (volutrauma), or both. Forms of pulmonary barotrauma include pulmonary interstitial emphysema, pneumomediastinum, pneumopericardium, pneumoperitoneum, and subcutaneous emphysema. Lung injury may also present as increased lung protein and fluid (edema) as a result of an increase in vascular filtration pressures.

When an overdistended alveolus ruptures, the escaped gas follows the path of least resistance. It moves centrally along perivascular sheaths toward the mediastinum, where it may rupture into the mediastinum or travel through pleural reflections of the great vessels into the pericardium. Alternatively, the air may dissect along fascial planes into the neck and torso, forming subcutaneous emphysema. Subcutaneous emphysema or pneumomediastinum is not likely to cause the patient a serious problem. Air in the pleural cavity (pneumothorax), however, causes varying degrees of lung collapse, adversely affecting ventilation. Progression to a tension pneumothorax may result in rapid cardiovascular decompensation. A pneumothorax must therefore be identified in a timely fashion and pleural decompression achieved through chest tube insertion (see Appendix III: Chest Drainage Systems).

High peak inspiratory pressure (PIP) is positively correlated with air leaks, which increase in frequency when the PIP is greater than 50 cm H_2O. Airway trauma occurs to a greater extent when gases are unevenly distributed in the lung. Gas flow is more turbulent under these conditions, creating greater shear forces. Predisposing factors for lung injury include high PIPs and volumes, a high mean airway pressure, preexisting lung disease especially emphysema and asthma, necrotizing pneumonia, and surfactant deficiency such as in adult respiratory distress syndrome (ARDS).

Lung damage may be minimized by preventing overdistention of alveolar units. Peak and mean airway pressures may be reduced by decreasing the tidal volume (VT), level of positive end-expiratory pressure (PEEP), and peak inspiratory flow rate; by altering the inspiratory-to-expiratory (I:E) ratio; and by eliminating the use of sigh volumes or end-inspiratory pauses. Gas distribution may be improved by using slower peak inspiratory flow rates, by using the decelerating flow waveform, and by administering bronchodilators when indicated. The use of prophylactic chest tubes for patients using high PEEP is an unresolved issue warranting further research. However, the clinician should be prepared for emergency chest tube insertion when the patient is at high risk of having barotrauma.

REDUCTION IN CARDIAC OUTPUT AND OXYGEN DELIVERY

PPV may result in hypotension and decreased cardiac output (CO). These complications are more pronounced when the lungs are compliant or when the chest wall is noncompliant because, under both conditions, more positive pressure is transmitted to the mediastinal structures. The hemodynamic effects of PPV are also more prevalent in the patient with hypovolemia, in the patient with poor cardiac reserve, and when PEEP is applied. Patients with high inflating pressures and on PEEP of 10 cm H_2O or greater should have CO and tissue oxygenation monitored through the use of a pulmonary artery catheter.

Three mechanisms are involved in the development of decreased CO under the condition of PPV:

1. Positive pressure increases lung volume, alveolar pressure, and pleural pressure. In the spontaneously breathing individual, venous blood return to the right side of the heart is promoted by negative pressure in the thorax on inspiration. With PPV, thoracic pressure rises above atmospheric pressure, resulting in decreased venous return to the right side of the heart (Fig. 8–1).

2. Pulmonary vascular resistance is increased as the increase in lung volume results in referred pressure to and possible compression of adjacent pulmonary capillaries. The right ventricular (RV) afterload is therefore increased, impeding the ability of this low-pressure, thin-walled chamber of the heart to eject its volume into the pulmonary vasculature and over to the left side of the heart.

3. Increased RV afterload may result in increased RV end-systolic volume, causing the interventricular septum to bulge into the left ventricle. This decreases the size, volume, compliance, and output of the left ventricle (Fig. 8–2).

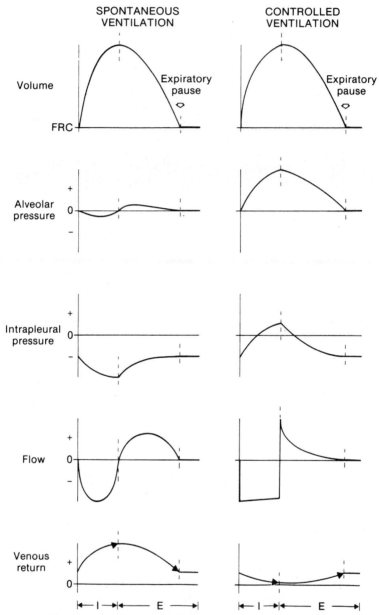

Figure 8-1 Physiologic differences in thoracic pressures under conditions of spontaneous versus positive-pressure ventilation. Flow = Pulmonary blood flow. (From Dupuis, YG: *Ventilators: Theory and Clinical Application.* 2nd ed. St Louis: Mosby–Year Book, 1992.)

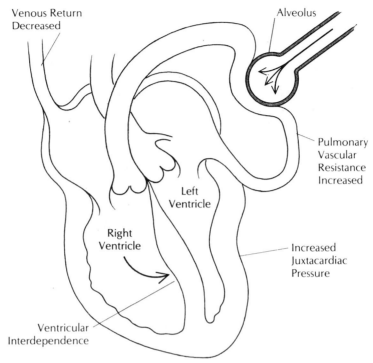

FIGURE 8–2 Factors responsible for a reduction of cardiac output during mechanical ventilation and PEEP. See text for details. (From Tobin, MJ: Update on strategies in mechanical ventilation. *Hosp Pract* 1986; 21(6):69–84. Illustration by Alan D. Iselin.)

Management of hypotension and decreased CO primarily involves the use of adequate volume to increase preload, followed by use of an inotropic agent as needed. Reduction of the mean airway pressure is also beneficial and may be achieved by using modes that allow more spontaneous breathing or lower peak inspiratory pressures.

Just as the application of positive thoracic pressure decreases venous return, its removal promotes return of fluid to the central veins. This may precipitate cardiac decompensation in patients with minimal cardiac reserve. Such an event could occur, for example, when a patient supported by ventilation in the assist/control (A/C) mode is disconnected from the ventilator for a T-piece weaning trial.

ALTERATION IN RENAL FUNCTION AND POSITIVE FLUID BALANCE

Under the conditions of PPV, renal blood flow may be decreased as a result of a reduction in CO. Furthermore, renal vein pressure may rise shifting blood flow from cortical to medullary areas, enhancing sodium reabsorption and decreasing filtration rate and therefore urine output. A decrease in renal perfusion, caused by a decrease in CO, "fools" the kidneys into thinking that there is an overall fluid deficit, with the result that the renin-angiotensin-aldosterone system is stimulated to retain additional sodium and water.

Fluid retention also results from a series of reactions that increase antidiuretic hormone (ADH) and decrease atrial natriuretic peptide (ANP). ADH promotes a decrease in urine output through fluid retention. ADH production by the posterior pituitary gland is stimulated by vagal receptors in the right atrium that sense the decreased venous return and interpret it as hypovolemia. ANP is a natural diuretic that also inhibits secretion of aldosterone and renin. When right atrial pressure rises with PPV (because pressure is referred back from the pulmonary circulation to the right side of the heart), secretion of ANP decreases. This results in less circulating natural diuretic and more aldosterone, and therefore sodium and water retention. Positive fluid balance is therefore primarily due to the kidneys' precipitating the conservation of salt and water through several mechanisms. Water can also be absorbed in the lung when inspired gases are highly saturated.

The patient's weight should be monitored frequently to allow fluid status trends to be determined. Diuretics should be administered as indicated. When peripheral edema is excessive, skin care must be meticulously performed.

IMPAIRED HEPATIC FUNCTION

Many factors may contribute to hepatic dysfunction in critically ill patients, prolonged application of positive pressure being only one of them. In the patient supported by mechanical ventilation, the downward movement of the diaphragm and impaired venous return to the right side of the heart may lead to an increase in portal vein pressure, followed by decreased portal venous blood flow to the liver and impairment of bile and hepatic vein flow. It is difficult, however, to discern adverse effects of PPV on hepatic function from manifestations of an underlying disease process.

INCREASED INTRACRANIAL PRESSURE

Persons who have had craniocerebral trauma, have cerebral tumors or vascular malformations, or have undergone neurosurgical procedures are at risk of having an increase in intracranial pressure (ICP) and/or a decrease in cerebral perfusion pressure (CPP) when PPV and PEEP are applied. Increases in superior vena cava and jugular vein pressure diminish cerebral venous outflow and as a result may increase the ICP. The CPP may be decreased if the CO and mean arterial pressure fall, as a result of increased intrathoracic pressures, when PPV is employed. Furthermore, the infusion of large amounts of volume to restore normal hemodynamics after the institution of PPV and PEEP should be avoided in patients with cerebral edema and increased ICP. Overall, high mean intrathoracic pressure should be avoided in the patient supported by mechanical ventilation who has an altered cerebrovascular status because ICP may increase or CPP decrease. PPV has no adverse effects on ICP in individuals with normal cerebrovascular hemodynamics.

VENTILATION/PERFUSION MISMATCH

Ventilation/perfusion ($\dot{V}/\dot{Q}$) mismatch may occur as a result of alveolar overdistention caused by elevated mean airway pressure, large tidal volumes, and use of PEEP. Alveolar overdistention results in compression of the adjacent pulmonary capillaries and regional hypoperfusion. This increase in dead space ventilation decreases CO_2 elimination.

Mechanical ventilation strategies should achieve optimal $\dot{V}/\dot{Q}$ matching, not worsen it. In nonuniform disease processes in which the VT is maldistributed, alveoli are especially vulnerable to overdistention. Strategies to reduce alveolar overdistention and iatrogenic $\dot{V}/\dot{Q}$ mismatch include use of low VT with high respiratory rate (RR) ventilation, reduction of PEEP as tolerated, and use of accelerating or decelerating inspiratory flow waveforms. In unilateral lung disease, independent lung ventilation may be indicated (see Chapter 11).

Problems Related to the Artificial Airway

To successfully manage the patient-ventilator system, one must pay detailed attention to the artificial airway. Complications related to artificial airways and the principles of airway management are outlined in Chapter 3.

Infection (Nosocomial Pneumonia)

Placement of an artificial airway provides a conduit for contamination of the lower airway. Bacterial contamination and infection may lead to pneumonia, especially in the presence of impaired host resistance. Factors contributing to infection in the patient supported by mechanical ventilation include poor oral hygiene; aspiration; contaminated respiratory therapy equipment; poor hand washing by caregivers; breach of aseptic technique during suctioning; impairment of the mucociliary system because of oxygen toxicity, inadequate hydration, suboptimal humidification, trauma during suctioning, or poor nutrition; and the decreased ability of the patient to produce an effective cough and remove secretions.

The principal mechanism for development of nosocomial pneumonia appears to be aspiration of gastric and oropharyngeal organisms, primarily colonized gram-negative bacteria, into the tracheobronchial tree. When these organisms overwhelm the patient's antibacterial defenses, pneumonia develops. Gram-negative colonization is known to occur rapidly in critically ill patients. Furthermore, gram-negative colonization is promoted by the presence of a nasogastric tube, enteral nutrition, patient position, and manipulation of the gastric pH with antacids or H_2 receptor blocking agents, common approaches to stress ulcer prophylaxis. Strategies aimed at reducing gram-negative colonization and nosocomial pneumonia include administration of aerosolized antibiotics, prophylactic parenteral administration of antibiotics, elevation of the head of the patient's bed to prevent reflux and aspiration of gastric contents, topical application of adhesive paste antibiotics to the oropharynx, gut decontamination with nonabsorbable antibiotics, and meticulous oral care. The role of each of these measures is not clear, and further controlled, prospective research is needed in this important area of pulmonary care.

Proper handling of condensate in the circuit tubing may prevent some infections. Circuit condensate should be viewed as infectious waste. It should always be emptied from the tubing and *never* drained back into the humidifier, because this action contaminates the entire water reservoir. Care should also be taken to avoid inadvertent washing of the condensate into the patient's airway. Respiratory therapy equipment must be adequately cleaned and decontaminated and equipment changes made as scheduled by protocol. Proper suctioning technique is essential, care should be taken to prevent aspiration, and proper hand washing must be performed. Aids to infection management and early detection include monitoring of vital signs and breath sounds, chest x-ray examination, observation of the character of the sputum, sputum culture and sensitivity, and leukocyte count. Prevention of all other contributing factors listed above should be attempted. Finally, the role of adequate nutrition in maintaining host defenses must not be minimized.

Patient Anxiety and Stress: Psychosocial Complications

The patient and family may demonstrate anxiety related to the disease process, diagnostic tests and procedures, and mechanical ventilation therapy. Some individuals may fear a grave prognosis associated with the use of an "artificial respirator." Their misconceptions may be a result of viewing television programs or reading books that are not factual in nature. Loss of hope may occur as the need for continued therapy becomes prolonged or if reintubation has been required. Alarms are also frightening to those who do not understand their function.

Patients have many reasons to be stressed and anxious. After all, they have lost autonomy over a vital body function: breathing. Their ability to communicate is also impaired. Disruption of sleep-wake cycles by procedures is common, and noise in the intensive care unit compounds sleep loss. The patient may be unable to determine day from night, the date, or the time. Position changes are limited by being attached to a ventilator, and physical restraint may be necessary to prevent self-extubation. Imposed immobility may create physical discomfort and frustration. The patient may experience pain from the endotracheal tube, from suctioning procedures, or from the tugging of the ventilator tubing on the airway.

The clinician should reduce anxiety by providing sufficient, which often means repetitive, realistic information relevant to the patient's and family's level of understanding. Periods of uninterrupted sleep should be arranged and meaningless noise and stimulation eliminated. A clock and a calendar should be placed within the patient's view. Frequent position changes are imperative, and the patient should be advanced to sitting in the chair or ambulating as tolerated. Whenever the patient is moved, the ventilator tubing should be supported to minimize discomfort and potential injury from tugging on the airway.

A means of communication, such as the use of a board with pictures or the alphabet, a magic slate, lipreading, gesturing, or pencil and paper, should be established. Reassure the patient that the loss of their voice is temporary and that speech will again be possible after the tube has been removed.

Gastric Distress

ABDOMINAL DISTENTION

Gastric distention may occur as air is swallowed or forced down into the stomach during use of a resuscitation bag and mask before insertion of an artificial airway. The stomach may become quite enlarged, and a gastric bubble may be evident on x-ray examination. A nasogastric tube should be inserted to decompress the stomach. Stool softeners should be administered as necessary because immobility and the inability to close the glottis may make defecation difficult.

STRESS MANIFESTATIONS: ULCERS AND GASTRITIS

Stress, anxiety, and critical illness may precipitate the formation of gastritis or gastric ulcers. Gastrointestinal (GI) bleeding is not directly related to the use of mechanical ventilation but more so to the severity of illness. Its incidence increases the longer mechanical ventilation continues and in severe respiratory disease such as ARDS.

Gastric pH and gastric mucosal blood flow are two important factors in the pathogenesis of stress ulceration. Manipulation of the gastric pH to greater than 3.5 markedly reduces the incidence of overt GI bleeding. The pH is generally manipulated with antacids or H_2 receptor antagonists. However, elevation of the gastric pH has also been associated with a higher incidence of gram-negative colonization of the stomach. Gastric organisms may be transmitted into the tracheobronchial tree, resulting in nosocomial pneumonia. The use of sulcralfate may lessen the incidence of gastric colonization and nosocomial pneumonia.

Gastric mucosal blood flow may be compromised if splanchnic blood flow is reduced during a hypotensive episode. This may result in gastric mucosal ischemia, tissue sloughing, and GI bleeding. The patient with inadequate perfusion pressure is therefore at higher risk of having GI bleeding.

The patient should be monitored for guaiac-positive nasogastric aspirate and stools. GI prophylaxis should be implemented early, and the gut should be used for feeding as soon as possible. The clinician should attempt to identify patient stresses and reduce them as much as possible, communicate with the patient in a calm and reassuring manner, and administer anxiolytic agents as necessary.

Complications Attributed to Operation or Operator of the Ventilator

Complications related to the operation or operator of the ventilator stem primarily from either carelessness or lack of knowledge of the ventilator's functioning. Examples of such errors are inaccurate settings, incompatible settings, incorrect assembly, and failure to set and activate all alarm systems correctly. The patient-ventilator system must be checked a minimum of every 4 hours, as described later in this chapter, and all alarm conditions must be investigated rapidly. Electrical and pneumatic failures can also result in failure to provide ventilation for the patient. A manual resuscitation bag with an O_2 flowmeter should be readily available at the bedside of each mechanically ventilated patient so that manual ventilation can be provided in the event of mechanical failure.

Accidental disconnection from breathing systems is a significant problem. The most common site of disconnection is the patient-machine interface. Disconnection from this site occurs more frequently in patients with a tracheostomy tube than in those with a nasotracheal or orotracheal tube. The likely explanation for the higher occurrence in patients with a tracheostomy is that the connection is made more gently at this site to minimize patient discomfort during manipulation. Other common disconnection sites include the exhalation line connection, the nebulizer connections, and the connections between the circuit tubing and the humidifier. Preventive measures include heightened awareness, consistent full use of alarm systems, rapid response to all alarm conditions, reduction of the weight and tension of the circuit tubing on the airway, and twisting of the component connections together, as opposed to pushing them together (twisting provides a stronger connection).

MONITORING THE PATIENT-VENTILATOR SYSTEM

The primary goals of continuous monitoring and frequent assessment of the patient and ventilator are to prevent complications and detect problems early, when they are easier to correct. The most efficient assessment is performed using a systematic approach. The patient-ventilator system should be checked (1) to evaluate the patient's response to the current level of ventilatory support, (2) to determine accuracy and appropriateness of the current ventilator settings, and (3) to ensure the presence and proper functioning of the necessary equipment at the bedside.

Monitoring the Patient

An understanding of the patient's medical history, current diagnosis, and clinical course is imperative in formulating a database that leads to sound clinical reasoning and decision making. Key components of monitoring the patient undergoing mechanical ventilation are identified below. The patient should be assessed at least every 2 hours and with any setting change, with the use of whatever portions of the examination are appropriate. The traditional techniques of the examination—inspection, palpation, percussion, and auscultation—are all performed. However, modifications of the traditional physical examination of the chest are required when the patient is undergoing mechanical ventilation. All findings should be described with terminology common to all caregivers. Furthermore, when the location of findings is described, the imaginary lines of the thorax are used (Fig. 8–3).

In the mechanically ventilated, versus the spontaneously breathing, patient *observation* of the ventilatory rate and pattern may not provide the same degree of information regarding disease severity. The reason is that varying amounts of ventilatory control are achieved by the ventilator, depending on the mode of ventilation used. Generally speaking, the more spontaneous breathing the patient is performing, the more useful are the rate and pattern indicators. Observation of the equality of chest excursion is best performed by observing the rise and fall of the exposed chest from the foot of the bed. Unequal chest excursion may be due to disorders or interventions resulting in unequal air distribution, such as

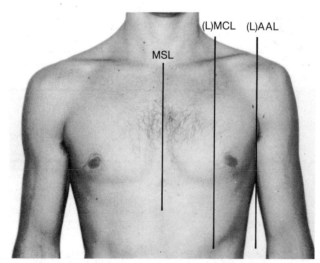

Figure 8–3 Imaginary lines of the thorax used to describe location of findings from physical examination techniques of observation, palpation, percussion, and auscultation. (A) Imaginary lines of the anterior chest. MSL = Midsternal line; (L)MCL = (left) midclavicular line; (L)AAL = (left) anterior axillary line.

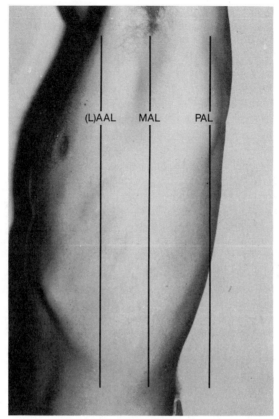

B

FIGURE 8-3 *Continued* *(B)* Imaginary lines of the lateral chest. (L)AAL = (Left) anterior axillary line; MAL = midaxillary line; PAL = posterior axillary line. (From Kersten, LD: *Comprehensive Respiratory Nursing.* Philadelphia: WB Saunders, 1989.)

TABLE 8-1 Percussion Sounds Over the Lung Fields

Sound	Description	Clinical Significance
Resonance	Drumlike, hollow, low-pitched sound	Normal air-filled lungs
Hyperresonance	Louder and lower pitched than resonant sound, somewhat musical or booming	Increased air in thorax, as in emphysema or pneumothorax
Flatness	Soft, higher-pitched, dull sound heard over very dense, almost airless tissue	Conditions replacing air with fluid or mucus: pneumonia, atelectasis, consolidation, pulmonary edema
Dullness	Soft, short, muffled thudlike sound heard over airless tissue	Lung tumor, pleural effusion; also heard over liver
Tympany	Loud, high-pitched sound heard over completely air-filled organ	Normally heard over stomach; large pneumothorax or herniated bowel

right main-stem intubation, pleural effusion, atelectasis, consolidation, lobectomy, pneumothorax, and pneumonectomy. Paradoxical chest wall motion is the sucking in of a portion of the chest wall on inspiration and its protrusion on expiration (the opposite of normal chest wall movement). This phenomenon is due to flail chest, in which several adjacent ribs have been broken in more than one location, creating a free-floating section of the chest wall.

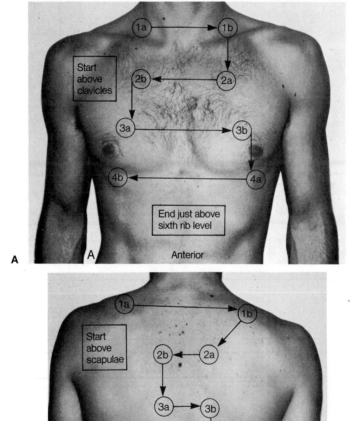

FIGURE 8-4 Sequence of systematic movements for auscultation, percussion, and palpation of the anterior (A), posterior (B), and lateral chest regions (C and D). Comparison of the right and left sides of the chest should be performed by moving from a to b, beginning proximally and moving distally down the chest wall. (From Kersten, LD: *Comprehensive Respiratory Nursing*. Philadelphia: WB Saunders, 1989.)

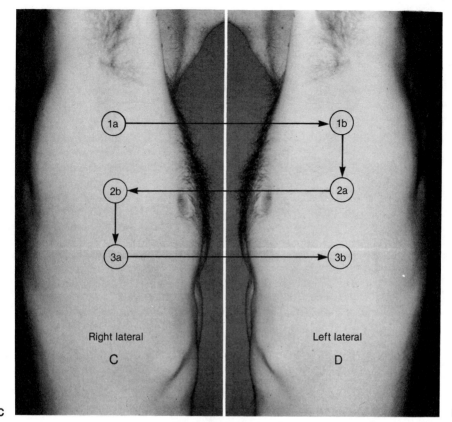

FIGURE 8–4 *Continued*

Palpation is useful in identifying the presence of subcutaneous emphysema or crepitus, which may indicate bony instability. The intubated patient is unable to perform the necessary maneuvers for eliciting tactile vocal fremitus or vocal resonance because the artificial airway courses through the glottis. Furthermore, in such a patient, palpation of the tracheal position will rarely elicit tracheal deviation because the endotracheal tube tends to splint the trachea. If the pathologic condition is severe, however, as in tension pneumothorax, the trachea may deviate, thus providing useful clinical information.

Percussion is limited by the ability to position the patient as needed and by the presence of wound and intravenous line dressings, incisions, electrocardiograph leads, and possibly braces or slings. Percussion may be used to gain further assessment data in a suspect area. Table 8–1 identifies the terms used to describe percussion notes and commonly associated pulmonary findings.

Auscultation is most often performed anteriorly and laterally in the mechanically ventilated patient, particularly in the critical care setting. Every opportunity to listen posteriorly should be seized. A systematic sequence should be used during auscultation, with sounds from one side of the chest wall compared with those from the other (Fig. 8–4). The clearest sounds, free of artifact, will be appreciated when all water is drained from the circuitry and when the artificial airway cuff is appropriately inflated. An air leak around a cuff may be misinterpreted as wheezing. The examiner should listen over the tracheal area for such a leak and correct it before completing the auscultatory portion of the examination. The stethoscope tubing should not touch the ventilator circuitry because air and water sounds in the circuitry will transmit to the examiner's ears. This artifact may be misinterpreted as adventitious sounds. Auscultation should not be performed over clothing because breath sounds, both normal and adventitious (Tables 8–2 and 8–3), will be more difficult to hear. The crackling sound of chest hair may be misinterpreted as adventitious sounds. Wetting the hair may reduce the amount of artifactual sound created.

TABLE 8–2 Normal Breath Sounds

Sound/ Description	Location	Cause	Clinical Significance
Bronchial—tubular, hollow, loud intensity, high pitched	Larynx, trachea	Turbulent flow of air through large airways	None unless heard over peripheral lung fields, which indicates consolidation. Normally, air-filled alveoli filter these sounds from reaching periphery. Consolidation creates more dense lung tissue, which transmits bronchial sounds to periphery.
Bronchovesicular	Main-stem bronchi; anteriorly at 1–2 ICS; posteriorly between scapulas	Turbulent flow in central airways; less intense and lower pitched than bronchial because of filtering of sound by chest wall tissue	None unless heard peripherally, which indicates consolidation.
Vesicular—soft, breezy, low pitched	Periphery of lung	Air movement through smaller airways	When diminished or absent, indicates decreased sound *production* (shallow breathing) or decreased sound *transmission* (less dense lung tissue, as in hyperinflation or partial physical obstruction such as with mucus). Absent vesicular sounds indicate that transmission is blocked, as in pleural effusion, pneumothorax.

ICS = intercostal space.

TABLE 8–3 Adventitious Breath Sounds

Sound/Description	Cause	Clinical Significance	Additional Descriptors/Comments
Crackles—discontinuous, explosive, bubbling sounds of short duration	Air bubbling through fluid or mucus, or alveoli popping open on inspiration	Atelectasis, fluid retention in small airways (pulmonary edema), retention of mucus (bronchitis, pneumonia), interstitial fibrosis	Fine: soft, short duration Coarse: loud, longer duration Wet or dry Other common (older) term: rales
Rhonchi—coarse, continuous, low pitched, sonorous or rattling sound	Air movement through excess mucus, fluid, or inflamed airways	Diseases resulting in airway inflammation and excess mucus (e.g., pneumonia, bronchitis, or excess fluid, as in pulmonary edema)	Inspiratory and/or expiratory May clear or diminish with coughing
Wheezes—high- or low-pitched whistling, musical sound heard during inspiration and/or expiration	Air movement through narrowed airway, which causes airway wall to oscillate or flutter	Bronchospasm, as in asthma, partial airway obstruction by tumor, foreign body or secretions, inflammation, or stenosis	High or low pitched; inspiratory and/or expiratory
Pleural friction rub—coarse, grating, squeaking, or scratching sound, as when two pieces of leather rub together	Inflamed pleura rubbing against each other	Pleural inflammation, as in pleuritis, pneumonia, tuberculosis, chest tube insertion, pulmonary infarction	Pleural rub occurs during breathing cycle and is eliminated by breath holding. Need to discern from pericardial friction rub, which continues despite breath holding.
Stridor—high pitched, continuous sound heard over upper airway; a crowing sound	Air flowing through constricted larynx or trachea	Partial obstruction of upper airway, as in laryngeal edema, obstruction by foreign body, epiglottitis	Potentially life threatening

Monitoring the Patient Undergoing Mechanical Ventilation: Key Components

VITAL SIGNS AND HEMODYNAMICS

Monitor blood pressure, heart rate and rhythm, temperature, and respirations, including patient and ventilator rates, pattern, and depth. Monitor volume status: pulmonary artery catheter readings, urinary output, intake and output, and weight. Monitor cardiac output. Finally, monitor the effect of the respiratory cycle on interpretation of hemodynamic parameters.

PHYSICAL EXAMINATION

Include in the physical examination patient comfort and work of breathing, use of accessory muscles, retractions, synchrony with the ventilator, and symmetry of chest wall excursion. Also observe skin color, temperature and moisture, and the presence or absence of crepitus or subcutaneous emphysema. Determine the presence and quality of pulses. Note the type, position, and stability of the artificial airway. Breath sounds are noted, including their presence and character and the presence of air leak around the cuff of the artificial airway. Monitor for air leak through the chest tube; the color, character, and amount of chest tube drainage; the color, amount, and character of secretions; the airway reflexes (cough, gag, and swallow); the presence of gastric distention; and the location, functioning and patency of gastric decompression and feeding tubes. Finally, determine nutrition status.

LABORATORY AND X-RAY FINDINGS

Monitor arterial blood gases (ABGs): oxygenation, ventilation, and acid-base status. Determine serum potassium, sodium, magnesium, and phosphorus concentrations. Determine end-tidal CO_2 value. Determine when the most recent chest x-ray film was done and its findings, the hemoglobin level, results of sputum cultures, and the leukocyte count. If resources are available, perform a more advanced assessment by determining the mixed venous O_2 saturation ($S\overline{v}O_2$), the arterial-venous oxygen content difference ($AVDO_2$), oxygen consumption ($\dot{V}O_2$), oxygen extraction, alveolar-arterial oxygen tension difference ($A\text{-}aDO_2$), percentage of shunt ($\dot{Q}s/\dot{Q}t$), and dead space/tidal volume ratio (V_D/V_T).

BEHAVIORS AND COMPLAINTS

Observe level of consciousness. Monitor for anxiety, fear, restlessness, agitation, confusion, disorientation, inappropriate behavior, somnolence, obtundation, dyspnea, degree of relaxion, sedation, pain, twitching and/or tetany, and psychologic wellness.

SAFETY

Provide appropriate application of restraints, secure airway safely, have spare airway of correct size readily available, and keep manual resuscitation bag and a mask at the bedside.

Monitoring the Ventilator: Key Components

The ventilator should be checked systematically on a scheduled, institution-specific basis, but usually no less often than every 4 hours. A check should also be performed before ABG values or bedside pulmonary function data are obtained, after any change in ventilator settings, as soon as possible after an event of patient deterioration, and at any time when the function of the ventilator is questionable. When caring for the patient, tune into the normal sounds of the ventilator and the patient's respiratory pattern as a means of providing constant patient monitoring.

SETTINGS
Check for correctness to prescribed order. Monitor information found on control panel: FIO_2; set rate; VT; mode; level of PEEP; level of pressure support or pressure control; peak inspiratory flow rate and waveform; I:E ratio or percentage of inspiratory and expiratory times; sensitivity; and sigh volume, interval, and multiples.

PATIENT DATA
Monitor the following information found on the display panel: peak, mean, and plateau airway pressures; PEEP; RR (ventilator and patient); exhaled VT (mandatory and spontaneous breaths); and minute ventilation ($\dot{V}E$). Measure compliance, resistance, vital capacity, and negative inspiratory force as indicated. Measure total PEEP as indicated to determine presence and amount of auto-PEEP formation. Monitor cuff pressure.

ALARMS
Ensure that all alarms are activated and appropriate alarm limits are set.

TECHNICAL CONSIDERATIONS
Secure all connections. Check system temperature and function of humidifier. Ensure patency of tubing and that water in tubing is properly drained by means of universal precautions.

TOUR OF ALARMS AND ALARM PARAMETERS AND TROUBLESHOOTING THEM

Alarms warn of technical or patient events that require the attention or action of the caregiver. They may provide audible and/or visual warnings depending on the severity of the condition but should never be viewed as being fail-safe. Though alarm systems on ventilators are becoming increasingly sophisticated, especially on microprocessor ventilators, they serve a purpose only if properly set. Furthermore, alarms are intended only as a backup to close patient observation.

In the intensive care unit there are many alarms. A ventilator alarm, however, may be the one with the highest priority. When it sounds, it may indicate a problem with the patient's airway or breathing, the two highest priorities in the ABCs (airway, breathing, and circulation). When any ventilator alarm sounds, the first thing to do is look at the patient. If the patient is disconnected from the ventilator, then reconnect the patient to the machine. If the patient is connected to the ventilator and is in distress and you cannot readily identify the cause, then disconnect the patient from the machine and provide manual ventilation while calling for help in troubleshooting the problem. Finally, if an alarm sounds and the patient is not in respiratory distress, determine which alarm is sounding and proceed with problem solving.

For rapid problem solving, clinicians must be familiar with the messages and keyboard on the ventilator with which they are working. In general, ventilator

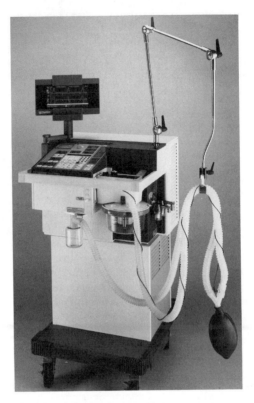

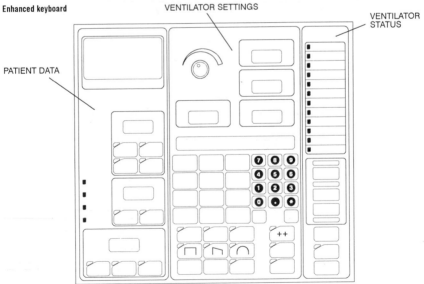

Enhanced keyboard

VENTILATOR SETTINGS

VENTILATOR
STATUS

PATIENT DATA

A

FIGURE 8-5 Rapid problem solving requires familiarization with the display and control panels of the ventilator in use. Several models are shown in Figures 8–5A to 8–5D. (A) Puritan Bennett model 7200ae ventilator (*top*). The basic keyboard (*bottom*) is divided into three fields: patient data (display panel), ventilator settings (control panel), and ventilator status (visual messages regarding alarm conditions). (Courtesy of Puritan-Bennett Corporation, Carlsbad, Calif.)

panels are divided into fields. A field contains dials that are grouped according to function. A field may be categorized further into an area of either display or control. The *control panel* is where ventilator settings and alarm parameters are established. The *display panel* provides patient information such as exhaled VT, minute ventilation, and peak inspiratory pressure. The control and display panels of several ventilators are shown in Figures 8–5A through 8–5D. The monitoring of the patient's ventilator in most settings is a collaborative function between the respiratory therapist/practitioner and the nurse. The respiratory therapist can also play an instrumental role in teaching the nurse how to quickly "read" the ventilator's messages.

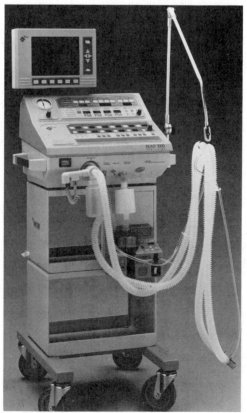

B

FIGURE 8–5 *Continued* (B) Bear 1000 ventilator. Display and control panels (*pp. 224 and 225*).

Continued on following page

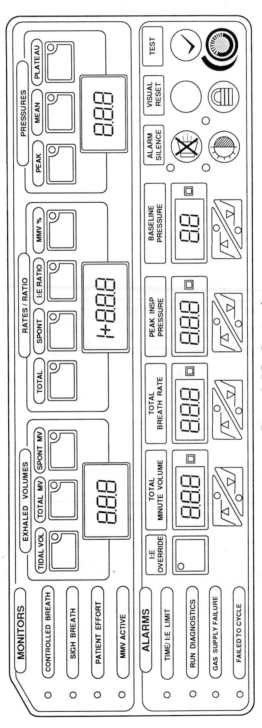

FIGURE 8-5 B *Continued.*

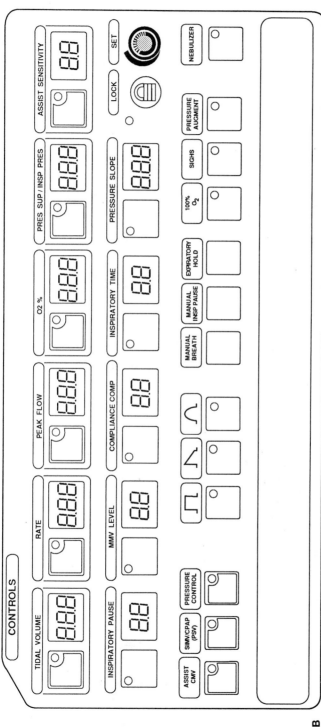

FIGURE 8-5 B *Continued* The control panel knobs have been logically grouped according to function (monitors, alarms, and controls) for simplification of operation and ease of use. (Courtesy of Bear Medical Systems, Riverside, Calif.)

Continued on following page

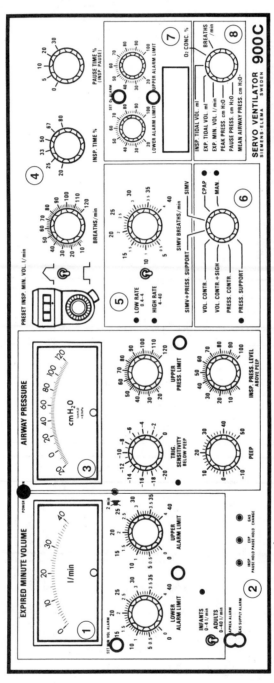

Figure 8–5 *Continued* (C) Servo 900C ventilator. The keyboard is divided into eight fields: *1*, expired minute volume; *2*, special functions; *3*, airway pressure; *4*, respiratory pattern; *5*, SIMV rate; *6*, mode selection; *7*, oxygen alarm; and *8*, parameter monitoring (digital readout of selected patient data). (Courtesy of Siemens Medical Systems, Electromedical Group, Danvers, Mass.)

Oxygen

Set above and below prescribed FIO_2. Alarm will sound if delivered FIO_2 deviates from the prescribed setting.

Cause	Assessment and Management
Set FIO_2 inadvertently changed	Return oxygen setting to prescribed value.
Intentional change in FIO_2 for delivery of 100% oxygen during suctioning	
Oxygen analyzer error	Calibrate analyzer.
Oxygen source failure	Correct failure (see low oxygen pressure, below).

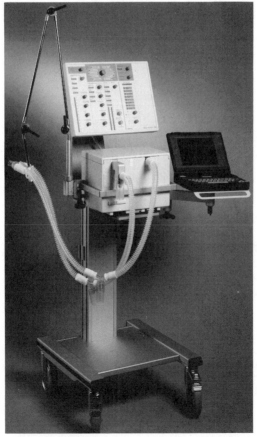

D

FIGURE 8–5 *Continued*   (D) Servo 300 ventilator. For easy and safe operation, the front panel (p. 228) is divided into eight fields.

Continued on following page

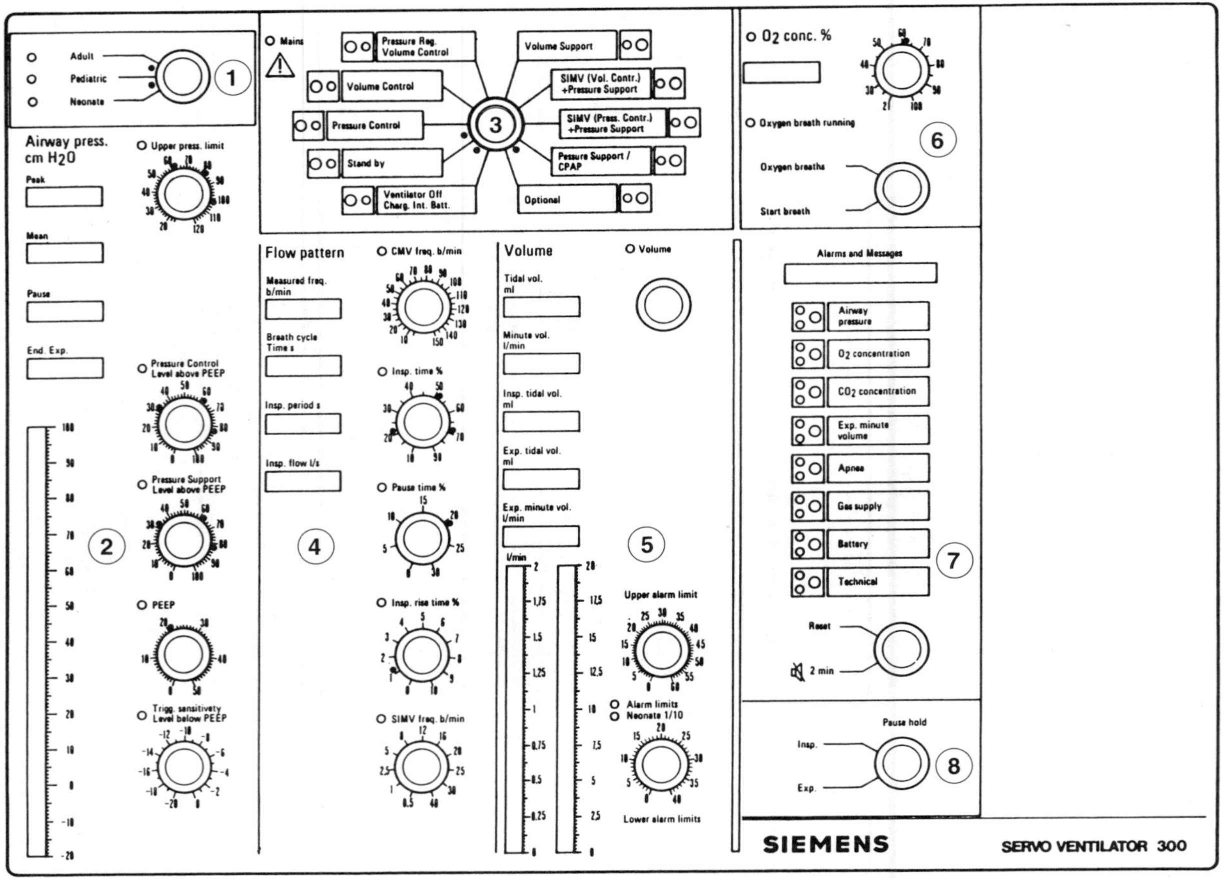

FIGURE 8–5 D *Continued 1*, patient range selection; *2*, airway pressures; *3*, mode selection; *4*, respiratory pattern; *5*, volumes; *6*, O₂ concentration; *7*, alarms and messages; and *8*, pause hold. (Courtesy of Siemens Medical Systems, Electromedical Group, Danvers, Mass.)

Pressure Alarms
HIGH PRESSURE LIMIT

The high pressure limit is usually set 10 cm H_2O above the patient's average peak inspiratory pressure (PIP). Alarm will sound if pressure increases anywhere in the circuit. When this alarm is activated, the ventilator terminates the inspiratory phase. Airway pressures are observed on a gauge on the ventilator display panel. The pressure gauge reflects, on a breath-to-breath basis, the peak inspiratory and end-expiratory airway pressures (Fig. 8–6). Normal PIP for a patient on a ventilator is between 20 and 30 cm H_2O. An increase in the PIP is due to changes in pulmonary compliance or airway resistance (see Chapter 2 for a detailed discussion of these essential physiologic principles). In general, airway pressure will rise more gradually if it is a problem with pulmonary compliance, the exception being the development of a tension pneumothorax. Changes in resistance to gas flow may cause the airway pressure to rise more suddenly. Compliance and resistance can be quantifiably measured, as explained in Chapter 2. Serial measurements may therefore be a part of troubleshooting the cause of high PIP and evaluating the effects of interventions designed to reduce the high pressure.

Cause	Assessment and Management
Increase in resistance to gas flow	Possible causes of airflow obstruction (increased resistance) include kinks or water in tubing, biting of tube by patient, secretions in airway, migration of airway into right main-stem bronchus, herniation of cuff over end of tube, and bronchospasm. Straighten airway and other tubing to eliminate kinks, drain water, place bite block or sedate patient, auscultate breath sounds for wheezes, and administer bronchodilator. Evaluate airway for change in placement; reposition if necessary. If unable to pass suction catheter or significant resistance is met during attempt to pass catheter, suspect cuff herniation. Deflate cuff and replace tube.
Decrease in pulmonary compliance	Pathologic conditions that cause the lungs to be "stiffer" such as atelectasis, pneumonia, ARDS, pulmonary edema, pulmonary fibrosis, and pneumothorax and hemothorax.
	Auscultate lungs for diagnostic clues such as crackles indicating edema, decreased breath sounds indicating atelectasis or infiltrate, and absent breath sounds indicating pleural space disease or consolidation.
	Assess chest x-ray film.
	Treat underlying pathologic condition with appropriate therapies: PEEP, mobilization of secretions with chest physiotherapy and suctioning, use of techniques that enhance ventilation such as turn cough and deep breathing, administration of diuretic for edema, evacuation of pleural effusion, pneumothorax or hemothorax.

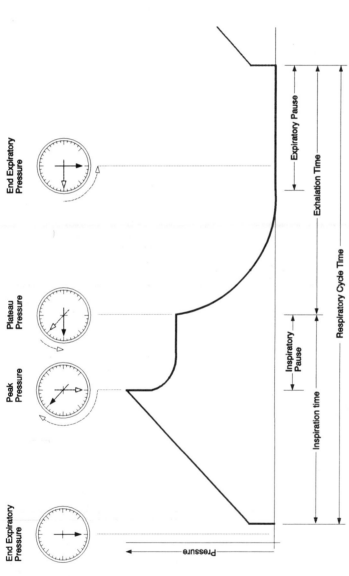

FIGURE 8–6 Peak airway pressure is a function of pressure created as a result of pulmonary compliance and airway resistance. When the PIP rises, a quick measurement of plateau pressure may assist in troubleshooting the cause of the elevation. The plateau pressure reflects alveolar pressure and therefore pulmonary compliance. The difference between the PIP and the plateau pressure, which is generally about 10 cm H_2O, reflects the pressure caused by airway resistance. If the difference is greater than 10 cm H_2O, the cause of high PIP is an increase in resistance to gas flow, that is, rising PIP with no change in the plateau pressure. If the PIP increases and the difference between peak and plateau pressures remains approximately 10 cm H_2O, then the cause of the elevated PIP is generally a reduction in compliance. (From Dupuis, YG: *Ventilators: Theory and Clinical Application.* 2nd ed. St. Louis: Mosby–Year Book, 1992.)

Cause	Assessment and Management
	Assessment findings accompanying a tension pneumothorax include a sudden increase in PIP, decreased to absent breath sounds, and hyperresonance on the affected side. The pulmonary artery and central venous pressures rise and acute cardiovascular decompensation occurs as a result of mediastinal shifting and kinking of the great vessels. Correct tension pneumothorax with needle thoracentesis, followed by chest tube insertion. Maintain chest tube drainage system.
	Correct causes of reduction in chest wall compliance: If patient is splinting respirations, then control pain, perform escharotomies on circumferential chest wall burns, and determine cause of patient's breathing out of synchrony with ventilator (see section entitled "Patient Fighting Ventilator or Breathing Out of Synchrony With Ventilator," below).
	Determine trend of serial measurements of static compliance. Adjust ventilator settings: decrease flow rate or V_T if possible, change flow pattern, or use pressure control mode.
Patient received sigh	Adjust pressure limit for sigh volumes.
Patient gagging, coughing, or attempting to talk	Determine what is causing gagging: for example, patient may be attempting to "tongue out" tube, tube may have been accidentally jarred or pulled, or patient may be vomiting.
	Correct problem, and reassure and calm patient. Suction as necessary. Explain to patient why they are unable to vocalize and that vocalization should be avoided. Develop alternative form of communication.
Patient "fighting" ventilator	See section entitled "Patient Fighting Ventilator or Breathing Out of Synchrony With Ventilator," below.

LOW INSPIRATORY PRESSURE

The low inspiratory pressure alarm is usually set 5 to 10 cm H_2O pressure below the patient's average PIP. Alarm will be activated if pressure in system has fallen and is not reaching the level that has generally been required for adequate ventilation in a particular patient.

Cause	Assessment and Management
Patient-ventilator disconnection, or leak in system	Determine cause of leak: patient-ventilator disconnection, loose connection in circuitry, site of in-line thermometer or airway pressure manometer, or leak around cuff of airway. Correct cause of leak.

Low Oxygen Pressure

The low oxygen pressure alarm warns of inadequate pressure in the oxygen lines supplying the ventilator.

Cause	Assessment and Management
Loss of oxygen source or loss of adequate pressure within oxygen source	May be due to accidental disconnection of oxygen line from O_2 outlet or to an array of problems generally handled by engineering department: for example, main oxygen line may have been interrupted because of construction occurring in another part of the facility. Check O_2 hose assembly for proper connection and reconnect if necessary. If main O_2 source is the problem, then quickly apply manual resuscitation bag to portable oxygen source and provide manual ventilation to patient.

Low Air Pressure

The low air pressure alarm warns of inadequate pressure in the air lines supplying the ventilator. If the air source is lost, most ventilators will provide 100% oxygen in an attempt to maintain an adequate source of fresh gas to the patient.

Cause	Assessment and Management
Loss of air source or loss of adequate pressure within air source	Check to see whether air hose assembly is properly connected. If ventilator becomes nonfunctional because its performance relies on high-pressure gas, then disconnect patient and provide manual ventilation until problem is corrected.

Low PEEP/CPAP

The low PEEP/CPAP (continuous positive airway pressure) alarm parameter is usually set 3 to 5 cm H_2O below the set PEEP/CPAP level. The alarm will be activated if the PEEP/CPAP level is not being maintained.

Cause	Assessment and Management
Usually a leak in the circuit	Systematically evaluate the circuitry for source of leak, make correction. Patient-related sources of leaks are around the artificial airway or through a pleural chest tube—because of a bronchopleural fistula, for example.

Volume Alarms

Low Exhaled Tidal Volume or Minute Ventilation

Volume alarm parameters are usually set 10% below the set tidal volume (VT) and the patient's average minute ventilation ($\dot{V}E$). Generally the low exhaled tidal volume (EVT) alarm is set 100 cc less than the prescribed VT. Some microprocessor ventilators will automatically set these alarms on the basis of measured parameters. These alarms are valuable for ensuring adequate alveolar ventilation, particularly in the patient whose respiratory status is frequently changing.

Cause	Assessment and Management
Patient disconnected, or possible air leak somewhere in the patient-ventilator system	Audible leak may come from mouth or circuitry connection. Patient may be able to phonate and may exhibit signs and symptoms of hypoxemia and hypercapnia.
	Systematically assess patient and circuit for source of air leak and correct. Common sites for a leak are at the patient-airway and circuit connection, connections in the circuitry such as at the humidifier, and at sites of in-line thermometers and airway pressure-monitoring devices.
	Air may need to be added to the cuff to reinstate seal (see Chapter 3 for technique). Leak may also be due to malposition of artificial airway.
	If leak is not immediately correctable, such as a large pleural air leak, then reset alarm parameters and adjust set V_T to compensate for volume loss.
Patient undergoing ventilation with pressure-cycled mode of ventilation and a decrease in compliance, increase in resistance, or patient fatigue occurs	Assess for and treat cause of decreased pulmonary compliance or increased airway resistance (see High Pressure Limit, under Pressure Alarms, above).
	Assess patient for other signs and symptoms of respiratory muscle fatigue: increased RR, irregular breathing pattern, use of accessory muscles.
	Provide additional ventilatory assistance by increasing inspiratory pressure assistance to achieve adequate V_T, providing an increased number of mandatory breaths, or placing patient on a volume-cycled mode of ventilation.
High-pressure alarm limit reached, causing ventilator to dump rest of V_T	Troubleshoot cause of high peak inspiratory pressure (see High Pressure Limit, under Pressure Alarms, above).
Wet flow sensor, which causes inaccurate measurement of exhaled volumes	Dry sensor and correctly reassemble.
Insufficient gas flow	Patient complains of not being able to "get enough air." Assessment findings include a prolonged inspiratory time in modes in which patient has control over inspiratory-to-expiratory (I:E) ratio. Correct by increasing the flow rate.

HIGH EXHALED TIDAL VOLUME OR MINUTE VENTILATION

Alarm parameters for high EV_T or $\dot{V}_E$ are set 10% to 15% above the desired V_T and $\dot{V}_E$. The alarm is activated when volumes of gas larger than the set alarm parameters are passing the flow sensor.

Cause	Assessment and Treatment
Increase in respiratory rate or tidal volume	Determine the reason that patient has increased $\dot{V}_E$: anxiety, pain, hypoxemia, or metabolic acidosis due to, for example, decreased tissue perfusion, fever, or loss of bicarbonate base through an abdominal drain.

Cause	Assessment and Management
	Determine cause of anxiety, reassure patient, and administer anxiolytic agents as necessary. Control pain. Determine cause of hypoxemia (see Low Pa_{O_2}, below) and correct.
	If patient has craniocerebral abnormality, the cause of hyperventilation may have a central neurogenic origin. Manage resulting respiratory alkalosis (see Respiratory Alkalosis, below).
Inappropriate or incompatible ventilator settings	Too high V_T, $\dot{V}_E$, or RR set on the ventilator, or alarm parameter not set appropriately for prescribed settings of V_T, RR, or $\dot{V}_E$.
Ventilator self-cycling because of incorrectly set sensitivity	Assist light is illuminated in the absence of patient inspiratory effort. Decrease sensitivity setting.
Excessive noise (water in tubing) as possible cause of false readings	Appropriately drain and discard all water from ventilator tubing.

Apnea

Alarm is activated when no exhalation is detected for an operator-selected period, usually set around 20 seconds. Some ventilators will automatically default to a safety mode of ventilation whenever apnea is detected. A message will appear on the ventilator stating that this function has been called into play.

Cause	Assessment and Management
No detectable spontaneous respiratory effort from the patient	Assess patient for respiratory excursion. If no spontaneous effort occurs, determine cause: lethargy, heavy sedation, respiratory arrest. Physically stimulate lethargic patient and instruct patient to take a breath. May need to use a mode that provides more support until patient is less lethargic. Weaning may have to be discontinued if apneic periods are frequent. Consider giving agents such as naloxone to reverse effects of narcotics.
	If patient is in respiratory arrest, remove from ventilator and provide ventilation manually with a manual resuscitation bag. If patient is pulseless, call for assistance and perform cardiopulmonary resuscitation.
Loose connection to exhalation flow sensor	Secure the connection.

I:E Ratio

Alarm for I:E ratio alerts caregiver when I:E ratio has exceeded 1:3 or is less than 1:1.5 (generally). Parameters may be altered when I:E ratios other than 1:2 are in use.

Cause	Assessment and Management
Incompatible V_T, peak inspiratory flow rate, and respiratory rate controls.	Check compatibility of V_T, peak inspiratory flow rate, and respiratory rate controls. Adjust as necessary. If V_T and RR are set correctly, adjust peak inspiratory flow rate to achieve desired I:E ratio.

Inoperative Ventilator/Machine Failure

A ventilator-inoperative alarm occurs when a fault is detected. A fault is a condition that jeopardizes the ventilator's ability to control the delivery of gas to the patient. When a ventilator is unable to reliably provide ventilation to a patient, the default response is usually either the opening of a safety valve to room air, enabling the patient to breathe unassisted by the ventilator, or the institution of a backup minimal ventilation mode. In addition, some microprocessor ventilators will perform a power-on self-test (POST) in an effort to detect and correct the cause of the internal problem. During the POST, one of the two methods of ensuring a source of fresh gas to the patient will be activated.

Cause	Assessment and Management
Loss of electrical power	Check electrical power cord for proper connection to working electrical outlet. The ventilator should always be plugged into an outlet that will be powered by a backup generator in the event of power outage. Provide manual ventilation until problem is corrected.
Loss of air or oxygen pressure	Check air and oxygen hose assemblies for proper connection and proper pressure. Provide manual ventilation until problem is corrected.
Internal hardware or microprocessor dysfunction	Provide manual ventilation and remove ventilator for servicing.

MORE TROUBLESHOOTING OF PATIENT PROBLEMS

Low Pao$_2$

A low PaO$_2$ is one that is less than 60 to 70 mm Hg with an O$_2$ saturation of 90% or less. The earliest warning signs of hypoxemia are changes in the clinical presentation of the patient. The patient may become restless, confused, and agitated; the heart rate, blood pressure, and respiratory rate may increase; dysrhythmias may develop; and the patient may complain of dyspnea. Ideally, this is the critical time to correct the hypoxemia, not when late signs and symptoms, such as cyanosis, bradycardia, and hypotension, have developed.

Objective early identification of oxygenation problems is most easily performed with a noninvasive monitor such as a pulse oximeter, especially in a patient with a tenuous oxygenation status. A change in the noninvasive value may be followed by rapid intervention to correct a readily identifiable cause of hypoxemia, or it may signal the need to obtain a blood gas. The PaO$_2$ and oxygen saturation are only part of an assessment of a patient's overall oxygenation status. To ensure adequate *tissue oxygenation*, one must achieve optimal oxygen delivery by ensuring an adequate hemoglobin and cardiac index, securing the physiologic states that promote the release of oxygen at the tissue level and reducing oxygen consumption.

Cause	Assessment and Management
Change in lung function, resulting in increased intrapulmonary shunt: for example, atelectasis, secretions, bronchospasm, pneumonia, ARDS, pulmonary edema	Rapidly assess patient for potential causes of hypoxemia that may be readily corrected, such as collected secretions, evident by coughing or increased rhonchi, or bronchospasm, evident by wheezing and elevated PIPs.
	Increase F_{IO_2} to prevent even transient hypoxemia until suctioning can be performed or a bronchodilator administered. To correct inadequate oxygenation, the primary two ventilator settings that are adjusted are the F_{IO_2} and the level of PEEP. (See discussion of pressure control–inverse I:E ratio ventilation, in Chapter 7, for further adjustments that can be made to achieve optimal oxygenation with this mode.) The F_{IO_2} is generally increased in increments of 0.1 to 0.2. PEEP should be added in increments of 2.5 to 5 cm H_2O if the hypoxemia is refractory and the F_{IO_2} is reaching a toxic level, i.e., >0.5.
	Alternatively, an inspiratory hold may be instituted to increase the mean airway pressure and thus improve oxygenation.
	Efforts to improve lung function, such as chest physiotherapy, suctioning, diuresis of edema, or administration of antibiotics, must be instituted simultaneously to making changes in the level of ventilatory support.
	Gather information to determine cause of increased shunting; for example, review the patient's history, perform a physical examination, obtain a chest x-ray film, and evaluate culture results.
	The hemoglobin should be checked for adequacy, and the patient should be prevented from fighting the ventilator.
Air leak, causing loss of PEEP	Low PEEP/CPAP alarm may sound. Utilize airway pressure manometer on ventilator to determine whether proper level of PEEP is being maintained. Troubleshoot source of air leak (around airway, ventilator circuitry, pleural space) and make correction.
Increase in intrapulmonary shunt as a result of a change in body position that places abnormal lung areas in the dependent position	Note body position in which decreased oxygenation became evident.
	Correlate patient history with chest x-ray findings of area of abnormality; for example, left chest wall bruising and rib fractures. Refrain from placing patient in "bad" lung-down position; use "good" lung down to achieve optimal ventilation/perfusion matching and thus oxygenation (see Chapter 2 regarding the effect of body position on $\dot{V}/\dot{Q}$ matching). Use pulse oximeter to determine trend in effect of body position on oxygenation.

Cause	Assessment and Management
Arterial blood gas error; sample drawn incorrectly or too soon after patient-ventilator disconnection	Wait at least 15 to 20 minutes after ventilator setting changes or after secretions have been suctioned before obtaining samples for ABG analysis. Eliminate excess heparin and air bubbles from specimen. Ensure that specimen container is capped tightly and kept on ice. Ensure that specimen is a pure arterial sample and contains no venous contamination.
Error in FiO_2, PEEP, inspiratory hold setting	Systematically check vent for correctness of settings and correct error.
Ventilator not delivering desired FiO_2	Low oxygen or low oxygen pressure alarms may activate. Assess air and oxygen lines for proper connection. If oxygen source has failed, provide oxygenation with portable oxygen source and manual resuscitation bag.
	Consider problems with oxygen blender, and utilize oxygen analyzer to confirm delivered FiO_2. Correct problem and reanalyze delivered oxygen.

High Pao$_2$

In general a PaO_2 of 100 mm Hg or greater is considered excessive and can be safely decreased.

Cause	Assessment and Management
Improvement in patient's lung function	Determination of whether to decrease the FiO_2 or the level of PEEP is based on the actual levels of these therapies being utilized. The FiO_2 should be decreased to nontoxic levels (i.e., 0.5 or less), followed by incremental decreases in the level of PEEP as described in Chapter 6 (withdrawal of PEEP).
	If a prolonged inspiratory time has been utilized, once the FiO_2 is 0.5 and the PEEP is 10 cm H_2O, the inspiratory time can be normalized. An inverse I:E ratio can be gradually reversed when the FiO_2 is 0.5, oxygenation is stabilized, and the underlying abnormality shows signs of resolution (e.g., improved chest x-ray findings, culture results, and measures of lung compliance).
Inaccurately high oxygen concentration setting on ventilator	High-oxygen alarm should sound. Correct setting.

Respiratory Alkalosis

Respiratory alkalosis is confirmed by blood gas findings of pH >7.45 with $PaCO_2$ <35 mm Hg. Because the $PaCO_2$ is inversely proportional to the alveolar minute ventilation, $PaCO_2$ is increased by manipulating factors that decrease alveolar $\dot{V}E$, as illustrated in the following formula:

$$\text{Alveolar } \dot{V}E = RR \times (V_T - V_D)$$

Where:
$\text{Alveolar } \dot{V}E = \text{alveolar minute ventilation}$
$RR = \text{respiratory rate}$
$V_T = \text{tidal volume}$
$V_D = \text{dead space volume}$

Therefore alveolar $\dot{V}E$ is decreased by decreasing the respiratory rate or tidal volume or increasing the dead space. Anatomic dead space remains relatively fixed in any given patient. Physiologic dead space is increased in pulmonary hypoperfusion, pulmonary embolus, ARDS, and by overdistention of the alveolus with excessive PEEP or tidal volumes. *Mechanical* dead space (the artificial airway and ventilator circuitry) may be manipulated during mechanical ventilation in an effort to alter the Pa_{CO_2}.

Cause	Assessment and Management
Factors that increase the respiratory rate (RR): anxiety, pain, hypoxemia, central nervous system abnormality	Confirm hyperventilation and respiratory alkalosis with ABG determinations. Reduce anxiety through calm, confident approach. Administer sedation and anxiolytic agent as needed. Assess and control pain. If problem is central neurogenic in origin, add mechanical dead space to circuitry between airway and ventilator wye.
Inappropriate ventilator settings of V_T, RR, or mode	Look at ventilator display panel for exhaled tidal volumes (EV$_T$). EV$_T$ should be 10 to 15 cc/kg for mandatory breaths and 5 to 8 cc/kg for spontaneous breaths. Decrease the EV$_T$ by decreasing the V_T in a volume-cycled mode (A/C or SIMV), or by decreasing the inspiratory pressure in a flow- or time-cycled mode (PS, PC). If SIMV and PS are in use, the EV$_T$ generated by each mode must be assessed and individually adjusted as necessary. If the ventilator's RR is too high, decrease the frequency of mandatory breaths in SIMV, A/C, or PC mode. If the A/C mode is in use and the patient is hyperventilating by breathing over the set rate, then the patient-related causes of increased RR must be ruled out and treated. If hyperventilation persists, then switch from A/C to SIMV mode.
Ventilator self-cycling	Spontaneous breath indicator flashes when patient shows no evidence of respiratory effort. Ventilator initiates inspiration before pressure manometer gauge reaches trigger level (2 cm H_2O below baseline pressure). Sensitivity is set too high. Adjust sensitivity to 2 cm H_2O below baseline pressure. Vibration of excess condensation in ventilator tubing may be read by the ventilator as patient effort. Discard excess condensation, using universal precautions.

Respiratory Acidosis

Respiratory acidosis is confirmed by blood gas findings of a pH <7.35 with a $PaCO_2$ >45 mm Hg. A rising $PaCO_2$ may cause the physical signs and symptoms of somnolence, obtundation, warm skin, vascular dilation, and headache. The $PaCO_2$ is determined by, and is inversely proportional to, the alveolar minute ventilation. Therefore the $PaCO_2$ is decreased by manipulating factors that increase $\dot{V}E$: increasing the RR or VT and decreasing the dead space. Anatomic dead space remains relatively fixed in any given patient. Physiologic dead space is increased in pulmonary hypoperfusion, pulmonary embolus, ARDS, and by overdistention of the alveolus with excessive PEEP or VT. *Mechanical* dead space (the artificial airway and ventilator circuitry) may be manipulated in the patient supported by mechanical ventilation in an effort to alter the $PaCO_2$.

Cause	Assessment and Management
Inadequate RR	Determine cause of decreased patient RR, such as acute neurologic event, oversedation, or metabolic alkalosis, and provide treatment. Increase RR setting on ventilator (assuming VT is set appropriately).
Inadequate VT	Monitor exhaled tidal volume (EVT) and compare with set VT. If deviation of 100 cc or greater exists in an adult, then evaluate cause of air loss, such as cuff leak, circuit leak, or pleural leak. Correct leak if possible. If leak is in pleural space, adjust VT to compensate for loss. If increasing the VT increases the air leak (by increasing bronchopleural pressure gradient), then increase the RR to increase the $\dot{V}E$.
	If EVT values are not 10 to 15 cc/kg for mandatory breaths and 5 to 8 cc/kg for spontaneous breaths, then (to increase VT) increase the VT setting in volume-cycled modes and increase inspiratory pressure in pressure- or flow-cycled modes.
Excess glucose loads in parenteral or enteral feeding solutions (As excess glucose is converted to fat, CO_2 production increases.)	Consider overfeeding as a potential cause of an unexplained, increased $\dot{V}E$ and/or failure of weaning. Patient who has limited ventilatory reserve will not be able to increase $\dot{V}E$ sufficiently to blow off excess CO_2 being produced; the result will be respiratory acidosis.
	Calculate nutritional needs. With assistance of dietitian, evaluate amount and source of nonprotein calories. Eliminate overfeeding. A high-fat, low-carbohydrate diet may be preferable for the patient with pulmonary disease because fat combustion yields less CO_2 than combustion of carbohydrates or protein.
Increased physiologic dead space	If caused by hyperinflation, chest x-ray film may show hyperinflation of nondiseased area of lung. Further evidence of increased physiologic dead space includes widened end-tidal to arterial CO_2 gradient and an increased CO_2 after increasing the VT or level of PEEP. Correct the problem by decreasing the VT or level of PEEP, if possible.

Cause	Assessment and Management
	If lung disease is unilateral and "good" lung is being hyperinflated, consider independent lung ventilation.
	If cause is worsening pathologic condition, such as ARDS, the caregiver may have to consider tolerating elevated CO_2 through use of permissive hypercapnia (see Chapter 11).
	Confirm suspicions of pulmonary embolus through diagnostic testing and treat on the basis of severity of embolus.
Increased mechanical dead space	Remove dead space tubing if present. Cut off excess endotracheal tube at $1\frac{1}{2}$ inches from teeth or nare after confirmation of placement by chest x-ray film. If increased mechanical dead space is potential cause of inability to wean patient from ventilator, then consider changing airway to a tracheostomy.

Patient Fighting Ventilator or Breathing Out of Synchrony With Ventilator

"Fighting the ventilator" is a phrase often used to indicate that the patient is having acute respiratory distress and the patient and ventilator are breathing out of synchrony with one another. Another common term used when the patient and ventilator are breathing out of synchrony with each other is that the patient is "bucking" the ventilator. Signs and symptoms of acute respiratory distress include dyspnea, agitation, use of accessory ventilatory muscles, nasal flaring or wide-open-mouth inspiratory efforts, tachypnea, abdominal paradox, tachycardia, hypertension, agitation, expression of fear, and diaphoresis. Multiple ventilator alarms, including high-pressure limit and low VT, may sound. A pulse oximeter may also warn of hypoxemia if the distress continues and cardiac monitors warn of hemodynamic instability and cardiac rhythm changes.

The primary goal of management of the patient in distress is to ensure adequate ventilation and oxygenation. The initial step is to disconnect the patient from the ventilator and provide manual ventilation with 100% oxygen. Rapid, systematic physical assessment and ventilator assessment should be performed to identify a cause of the distress. Acute distress in the patient usually involves the sensation of dyspnea, which needs to be explored by the clinician, using direct questions that the patient can answer with head nodding or pointing. Be cautious about releasing the restrained hand of a patient who is fighting the ventilator, because self-extubation may occur if the patient believes that the airway is the cause of the sensation of dyspnea. Call for assistance as needed in maintaining patient stability, assessing the cause of distress, and implementing appropriate measures to alleviate distress.

If the initial step of disconnecting the patient from the ventilator and providing manual ventilation relieves the respiratory distress, then the cause of the problem was likely within the ventilator. If the distress continues, then the problem is probably patient based. Table 8–4 delineates some of the most common ventilator- and patient-related causes of patient-ventilator asynchrony.

TABLE 8–4 Potential Reasons for Patient to Have Acute Respiratory Distress and to "Fight the Ventilator"

Patient-based Causes	Ventilator-based Causes
Artificial airway problems	Sensitivity set too high or too low
• Cuff herniation	Inadequate peak inspiratory flow
• Upward migration	rate setting
• Main-stem intubation	Inadequate ventilatory support or
Sudden increase in airway resistance:	inadequate delivery of oxygen
• Bronchospasm	Large air leak in circuitry or pa-
• Secretions	tient-ventilator disconnection
Acute change in lung compliance:	
• Tension pneumothorax	
• Pulmonary edema	
Acute agitation and anxiety, possibly because of inadequate sedation, emergence from street drugs, alcohol withdrawal, or pain	
Change in respiratory drive:	
• Central neurogenic hyperventilation	
• Fatigue	
Unknown development of auto-PEEP, which creates need for increased inspiratory effort, and thus work of breathing, to trigger ventilator	
Acute change in ventilation/perfusion matching:	
• Pulmonary embolus	
• Change in body position that leads to hypoxemia (e.g., lung with greatest abnormality placed in dependent position)	

RECOMMENDED READINGS

Ahrens, T.S. (1991). Effects of mechanical ventilation on hemodynamic waveforms. *Crit Care Nurs Clinics North Am* 3(4), 629–639.

American Association of Respiratory Care Mechanical Ventilation Guidelines Committee (1992). AARC clinical practice guideline: Patient-ventilator system checks. *Respir Care* 37(8), 882–886.

Campbell, R.S. (1994). Managing the patient-ventilator system: System checks and circuit changes. *Respir Care* 39(3), 227–236.

Fulkerson, W.J., and Piantadosi, C.A. (1993). Hemodynamic effects of mechanical ventilation. In R.W. Carlson and M.A. Geheb (Eds.). *Principles and Practice of Medical Intensive Care* (pp. 944–949). Philadelphia: W.B. Saunders.

Grossbach, I. (1986). Troubleshooting ventilator- and patient-related problems. Part I. *Crit Care Nurse* 6(4), 58–70.

Grossbach, I. (1986). Troubleshooting ventilator- and patient-related problems. Part II. *Crit Care Nurse* 6(5), 64–79.

Janowski, M.J. (1984). Accidental disconnections from breathing systems: What FDA found and what you can do about it. *AJN* 84(2), 241–244.

Johanson, W.G. (1982). Infectious complications of respiratory therapy. *Respir Care* 27(4), 445–452.

Johnson, M.M., and Sexton, D.L. (1990). Distress during mechanical ventilation: Patient's perceptions. *Crit Care Nurse* 10(7), 48–57.

Kersten, L.D. (1989). *Comprehensive Respiratory Nursing: A Decision-making Approach* (pp. 700–750). Philadelphia: W.B. Saunders.

MacIntyre, N.R., and Day, S. (1992). Essentials for ventilator alarm systems. *Respir Care* 37(9), 1108–1112.

Meijer, K., van Saene, H.K.F., and Hill, J.C. (1990). Infection control in patients undergoing mechanical ventilation: Traditional approach versus a new development—selective decontamination of the digestive tract. *Heart Lung* 19(1), 11–20.

Parker, J.C., Hernandez, L.A., Peevy, K.J. (1993). Mechanisms of ventilator-induced lung injury. *Crit Care Med* 21(1), 131–143.

Pierson, D.J. (1992). Complications of mechanical ventilation. In D.J. Pierson and R.M. Kacmarek (Eds.). *Foundations of Respiratory Care* (pp. 999–1006). New York: Churchill Livingstone.

Pilbeam, S.P. (1992). *Mechanical Ventilation: Physiological and Clinical Applications*. St. Louis: Mosby–Year Book.

Pingleton, S.K. (1994). Complications associated with mechanical ventilation. In M.J. Tobin (Ed.). *Principles and Practice of Mechanical Ventilation* (pp. 775–792). New York: McGraw-Hill.

Silver, M.R., and Bone, R.C. (1993). Selective digestive decontamination in critically ill patients. *Crit Care Med* 21(10), 1418–1420.

Strieter, R.M., and Lynch, J.P. (1988). Complications in the ventilated patient. *Clin Chest Med* 9(1), 127–139.

Task Force on Guidelines, Society of Critical Care Medicine (1991). Guidelines for standards of care for patients with acute respiratory failure on mechanical ventilatory support. *Crit Care Med* 19(2), 275–278.

Tobin, M.J. (1986). Update on strategies in mechanical ventilation. *Hosp Pract* 21(6), 69–84.

Tobin, M.J. (1991). What should the clinician do when a patient "fights the ventilator"? *Respir Care* 36(5), 395–406.

van Saene, H.K.F., Stoutenbeek, C.C., and Stoller, J.K. (1992). Selective decontamination of the digestive tract in the intensive care unit: Current status and future prospects. *Crit Care Med* 20(5), 691–703.

Noninvasive Respiratory Monitoring and Invasive Monitoring of Direct and Derived Tissue Oxygenation Variables

Monitoring the patient's respiratory status is one of the primary functions of critical care practitioners. The previous chapter discussed many aspects of monitoring data provided by the patient-ventilator system. This chapter will examine noninvasive and invasive methods for monitoring the patient's oxygenation and ventilation. The clinician must become thoroughly familiar with these commonly used techniques. When utilizing a pulse oximeter or end-tidal CO_2 monitor, one must know how to correctly apply and troubleshoot the monitors, interpret the data they provide, and respond appropriately to achieve optimal patient outcome. Blood gas interpretation extends from analysis of the direct variables provided by the arterial and the mixed venous samples to the derived variables obtained with one or both of the samples. Invasive methods of monitoring tissue oxygenation with a variety of configurations of the pulmonary artery catheter are in widespread use. Understanding the direct and derived variables that these catheters provide is essential to reaching the ultimate goal: preservation of *tissue oxygenation*.

Ideally the best methods of monitoring, whatever techniques are employed, provide the greatest accuracy with the least risk to the patient. Risk to the patient is minimized when the monitor is managed by a knowledgeable practitioner.

PULSE OXIMETRY: MEASURING OXYGEN SATURATION

Principles of Operation

Pulse oximetry is the continuous, noninvasive measurement of arterial oxygen saturation (SaO_2), which is the amount of oxygen carried by hemoglobin. When the SaO_2 is measured with a pulse oximeter, the abbreviation is SpO_2.

SpO_2 is measured by placing a probe on a finger, bridge of the nose, earlobe, or other translucent body part in which the pulsating arterial bed can be detected. The probe emits two wavelengths of light, red and infrared, from light-emitting diodes (LED). The light is transmitted through the body part and received by a photodetector (PD) on the other side. The PD utilizes the principles of spectrophotometry to determine the amount of light absorbed as it passes through the body part (Fig. 9–1). The red light is readily absorbed by deoxygenated (reduced) hemoglobin, and the infrared light is absorbed by the oxyhemoglobin (HbO_2). This information is then carried to the pulse oximeter monitor which performs a logarithmic computation and displays a digital readout of the ratio of saturated hemoglobin to total hemoglobin as illustrated in the following formula:

$$SpO_2 = \frac{HbO_2}{Hb + HbO_2}$$

The pulse oximeter measures the amount of deoxygenated hemoglobin (Hb) and oxygenated hemoglobin (HbO_2). Total Hb is the sum of Hb and HbO_2. The SpO_2 value is the percentage of total hemoglobin that is hemoglobin saturated with oxygen.

To differentiate arterial from venous blood, the pulse oximeter utilizes the principles of plethysmography to measure a change in volume. Identification of the arterial blood is accomplished by the recognition that arterial blood pulsates, whereas other optical components such as venous blood and tissue do not. The pulsating arterial bed dilates at systole, the blood volume increases, and so does the light absorption. Light absorbed by skin, bone, tissue, and venous blood is constant and therefore represents a baseline (Fig. 9–2). The pulse oximeter assumes that only pulsatile absorbance is arterial blood.

Most pulse oximeters have features that provide graphic information about the amplitude of the pulse signal being received. Many oximeters provide a real-time waveform that confirms reception of the arterial pulsation. Some oximeters feature a lighted, segmented vertical column. The height of the light on the column will rise with increases in the pulse amplitude, thus providing the operator with a visual cue as to pulse amplitude. Other oximeters provide auditory cues about pulse amplitude. The intensity, or pitch, of a beep tone will vary to correspond with pulse amplitude. Both methods, auditory and visual, may be present on some models. Verification of the adequacy of the pulse amplitude is essential for ensuring the accuracy of the SpO_2 value.

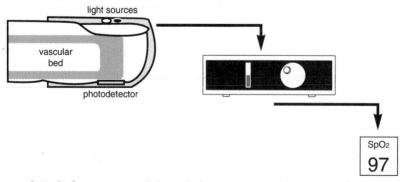

FIGURE 9–1 Light is transmitted through the translucent body part from light-emitting diodes (LEDs). A photodetector opposite the LEDs detects how much light passes through, unabsorbed by Hb or HbO_2. See text for further explanation. (Reprinted with permission. Copyright Nellcor Incorporated, Pleasanton, Calif.)

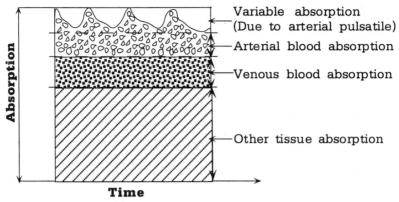

FIGURE 9-2 Absorption of light is translated into a plethysmographic waveform. Light absorption by venous blood and tissues is constant. Absorption of light by the arterial bed is variable because of the expanding vascular volume during systole. (From Petty, TL: *Clinical Pulse Oximetry.* Monograph of the Webb-Waring Lung Institute, Denver, Colo., 1986. Sponsored by Ohmeda.)

Accuracy

Investigators focusing on critically ill patients have concluded that pulse oximeters are accurate within 2% in the saturation range of 70% to 99.9%. Accurate oximeter readings can be obtained through dirty or burned skin.

Errors in SpO_2 measurement are introduced by several factors that either exceed the capabilities of, or interfere with, the instrument's two wavelengths of light or its spectrophotometric analysis. The presence of dysfunctional hemoglobins, notably carboxyhemoglobin (COHb) and methemoglobin, leads to falsely high and low SpO_2 values, respectively, as compared to co-oximeter assessed SaO_2. These hemoglobins are not detected by the two-wavelength system; therefore the total hemoglobin is incorrectly calculated. An instrument with four wavelengths of light is required to detect these abnormal hemoglobins. Clinically the amount of dysfunctional hemoglobins is usually negligible, and therefore a two-wave length analysis is generally sufficient. In cases of inhalation injury, however, when the amount of COHb can be significant, the pulse oximeter while accurately calculating SpO_2 may not be a reliable indicator of total oxygen saturation. When COHb is present, SpO_2 can be used to determine how well normal Hb is saturated and whether it is functioning optimally. A co-oximeter SaO_2, however, must be intermittently assessed to determine the total Hb saturation.

Several other factors may affect light transmission, absorption, or analysis. Three vascular dyes—methylene blue, indigo carmine, and indocyanine green—have all been reported to cause abrupt, transient decreases in SpO_2 measurements. In individuals with deeply pigmented skin, oximeter readings have been found to be slightly less accurate and more technical problems may occur. Most nail polishes have no effect on oximeter readings, with the exception of black, blue, green, and frosted, which cause erroneously low readings. Synthetic fingernails that are very thick may also adversely affect oximeter accuracy.

Error in SpO_2 measurement is also introduced by factors that dampen the phethysmographic signal. Any event that significantly reduces vascular pulsations will reduce the instrument's ability to perform plethysmographic analysis.

Such events include significant hypothermia, hypotension (mean blood pressure less than 50 mm Hg), infusion of vasoconstrictive drugs at high doses, and direct arterial compression, such as with application of a blood pressure cuff.

Advantages and Limitations of Pulse Oximetry

Some advantages of the pulse oximeter are as follows: It is noninvasive and therefore painless. It requires no calibration and minimal site preparation, making it quick and easy to apply. The measurement of SpO_2 is in real time and continuous, and therefore the time delay and sporadic monitoring associated with arterial blood gas determination are eliminated. Pulse oximetry is a valuable tool for routine monitoring of the patient at risk of having hypoxemia.

The biggest dangers in applying pulse oximetry are in misinterpreting the value and in using it as a monitor of ventilation status. The relationship of SpO_2 to PaO_2 is expressed in the oxygen hemoglobin dissociation curve (Fig. 9–3). This is a sigmoid-shaped curve, and therefore SpO_2 and PaO_2 are not linearly related (see Chapter 2). One must recognize that when the SpO_2 is 90%, the PaO_2 is around 60 mm Hg under conditions of normal body temperature, pH, $PaCO_2$, and blood levels of 2,3-diphosphoglycerate (2,3-DPG). Changes in these factors cause the curve to shift to the right or left. This increases or decreases, respectively, the affinity of oxygen to hemoglobin and therefore the relationship of SaO_2 to PaO_2. Correct interpretation of SpO_2 requires taking into consideration all factors present in the patient that may cause a shift in the oxyhemoglobin dissociation curve.

The pulse oximeter can be used for patients of any age. SpO_2 monitoring is useful during anesthesia, during transport of patients from the operating room to the recovery room or from the intensive care unit to a procedure site or another

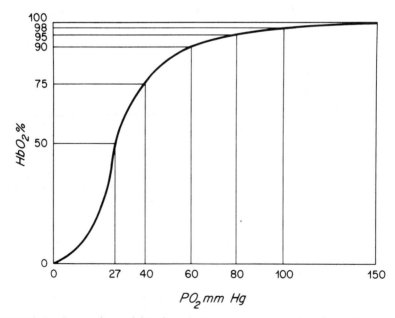

FIGURE 9–3 Oxygen-hemoglobin dissociation curve expresses the relationship between SaO_2 and PaO_2. (From Kacmarek, RM, and Stoller, JK: *Current Respiratory Care*. Toronto: BC Decker, 1988.)

nursing unit. In the critical care unit, pulse oximetry is useful in determining a patient's oxygenation status during procedures such as bronchoscopy, suctioning, and turning, or while patients are undergoing oxygen therapy with low- or high-flow systems or mechanical ventilation. It must be recognized that pulse oximetry alone may not be useful during the process of weaning from mechanical ventilation because it does not reflect changes in ventilation ($PaCO_2$). It is also useful for evaluation of patients with sleep-disordered breathing, in emergency medicine, and in dental and outpatient surgical settings. Pulse oximeters may also be used to monitor the adequacy of perfusion distal to a surgical or traumatic injury such as after digit or extremity reimplantation surgery.

Technical Limitations and Suggestions for Their Alleviation

There are technologic limitations to pulse oximeters, just as with any technology utilized in the intensive care unit (ICU). Therefore it is important for the clinician to be able to troubleshoot problems that may occur and thus to maintain accuracy of the values obtained.

Optical interference occurs when ambient light is allowed to reach the PD. Ambient light detection by the PD creates inaccuracies or, sometimes, complete loss of measurement. Most oximeters are designed to reject ambient light; however, when the intensity of ambient light is high (as from a heat lamp or from sunlight), the photodetector cannot sense the light transmitted through tissue or calculate SpO_2. The digital display may remain blank, the unit may show a falsely low pulse rate or SpO_2, or the unit may show by activation of an alarm that there has been a loss of signal. Protecting the PD from bright light sources (such as procedure or bilirubin lights, direct sunlight, or heating lamps) by covering it with an opaque material will obviate the problem. Optical interference can also occur when the sensor's optical components are misplaced, such as when the sensor has been applied too loosely.

Another technical problem that may occur during use of an oximeter is *optical shunting*. This occurs when part of the light from the light-emitting diodes reaches the photodetector without passing through the finger (i.e., it travels around the finger to the PD). The displayed saturation is a combination of the patient's actual saturation and the value the oximeter calculates when light directly travels from the LED to the PD. Correct alignment of the LED and the PD, so that they are opposite each other and flush to the skin, will eliminate optical shunting.

Incorrect choice or application of the oximeter probe may also lead to technical problems. Choosing the proper size and type of sensor for the patient helps eliminate optical interference, optical shunting, and loss of signal. Sensors may be reusable (durable) or single use (disposable) (Fig. 9–4). Cost, setting, and patient size are factors to consider when choosing a sensor. When applying the sensor, the clinician must be sure that it is free of body oils or dirt that will affect its sensing capability. The sensor may be cleaned with alcohol as necessary.

Factors that lead to venous congestion or venous pulsation cause erroneously low SpO_2 values to be reported because the venous bed is misinterpreted as arterial. The sensor should be applied snugly, but not too tightly, around the monitoring site. Ensure that the sensor is not constrictive, prevent dependent positioning of the monitored site, and avoid tight-fitting garments on a monitored extremity.

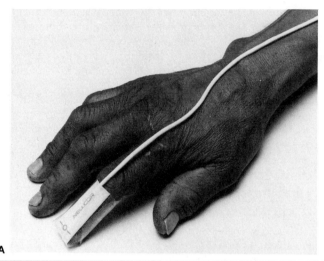

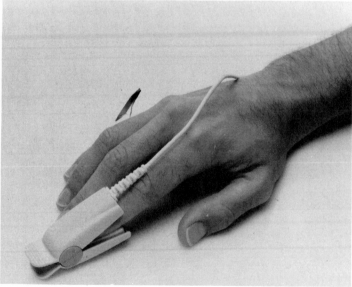

FIGURE 9–4 Reusable and disposable pulse oximeter sensors. (A) Disposable, adult sterile adhesive sensor. (B) Reusable clip-style finger sensor.

Instituting Pulse Oximetry

After correctly choosing and applying the sensor probe, perform auditory and/or visual verification of the arterial signal to confirm that the pulse signal is adequate to provide accurate optical measurements. Obtain an arterial blood gas (ABG) and compare the SpO_2 reading taken concurrently with the laboratory-determined SaO_2 to determine an acceptable correlation. To be considered accurate, the SpO_2 and SaO_2 values should be within 2% of each other. Troubleshoot >2% disparities by checking the monitor for proper function and searching for the presence of factors that cause erroneous SpO_2 values. Set HIGH and LOW pulse

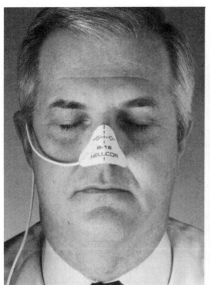
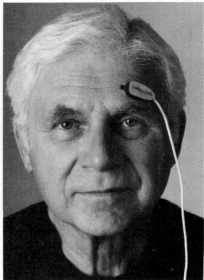

C

D

FIGURE 9–4 *Continued* (C) Disposable, adult nasal sensor. (D) Limited-reuse adult reflectance sensor. Application of sensor is to forehead or temple. The manufacturer's directions for use of each sensor should be carefully followed for optimal performance. (Photos courtesy of Nellcor Incorporated, Pleasanton, Calif.)

and SpO_2 alarm parameters and alarm volume. Pulse alarms, if present, should be set at 10 beats/min above and below the patient's heart rate. The SpO_2 high alarm should be set at 100%, and the low alarm at the minimum acceptable SpO_2 as determined by the physician's order or by institution protocol.

END-TIDAL CO₂ MONITORING

End-tidal CO_2 (etCO_2) monitoring is the noninvasive, trend measurement of alveolar CO_2 at the end of exhalation, when CO_2 concentration is at its peak. It can be measured at the bedside with a monitor that both numerically and graphically displays values of exhaled carbon dioxide (CO_2). The measurement and numeric display of the amount of CO_2 in respired gases is known as capnometry, whereas capnography is the measurement and graphic display of respired gases in a waveform known as a capnogram. Primary application of etCO_2 monitoring is in the monitoring of the patient's ventilatory ($PaCO_2$) status.

Principles of Operation

Monitors that measure etCO_2 utilize either of two methods of analyzing exhaled gases for CO_2 concentration: mass spectrometry or infrared absorption spectrophotometry. A mass spectrometer is an instrument capable of analyzing a gas sample for its concentrations of oxygen, carbon dioxide, nitrogen, and even anesthetic gases. Because mass spectrometers are highly sophisticated and expensive systems, they are usually used to monitor more than one patient. Gases are therefore sampled at the patient's airway and travel through special plumbing to the mass spectrometer for analysis. Since many patients may be monitored with one system, gas samples are typically taken from patients in a sequential fashion. Therefore no patient is continuously monitored.

Infrared absorption spectrophotometry, the alternative to mass spectrometry, utilizes infrared light absorption to determine the concentration of CO_2 in the respired gases. The CO_2 concentration is determined by comparing the amount of light absorbed by the CO_2 in the exhaled sample with that absorbed by a reference sample that is free of CO_2. Infrared analyzers are portable, are less expensive to purchase and maintain, and may provide continuous monitoring. For these reasons they are more commonly used in the intensive care setting (Fig. 9–5).

End-tidal CO_2 monitors are further categorized by gas sampling technique as sidestream, mainstream, or proximal diverting (Fig. 9–6). *Mainstream* analyzers measure CO_2 directly at the airway. Analyzing CO_2 in this fashion requires that the infrared device attached to the airway be heated to avoid condensation on the sensor cells. The presence of condensation on the sensor cell can lead to erroneously high readings. Two of the advantages of mainstream analyzers are that they provide continuous monitoring of one patient and that testing of exhaled CO_2 is more rapid because transport of the gas sample to another site for analysis is avoided. Disadvantages are that placing the analyzer in-line creates mechanical dead space and extra weight, and thus traction, on the patient's airway. A *proximal diverting* system transports the gas sample a short distance from the airway to a site where the CO_2 sensor is housed. This method reduces bulk at the airway. A *sidestream* analyzer aspirates a gas sample through small-bore tubing and transports it to the CO_2 sensor for analysis. An advantage is that no additional dead space or weight is added by the CO_2 sensor at the airway. Disadvantages include a time delay that occurs as the gas travels from the sample site to the analyzer; volume loss because the sample is aspirated from the airway, which affects measurement of total exhaled minute volume; and falsely low measurements because of potential moisture collection in the sample tubing. Some sys-

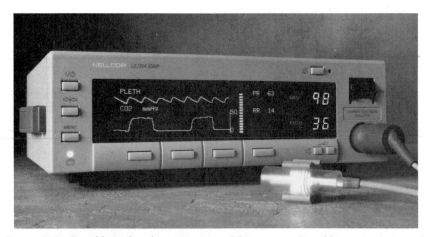

FIGURE 9-5 Portable, infrared mainstream etCO$_2$ monitor. Portable monitors expand use of etCO$_2$ monitoring beyond the operating room or intensive care setting into the emergency department and recovery room and during transport. The monitor shown also performs the dual function of pulse oximetry. (Photo courtesy of Nellcor Incorporated, Pleasanton, Calif.)

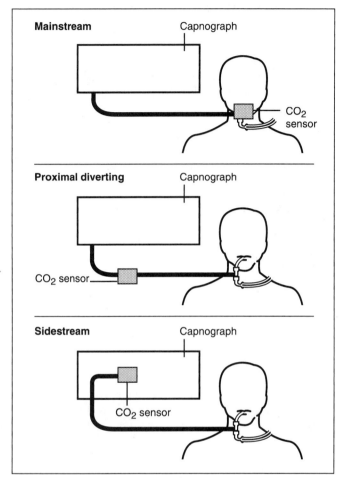

FIGURE 9-6 End-tidal CO_2 monitors may be categorized by gas sampling technique as mainstream, proximal diverting, or sidestream. See text for complete discussion. (Reprinted with permission. Copyright Nellcor Incorporated, Pleasanton, Calif.)

tems contain water traps or a purging mechanism to alleviate the latter problem. Regardless of the system in use, technical problems that obviate accurate gas sampling must be eliminated by the clinician. These problems include gas leaks caused by poor connections, partial to complete obstruction of the gas sampling lines or sensors, and incorrect circuit assembly.

CO_2 Physiology

Essential to understanding the indications and uses of $etCO_2$ monitoring and interpretation of the $etCO_2$ variable is an understanding of the physiology of CO_2 elimination. CO_2 is produced by the cells as a by-product of metabolism, diffuses from the cells into the blood, and is then carried to the lungs for elimination (Fig. 9–7). At the level of the lung the CO_2 readily diffuses from the pulmonary capillaries into the alveoli, and therefore the amount of CO_2 in these two compartments reaches near equilibrium. CO_2 is then eliminated

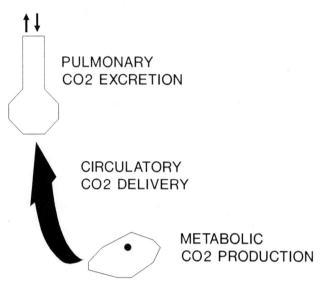

PULMONARY
CO2 EXCRETION

CIRCULATORY
CO2 DELIVERY

METABOLIC
CO2 PRODUCTION

FIGURE 9-7 The amount of carbon dioxide in the exhaled gases is determined by metabolic rate, perfusion status, and alveolar ventilation. (From Hess, D: Noninvasive respiratory monitoring during ventilatory support. *Crit Care Nurs Clin North Am* 1991; 3(4):565–574.)

from the body during the exhalation phase of the respiratory cycle (Fig. 9–8). At the beginning of exhalation, gases from the anatomic dead space that are free of CO_2 are exhaled. CO_2 elimination rapidly rises, reaching a plateau as alveolar gases are exhaled. At the end of a tidal breath the concentration of exhaled CO_2 is at its highest. Therefore the measurement of the concentration of CO_2 at the end of a tidal breath provides a reflection of the alveolar CO_2 ($P_{A}CO_2$), which in turn reflects the arterial CO_2 ($P_{a}CO_2$). Accordingly, $etCO_2 \sim P_{A}CO_2 \sim P_{a}CO_2$.

Normally, $P_{a}CO_2$ is 35 to 45 mm Hg. Typically $etCO_2$ values average 2 to 5 mm Hg less than the $P_{a}CO_2$ in individuals with normal ventilation and perfusion to the lung. Therefore, if the $etCO_2$ is measured at the same time that a blood gas value is obtained, the $etCO_2$ can be subtracted from the $P_{a}CO_2$, providing an index known as the $P_{a}CO_2$-$etCO_2$ gradient, or a-$ADCO_2$. For example, if a blood gas is obtained and the $P_{a}CO_2$ is 39 and simultaneously the $etCO_2$ is noted to be 35, the $P_{a}CO_2$-$etCO_2$ gradient is +4. Knowing this gradient allows for noninvasive monitoring of the patient's ventilation by monitoring the $etCO_2$ trend and by inferring the $P_{a}CO_2$ with the use of the gradient.

Circumstances that widen the a-$ADCO_2$ gradient ($P_{a}CO_2$ rises, whereas $etCO_2$ stays the same or decreases) are clinically significant. Knowing the factors that can alter the a-$ADCO_2$ will alert the clinician to recheck the gradient when one of these conditions arises so that accurate trend monitoring can be maintained. Conversely, understanding what causes a widened a-$ADCO_2$ will assist in interpreting what is occurring physiologically in a patient when a widened gradient is identified. The a-$ADCO_2$ may be widened with increasing physiologic dead space because perfusion of the mixed venous, CO_2-rich blood to some of the ventilated alveoli is decreased or absent (Fig. 9–9). Exhaled gases from CO_2-"free" dead

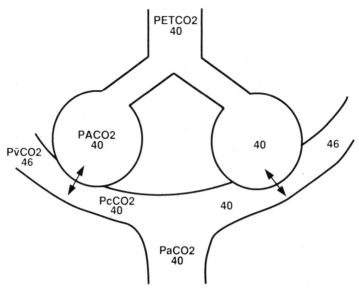

FIGURE 9-8 Normal partial pressure of CO_2 in the mixed venous ($P\bar{v}CO_2$) and arterial ($PaCO_2$) blood, the alveolus ($PACO_2$), and the exhaled gases ($PetCO_2$). $PcCO_2$, Partial pressure of CO_2 in capillary blood. (From Szaflarski, NL, and Cohen, NH: Use of capnography in critically ill adults. *Heart Lung* 1991; 20(4):363–372.)

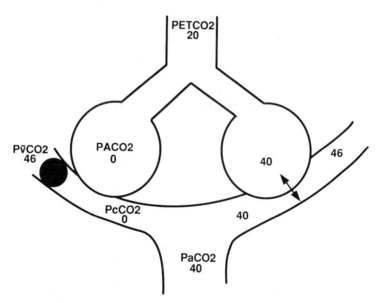

FIGURE 9-9 Model of lung unit with dead-space ventilation (left) demonstrates how the arterial-to-alveolar gradient for CO_2 widens under these conditions. $PetCO_2$ is significantly lowered. $PcCO_2$, Partial pressure of CO_2 in capillary blood. (From Szaflarski, NL, and Cohen, NH: Use of capnography in critically ill adults. *Heart Lung* 1991; 20(4):363–372.)

Box 9–1 Causes of a Widened Arterial (Pa_{CO_2}) to Alveolar (PA_{CO_2}) Gradient (a-$ADco_2$)

Increased physiologic dead space
    Pulmonary embolus (thromboembolic, fat, or air)
    Pulmonary hypoperfusion (hypotension $\rightarrow$ cardiac arrest)
    Excessive tidal volume or PEEP ventilation
    Adult respiratory distress syndrome (ARDS)
Incomplete alveolar emptying
    Severe hypoventilation
    High rate/low tidal volume ventilation
Poor sampling technique
    Dilution of gas sample with CO_2 free gas (poorly fitting mask or mouth breathing when sampling is performed via nasal cannula setup, or sample site too far from airway and too close to fresh gas inlet)
    Leakage of exhaled gas into the atmosphere (ETT cuff leak)

ETT = Endotracheal tube.

space units mix with those from lung units with a normal ventilation/perfusion ratio, "diluting" the $etCO_2$ value. Box 9–1 further delineates causes of a widened a-$ADco_2$.

The most common pitfall of $etCO_2$ monitoring is believing that $etCO_2$ reflects the patient's ventilatory status alone. As shown in Table 9–1, changes in exhaled CO_2 levels may occur because of changes not only in ventilation but also in CO_2 production (metabolism), transport of CO_2 to the lung (pulmonary perfusion), and accuracy of equipment. If any three of these variables are held constant, a change in the CO_2 value reflects an alteration in the remaining variable. For example, if metabolism, cardiac output, and accuracy of monitoring are all held constant, the $etCO_2$ concentration is inversely related to alveolar ventilation. An increase in the $etCO_2$ value would indicate hypoventilation, and a decrease in the value would indicate hyperventilation.

Graphing the Exhaled CO_2 Waveform: Capnography

The capnogram is a tracing of the inhaled and exhaled concentrations of CO_2 with time (Fig. 9–10). In the normal capnogram, at the beginning of exhalation the CO_2 value is zero as gas from the anatomic dead space leaves the airway (A-B). A sharp rise in the waveform, and thus in CO_2 elimination, occurs as alveolar air mixes with dead space gas (B-C). Most of exhalation is represented by a leveling of the curve known as the alveolar plateau, which represents gas flow from the alveoli (C-D). The Pco_2 at the end of the plateau (D) is known as the end-tidal CO_2 ($etCO_2$). The $etCO_2$ is the highest concentration of exhaled, alveolar CO_2. The curve then takes a rapid, sharp downstroke as inspiration of CO_2-free gas occurs (D-E). It is notable that on a capnogram, positive deflections represent expiration, whereas negative deflections represent inspiration (which is the opposite of most respiratory waveforms). The shape of the capnogram can be diagnostic of abnormal lung function or may indicate technical problems (Fig. 9–11A-J).

TABLE 9-1 Causes of Alterations in End-tidal CO_2 (etCO$_2$)

Increased etCO$_2$	Decreased etCO$_2$
Ventilation	
Mild hypoventilation	Moderate to extreme hypoventilation
Rebreathing, as when mechanical dead space is added to circuitry	Hyperventilation
	Airway obstruction
	Increased physiologic dead space (increase in amount of exhaled gas that has not interfaced with CO$_2$-laden blood)
Perfusion	
Increased transport of CO$_2$ to lungs after perfusion has been impaired (e.g., after cardiopulmonary bypass, after arrest, or post shock state)	Impaired pulmonary perfusion (e.g., pulmonary embolus, state of decreased cardiac output up to and including cardiac arrest)
Metabolism	
Increased CO$_2$ production, as in fever, pain, a hypermetabolic state such as after trauma, or increased muscle activity caused, for example, by seizures or shivering	Decreased CO$_2$ production, as in hypothermia, or decreased muscle activity caused, for example, by heavy sedation and/or paralytic agents
Injection of sodium bicarbonate (transient rise)	
Malignant hyperthermia	
Equipment	
Leak in ventilator circuit, resulting in reduced tidal volume delivery to patient	Poor sampling, such as when water is in sample line of sidestream system
Exhausted CO$_2$ absorber (anesthesia system)	Leak around endotracheal tube cuff, resulting in loss of exhaled gas to atmosphere
Reduced ventilation due to partially obstructed airway	Ventilator disconnect
	Esophageal intubation or dislodged artificial airway
	Obstructed or kinked endotracheal tube

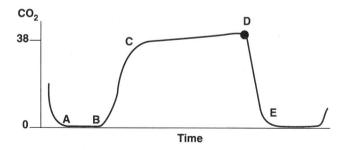

- Zero baseline (A-B)
- Rapid, sharp rise (B-C)
- Alveolar plateau (C-D)
- End-tidal value (D)
- Rapid, sharp downstroke (D-E)

FIGURE 9-10 Normal capnogram. See text for explanation. (Reprinted with permission. Copyright Nellcor Incorporated, Pleasanton, Calif.)

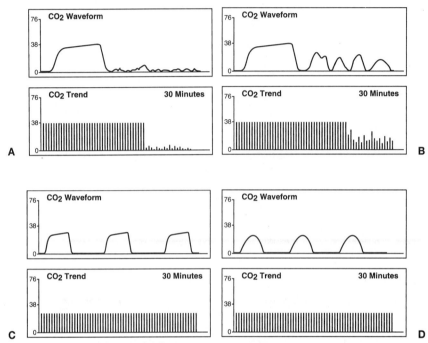

FIGURE 9-11 Abnormal capnographic waveforms: (A) Sudden decrease in etCO₂ to zero or near-zero value. Possible causes include airway disconnection; esophageal intubation; and dislodged, totally obstructed, or kinked ETT. (B) Sudden decrease in etCO₂ to low, nonzero value. Decrease may be due to air leak in the system, such as around the mask or endotracheal tube or in the ventilator circuitry, or to partial airway obstruction. (C) Persistent low etCO₂ with good alveolar plateau. Possible causes include hyperventilation, hypothermia, sedation, anesthesia, and increased dead space ventilation. (D) Persistent low etCO₂ without alveolar plateau. Possible causes include incomplete exhalation caused by kinking of the airway, bronchospasm, or mucous plugging, and poor sampling technique. (E) Exponential decrease in etCO₂. Possible causes include factors that decrease pulmonary blood flow, such as cardiac arrest, pulmonary embolus, and hypotension. (F) Elevated etCO₂ with good alveolar plateau. Possible causes include inadequate minute ventilation, combined with tidal volume sufficient to empty alveolar gas, and factors that increase the metabolic rate such as fever, pain, and shivering. (G) Gradually increasing etCO₂. Possible causes include hypoventilation, factors that increase the metabolic rate such as a rising body temperature or malignant hyperthermia. (H) Rise in baseline and etCO₂. Possible causes include rebreathing of exhaled CO₂, as in increased mechanical dead space; exhausted CO₂ absorber; and defective exhalation valve. (I) Capnographic waveform, showing alveolar cleft, indicates inadequate neuromuscular blockade or emergence from blockade. (J) Spontaneous breathing during mechanical ventilation. Spontaneous breaths of patient shown on *top* are more shallow than those of patient shown on *bottom*. (Reprinted with permission. Copyright Nellcor Incorporated, Pleasanton, Calif.)

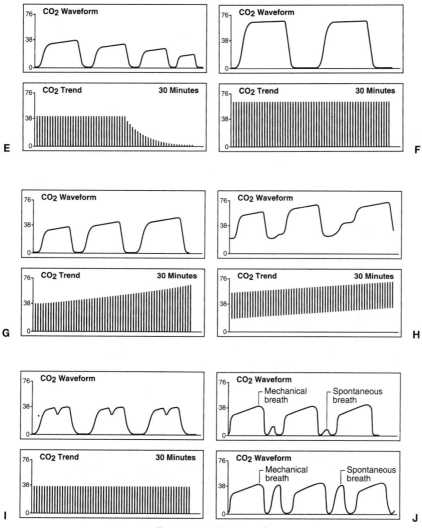

FIGURE 9-11 Continued

Applications of etCO$_2$ Monitoring

In addition to providing a reflection of the PaCO$_2$ in patients with a stable respiratory pattern and perfusion status, other uses for etCO$_2$ monitoring have been identified. Detection of esophageal intubation may be achieved with the use of a disposable CO$_2$ detector. The etCO$_2$ detector is a device that attaches between the manual resuscitation bag and the endotracheal tube (ETT). The instrument detects, and in some cases provides an estimated measure, of exhaled CO$_2$ (Fig. 9–12). These disposable devices assist in determining correct placement of the ETT in patients in whom perfusion is present. They are useful, but not specific, for determining correct ETT placement in patients with cardiopulmonary arrest because, if circulation has not been established, lack of CO$_2$ detection does not necessarily mean esophageal intubation. A further caution is in regard to esophageal intubation in a patient who has consumed carbonated beverages. The result will be positive CO$_2$ detection, which may be erroneously interpreted as correct ETT placement. It is suggested that CO$_2$ be monitored for 20 to 30 seconds after intubation; this period should be adequate for gastric CO$_2$ to be washed out.

The main use of etCO$_2$ monitoring is to determine the adequacy of ventilation in the patient supported by mechanical ventilation, especially during manipulation of the ventilator settings. Acute increases in PaCO$_2$, requiring adjustments in the ventilator settings, may occur in patients who are unable to increase their minute ventilation—for example, in the patient who is being rewarmed after cardiopulmonary bypass or in the patient whose perfusion is improving after a shock episode. Monitoring of etCO$_2$ also provides continuous, noninvasive assessment of the patient for whom controlled hypocapnia is being utilized as a measure to decrease intracranial pressure.

In the operating room the etCO$_2$ monitor is very useful as an indicator of accidental ventilator disconnection. In the ICU, however, ventilators have so-

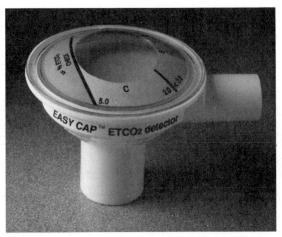

FIGURE 9–12   Disposable colorimetric CO$_2$ detector, used to verify CO$_2$ in exhaled gases and assist in confirmation of correct endotracheal tube placement. Device contains a pH-sensitive membrane that changes hue as the exhaled gases pass through. (Photo courtesy of Nellcor Incorporated, Pleasanton, Calif.)

phisticated alarm systems that warn of disconnections, making the $etCO_2$ an expensive additional alarm if it is being used only for this purpose. There are many uses for $etCO_2$ monitoring in the postanesthesia recovery unit, including its use as an indicator of hypoventilation and apnea.

It is very important to understand that $etCO_2$ monitoring is not very useful as a monitor for weaning a patient from a ventilator. Many factors that can alter the $etCO_2$ variable, such as changes in metabolic rate, may be present during a weaning trial. Therefore $etCO_2$ will not always accurately reflect the patient's $PaCO_2$ during ventilator weaning.

Monitoring of exhaled CO_2 to assess the patient for the presence of perfusion has been shown to be extremely valuable during cardiopulmonary resuscitation (CPR). At the time of cardiac arrest, the $etCO_2$ value falls to zero because there is a lack of pulmonary perfusion. The detection of exhaled CO_2 provides an indication of the adequacy of cardiac compressions and the return of spontaneous circulation.

To ensure accurate monitoring of $etCO_2$ when it is first being instituted, the practitioner must perform the required calibration routines as described in the operator's manual. Correct assembly of the airway adapter, CO_2 sensor, and display monitor is essential to prevent sampling errors. Proper connection to the patient's airway minimizes error caused by gas leaks. In a sidestream sampling device, to decrease fluid accumulation in the sample line, ensure that the sampling port is placed at a right angle to the patient's airway. After correctly setting up and connecting the $etCO_2$ monitor, obtain an arterial blood gas (ABG) to compare the initial $etCO_2$ reading with the laboratory-determined $PaCO_2$. Troubleshoot >5 mm Hg disparities by checking the monitor for proper function and searching for the presence of factors that can cause erroneous $etCO_2$ values. Determine and document the a-ADCO_2. Set HIGH and LOW $etCO_2$ alarm parameters and alarm volume.

BLOOD GASES

Arterial Blood Gas

TECHNIQUE

Normal values and the method of interpreting ABG values were previously discussed in Chapter 2. This section will present the proper technique of obtaining the ABG sample so that the patient has no complications and errors are not entered into the results.

The most common site for obtaining an ABG sample is the radial artery. In the adult, other sites are the brachial and femoral arteries, the latter being the most commonly used site in emergency settings because of its accessibility and relative ease of palpating a weak pulse. Before an arterial puncture (arteriotomy) is performed, an assessment should be made of the adequacy of collateral circulation, because if vessel disruption or hematoma formation leads to circulatory compromise, the result could be loss of the limb. Collateral hand circulation is assessed with a modified Allen test (Fig. 9–13).

Coagulopathy or medium- to high-dose anticoagulation therapy is a relative contraindication to arterial puncture. If necessary, then, adequate time should be allotted for the application of pressure to achieve hemostasis. Arterial puncture should not be performed distal to a surgical shunt or through an infected lesion. Repeated puncture of a single site should also be avoided because it increases

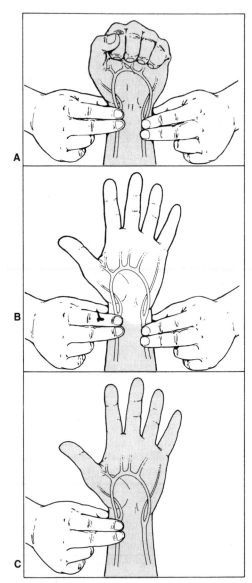

Figure 9-13 Modified Allen test used to assess adequacy of collateral circulation in the hand, via the ulnar artery, before performance of a radial arteriotomy. (A) Elevate the hand, and compress radial and ulnar arteries while the patient opens and closes his fist until (B) the hand blanches. (C) Release pressure from ulnar artery and evaluate for return of normal hand color. An erythematous blush is a positive Allen test result, whereas pallor is a negative result and indicates poor collateral circulation. Therefore arterial puncture should not be performed. (From Weilitz, PB: *Pocket Guide to Respiratory Care*. St. Louis: Mosby–Year Book, 1991.)

Box 9–2   Procedure for Arterial Puncture

1. Wash hands. Prepare heparinized syringe with a 22-gauge (or smaller) needle. Don clean gloves.
2. Place the patient's wrist (for arterial puncture) or arm (for brachial puncture) in a hyperextended position.
3. Clean the skin with alcohol or povidine-iodine.
4. Palpate the pulse and insert the needle, bevel up, at a 45-degree angle to the skin (90 degrees for femoral puncture).
5. Observe for flash of blood at hub of needle. Pressure within the arterial system should allow the syringe to fill passively without aspiration. Withdraw approximately 3 ml of blood. Amount of blood needed depends on method of analysis.
6. Remove the needle and apply direct pressure for at least 5 minutes, longer if the patient has a history of anticoagulant therapy or coagulopathy.
7. While applying pressure, remove any bubbles from the syringe by holding it upright, allowing the air to float to the top, where it can be easily expelled.
8. Cap the syringe and immediately place it on ice.
9. Properly dispose of equipment and wash hands.

---

the likelihood of hematoma formation, scarring, or laceration of the artery (see Box 9–2).

If frequent ABG analysis or continous monitoring of blood pressure is required, arterial cannulation should be performed. Patency of the arterial catheter is achieved with a continuous-flush device. All connections of such a device must be carefully secured because a loose connection could result in rapid blood loss.

When the specimen is obtained, precautions must be taken to handle it correctly for prevention of inaccurate results (see Box 9–3). For prevention of clotting, liquid or powdered (lyophilized) heparin must be added to the syringe. Only a small amount of heparin should be utilized (the barrel of the syringe should be wet slightly and any excess heparin removed), or it may produce acidification of the sample because the pH of heparin is 7.0. The sample should be placed immediately in an ice bath to slow metabolism; otherwise, O_2 levels will be lowered and CO_2 levels elevated. If the specimen is held at 4° C, analysis may be performed for up to 1 hour. If it is held at room temperature, analysis should be performed within 15 minutes. The sample must be obtained anaerobically and any air bubbles rapidly expelled. Air bubbles will cause O_2 levels to be elevated and CO_2 levels to be lowered. The patient's body temperature should be taken at the time the specimen is obtained and recorded on the laboratory requisition. When ABGs are analyzed, a normal body temperature of 37° C is assumed. Temperature correction of the results can be performed by the laboratory if personnel are alerted to an abnormal body temperature. Temperatures >37° C result in higher O_2 and CO_2 values, whereas temperatures <37° C have the opposite effect (recall the concepts of the oxyhemoglobin dissociation curve). After the sample is

---

Box 9–3   Procedure for Obtaining an ABG Specimen From an Indwelling Arterial Catheter

1. Wash hands. Prepare heparinized syringe. Don clean gloves.
2. Remove dead-end cap from stopcock. Prevent contamination of cap.
3. Place nonheparinized syringe on stopcock.
4. Turn stopcock off to the flush device and open to the artery. Withdraw a sufficient amount of blood to ensure that line is free of flush solution, usually 2 to 3 ml. Conserve as much of the patient's blood as possible. Some systems are closed systems, avoiding the need to discard any blood.
5. Turn stopcock partially off to artery.
6. Remove syringe and discard blood and flush properly.
7. Place heparinized syringe on stopcock, open stopcock to artery, and withdraw approximately 3 ml of arterial blood. Amount of blood needed depends on method of analysis.
8. Turn stopcock off to artery, remove syringe, debubble, cap syringe, and immediately place syringe in ice bath.
9. Flush arterial line until free of blood. Always flush stopcock of residual blood and replace protective dead-end cap. Blood in line or stopcock provides an excellent culture medium for the growth of pathogens.

---

obtained, pressure should be applied to the vessel for 5 minutes to achieve hemostasis.

Mixed Venous Blood Gas

TECHNIQUE

Mixed venous blood gas analysis is performed to determine the adequacy of tissue oxygenation. The partial pressure of O_2 in mixed venous blood ($P\bar{v}O_2$) and saturation of hemoglobin with O_2 in mixed venous blood ($S\bar{v}O_2$) are also utilized to calculate additional tissue oxygenation variables (to be discussed in the following sections). Mixed venous blood can be obtained *only* from the distal port of a pulmonary artery (PA) catheter (see Box 9–4). It is at this point in the vasculature that the blood returning from all the venous beds of the body has been thoroughly "mixed" in the right ventricle and therefore represent total-body venous blood (Fig. 9–14). Blood from the proximal port of the PA catheter, the right atrial (RA) port, is not true mixed venous blood because blood from the superior vena cava and that from the inferior vena cava have not yet adequately blended. Furthermore, blood from the coronary sinuses (which has a $P\bar{v}O_2$ of 23 mm Hg) empties into the RA; therefore, if the proximal sampling port were lying close to the coronary sinus, then the sampled blood would be tainted and would certainly not reflect total-body venous oxygen values.

The same handling precautions that apply to arterial samples applies to mixed venous samples: ensure that the specimen is free of bubbles, obtained anaerobically and capped, immediately placed on ice to slow metabolism, and analyzed with the use of the patient's body temperature at the time of sampling. Several calculations discussed in the following section will require both an arterial

Box 9–4 Procedure for Obtaining a Mixed Venous Blood Gas Specimen From a Pulmonary Artery Catheter

1. Wash hands. Prepare heparinized syringe. Don clean gloves.
2. Remove dead-end cap from stopcock. Prevent contamination of cap.
3. Place nonheparinized syringe on stopcock. Turn stopcock off to the flush device and slowly withdraw 3 ml of flush solution and blood for discard.
4. Turn stopcock partially off to pulmonary artery.
5. Remove syringe, and discard blood and flush properly.
6. Attach heparinized syringe, turn stopcock off to flush device, and *slowly* withdraw (over 1 minute) 1 to 3 ml of mixed venous blood. Too rapid withdrawal of blood may cause arterialized pulmonary capillary blood to flow retrograde, contaminating the sample. This would lead to $P\overline{v}O_2/S\overline{v}O_2$ readings higher than that of the true mixed venous blood.
7. Turn stopcock off to the sampling port and remove syringe. Debubble specimen, cap syringe, and immediately place syringe in ice bath.
8. Flush pulmonary artery catheter until free of blood. Always flush stopcock of residual blood and replace protective dead-end cap. Blood in line or stopcock provides an excellent culture medium for the growth of pathogens.

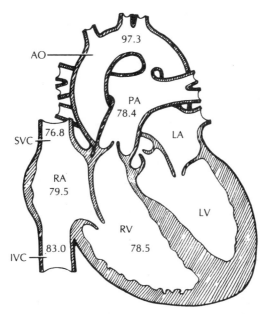

FIGURE 9–14 Normal values for oxygen saturation in the chambers of the heart and great vessels. *IVC,* Inferior vena cava; *SVC,* superior vena cava; *PA,* pulmonary artery; *AO,* aorta; *RA,* right atrium; *LA,* left atrium; *RV,* right ventricle; *LV,* left ventricle. (From Quan, SF: Mixed venous oxygen. *Am Fam Physician* 1983;27(2):211. Published by the American Academy of Family Physicians.)

TABLE 9-2   Normal Values for Arterial and Mixed Venous Blood Gases

Component	Arterial	Mixed Venous
pH	7.35–7.45	7.30–7.37
P_{O_2} (mm Hg)	80–100	36–42
P_{CO_2} (mm Hg)	35–45	42–46
%Saturation	92–100	60–80
HCO_3^- (mEq/L)	22–26	24–28
Base excess (mEq/L)	−2 to +2	

and a mixed venous sample; therefore the samples should be obtained in as close a time frame to each other as possible so that changes in the patient's condition do not confound the results. Normal values for each sample are delineated in Table 9–2.

INTERPRETATION OF MIXED VENOUS BLOOD GAS VALUES

Mixed venous blood samples are primarily used to determine the adequacy of tissue oxygenation in relation to tissue oxygen demand. The heart and lungs work together to deliver oxygenated blood to the tissues. At the tissue level, oxygen is normally consumed at a relatively constant rate. This relatively constant rate of consumption is maintained by a tissue extraction of ∼ 25% of the oxygen delivered. If cardiac output falls, or if it fails to increase when arterial oxygen saturation decreases, then >25% of delivered oxygen will have to be extracted to maintain a constant rate of tissue oxygen consumption ($\dot{V}_{O_2}$). Therefore, $P\bar{v}_{O_2}$ and $S\bar{v}_{O_2}$ values lower than normal, <35 mm Hg and <60%, respectively, are indicative of oxygen delivery that is inadequate in relation to oxygen demand. $P\bar{v}_{O_2}$ values <30 mm Hg are usually associated with lactate formation, an indication that tissue oxygenation is reaching critical levels and anaerobic metabolic pathways are being utilized. The clinician must then determine whether the oxygen delivery problem is cardiac or pulmonary in origin by systematically evaluating the adequacy of arterial oxygenation, hemoglobin, and cardiac output (heart rate, preload, afterload, and contractility).

$P\bar{v}_{O_2}$ and $S\bar{v}_{O_2}$ values that are higher than normal do not necessarily mean that tissue oxygenation is adequate. In fact, tissue hypoxia may be severe because of impaired *tissue utilization* of oxygen, as in severe sepsis. Therefore the monitoring of $P\bar{v}_{O_2}$ and $S\bar{v}_{O_2}$ alone may be inadequate in complex critical illness, and more sophisticated indices of tissue oxygenation may be necessary to complete the picture. These concepts will be further expanded in subsequent sections.

Mixed venous blood gas values may also be utilized to evaluate whether an atrial or ventricular septal defect is present. When these clinical conditions are present, arterial blood from the higher-pressure left side of the heart combines with blood in the right side of the heart, resulting in higher than normal values for mixed venous oxygen saturation. As a standard PA catheter is passed, blood samples are obtained from the right atrium (RA), right ventricle (RV) and pulmonary arteries. As the fiberoptic $S\bar{v}_{O_2}$ PA catheter is passed, venous blood saturation in each chamber of the heart is recorded. An abnormal increase in mixed venous oxygen saturation as the catheter is passed into the RA or RV (abnormal "step-up") indicates a patent defect.

CONTINUOUS MONITORING OF MIXED VENOUS OXYGEN SATURATION: S$\bar{\text{v}}$O$_2$ MONITORING

Mixed venous oxygen saturation (S$\bar{\text{v}}$O$_2$) is the flow-weighted average of the saturation of venous effluents from all the body's perfused vascular beds. It does not reflect perfusion of any one organ but, rather, reflects the balance of oxygen supply to oxygen demand within the entire organism. It is a cardiopulmonary variable, utilized to determine the adequacy of tissue oxygenation. S$\bar{\text{v}}$O$_2$ may be continuously monitored through the use of a fiberoptic pulmonary artery catheter. The catheter does not provide any additional information about tissue oxygenation than the intermittent mixed venous blood sample does; however, continuous S$\bar{\text{v}}$O$_2$ monitoring provides real-time data reflecting the often ever-changing status of the critically ill adult.

Components of an S$\bar{\text{v}}$O$_2$ Monitoring System

The three components of an S$\bar{\text{v}}$O$_2$ monitoring system are the fiberoptic PA catheter, the optical module, and an accompanying monitor (Fig. 9–15). The fiberoptic PA catheter utilizes the principles of reflectance spectrophotometry to determine S$\bar{\text{v}}$O$_2$ (Fig. 9–16). Multiple wavelengths of light from light-emitting diodes in the optical module are transmitted into the PA blood through fiberoptic bundles. The amount of light reflected by oxygenated versus deoxygenated blood is carried back to a photodetector in the optical module via another fiberoptic filament. The microprocessor-based monitor than derives the oxy-

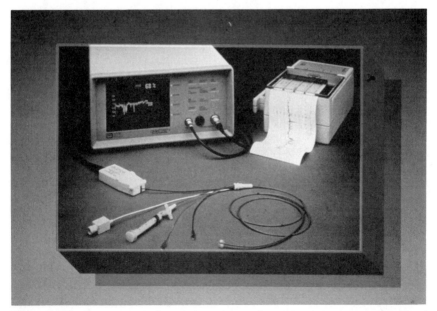

FIGURE 9–15 Components of a continuous mixed venous oxygen saturation (S$\bar{\text{v}}$O$_2$) monitoring system: pulmonary artery catheter, optical module, and microprocessor-based monitor. Also shown is a strip-chart recorder, an optional feature. (Courtesy of Abbott Critical Care Systems, Mountain View, Calif.)

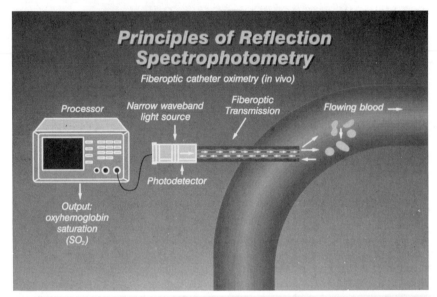

FIGURE 9–16 Principles of reflectance spectrophotometry. Fiberoptics transmit two or three wavelengths of light from light-emitting diodes. Another fiberoptic bundle sends information back to the photodetector about the amount of light reflected by the oxygenated and deoxygenated hemoglobin. The microprocessor then calculates the percentage of hemoglobin saturated with oxygen. (Courtesy of Abbott Critical Care Systems, Mountain View, Calif.)

hemoglobin saturation by evaluating the ratio of transmitted to reflected light. In addition to containing fiberoptics, the $S\bar{v}O_2$ PA catheter has PA and RA lumens for pressure readings, sampling, or infusion; a thermistor for thermodilution measurement of cardiac output; and a balloon lumen for measuring pulmonary capillary wedge pressure.

The microprocessor monitor continuously displays the $S\bar{v}O_2$ value and is generally capable of providing a trend graph of data during various time frames. Some monitors are capable of providing a printout of the trend data. Visual and audible alarms are available for low and high $S\bar{v}O_2$ values, with some systems providing additional alarm messages. The monitor also provides a display of intensity of the reflected light signal, which serves as a source of information about catheter position and system integrity and therefore about the accuracy of the reported $S\bar{v}O_2$ value. Light intensity problems should be corrected before the reported $S\bar{v}O_2$ value is accepted or calibration procedures are performed (Table 9–3). Accuracy is also determined by proper system calibration. There are two calibration methods: preinsertion and in vivo. Preinsertion calibration is performed to an optical reference and should always be performed. In vivo calibration should be performed if preinsertion calibration was inadvertently omitted, there is reason to suspect that the oxygen saturation reading is incorrect, or system integrity has been disrupted.

Two catheter designs are currently available, one with two reference wavelengths of light and the other with three reference wavelengths. Research has shown that three-wavelength $S\bar{v}O_2$ systems more closely approximate actual

TABLE 9–3 Troubleshooting Continuous $S\bar{v}O_2$ Monitoring Light Intensity Problems

Problem	Potential Cause	Check and Adjust
High intensity	Catheter tip may be against vessel wall.	Check PA pressure waveform for catheter position. Reposition catheter if it appears to be wedged. To move tip away from vessel wall, inflate balloon, flush catheter (with balloon down), or twist the catheter a one-fourth turn.
Low intensity	Loose connection at optical module, kink in catheter, clot at catheter tip, or break in fiberoptics may have occurred.	Secure connection between optical module and PA catheter. Straighten out any kinks. Ensure that distal lumen is patent by first aspirating blood to remove any clot and then flushing catheter. If fiberoptics are broken, catheter will have to be replaced.
Dampened or erratic intensity	Catheter has floated out too far or is in a wedged position, or clot is forming on the tip.	Check PA waveform for catheter position; reposition as necessary. Ensure that balloon is completely deflated. Ensure that distal lumen is patent by first aspirating blood to remove any clot and then gently flushing catheter.

$S\bar{v}O_2$ values. Increased reliability of the $S\bar{v}O_2$ value provides more accurate assessment data and decreases the number of mixed venous blood samples necessary for machine calibration. Therefore the three-wavelength system is probably more cost-effective because of its saving of practitioner time in obtaining samples and recalibration procedures, its saving of laboratory fees for analysis of mixed venous samples, and its overall accuracy.

Indications for Using Continuous $S\bar{v}O_2$ Monitoring

Monitoring of $S\bar{v}O_2$ is useful in that it provides an early warning of cardiopulmonary insufficiency, often before changes in the patient's hemodynamic status become evident. Interventions designed to achieve optimal tissue oxygen delivery or to decrease tissue oxygen demand can then be initiated before impairment in tissue oxygenation occurs. $S\bar{v}O_2$ monitoring is also useful as a patient management tool to monitor the effects of various interventions designed to increase tissue oxygen delivery or decrease tissue oxygen demand, such as volume loading, titration of vasoactive agents, or administration of sedation to reduce agitation. Furthermore, cardiorespiratory tolerance of routine care such as positioning and various treatments (e.g., suctioning, turning, chest physiotherapy) can be assessed on a real-time basis so that the plan of care can be altered immediately if necessary.

Despite the benefit of providing continuous insight into the patient's tissue oxygenation status, continuous $S\bar{v}O_2$ monitoring is not indicated in all critically ill patients. The risk/benefit ratio for invasive monitoring and the high cost associated with $S\bar{v}O_2$ monitoring must be factored into the decision to utilize this technology. In general, if it is anticipated that mixed venous blood gases will be drawn several times a day for evaluation of tissue oxygenation, then the use of an $S\bar{v}O_2$ catheter may be cost-effective. Each institution should develop indications for use of continuous $S\bar{v}O_2$ monitoring on the basis of its patient population. The following are examples of types of patients who may benefit from continuous $S\bar{v}O_2$ monitoring:

- Patients with severely compromised pulmonary function who require high levels of ventilatory support (e.g., >10 cm H_2O PEEP, FIO_2 >0.6) or who are undergoing modes of ventilation known to affect tissue oxygen delivery, such as pressure-control inverse inspiratory-to-expiratory (I:E) ratio ventilation
- Patients with severely compromised cardiac function, such as hemodynamically unstable patients receiving multiple vasopressor/inotropic agents, or frequent titration or high doses of such agents, and patients undergoing massive volume resuscitation
- Patients with multiple organ dysfunction syndrome (MODS)
- Patients with systemic inflammatory response syndrome (SIRS), with sepsis, or in whom sepsis is suspected

Interpreting Changes in $S\bar{v}O_2$

NORMAL $S\bar{v}O_2$

The heart and lungs work together to deliver adequate, well-oxygenated blood to the tissues. Normal arterial oxygen saturation (SaO_2) is 95% to 100%, and normal $S\bar{v}O_2$ is 75%. These values indicate that 25% of all oxgyen delivered is used by the tissues to maintain a constant state of $\dot{V}O_2$ via aerobic metabolic pathways (Fig. 9–17). Because 75% of the hemoglobin returning to the right side of the heart is still saturated with O_2, some O_2 reserve is available for times of increased need, such as during increased patient activity, episodes of fever, or administration of treatments such as suctioning or bathing.

The $S\bar{v}O_2$ value can be utilized as an indicator of available O_2 reserve. It is important to note that some tissue beds, such as the brain and heart, utilize more oxygen than others; the result is a much lower $S\bar{v}O_2$ value for these specific organs and therefore little oxygen reserve. Because present technology does not allow for monitoring the $S\bar{v}O_2$ of specific organs, we must rely on the $S\bar{v}O_2$ value, which reflects total body tissue utilization of oxygen, for clinical decision making about the adequacy of tissue oxygenation. An $S\bar{v}O_2$ greater than 65% indicates adequate reserve, 50% to 65% limited reserve, 35% to 50% inadequate reserve, and <35% inadequate tissue oxygenation.

Prerequiste knowledge to an interpretation of a lower-than-normal $S\bar{v}O_2$ value (<60%) is an understanding of how the body responds when tissue O_2 needs exceed O_2 supply. Initially, tissue PO_2 will fall, resulting in a widened diffusion gradient between tissue and capillary, and promoting O_2 diffusion out of the capillary and into tissue. The falling PaO_2 then prompts hemoglobin to begin unloading more O_2. The increased use of oxygen by tissues is termed *increased extraction* or *increased utilization*. Its purpose is to maintain a level of $\dot{V}O_2$ that can maintain metabolic processes aerobically. An increase in the acidic chemical by-product of aerobic metabolism, CO_2 (or lactate with anaerobic metabolism), stimulates chemoreceptors in the central nervous system to prompt a higher cardiac output (CO). This higher CO is mediated through the sympathetic nervous system. The goal is to deliver more oxygen to meet the increased

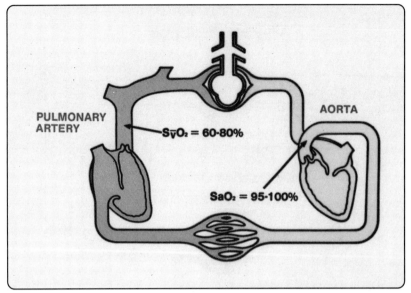

FIGURE 9-17 Normal arterial and mixed venous blood oxygen saturations. Normally 25% of the available O_2 is utilized by the tissues, leaving an O_2 reserve for times of increased demand or physiologic stress. (Courtesy of Baxter Healthcare Corp., Edwards Critical-Care Division, Santa Ana, Calif.)

demand. If the CO delivers enough oxygen each minute, an adequate capillary Po_2 will be ensured and normal diffusion gradients maintained. If the CO is not sufficient to deliver enough oxygen each minute, capillary Po_2 will fall, prompting hemoglobin to unload more oxygen and leaving a lower-than-normal $S\bar{v}o_2$ (Fig. 9–18). Hence a decreased $S\bar{v}o_2$ means that oxygen demand has exceeded the supply.

DECREASED S$\bar{v}$O$_2$

When a *decreased* $S\bar{v}o_2$ (<60%) is detected, the clinician must differentially determine, in a systematic fashion, whether the problem is cardiac or pulmonary in origin. If a pulse oximeter is in use, a quick look at the Sao_2 will rule out a pulmonary cause for a decrease in tissue oxygen delivery. If the Sao_2 is low, potential causes include a change in the underlying lung condition or a technical problem with the ventilator system, such as disconnection, loss of tidal volume or PEEP, or inaccurate setting of Fio_2. If the pulmonary system is ruled out as the cause of inadequate oxygen transport, then the cardiac system is systematically evaluated. A thermodilution CO is performed. If the CO is low, then analysis of the components of the CO—heart rate and stroke volume, specifically, preload, afterload, and contractility—will determine the cause of the low CO and necessary corrective action.

The low $S\bar{v}o_2$ state must be corrected or the body will convert to utilization of the much less efficient anaerobic metabolic pathways, resulting in lactic acid production. Metabolic acidosis will develop and variable amounts of tissue ischemia will occur. What tissue beds in the body will experience hypoxia depends on the vulnerability of specific organs in regard to their need for O_2.

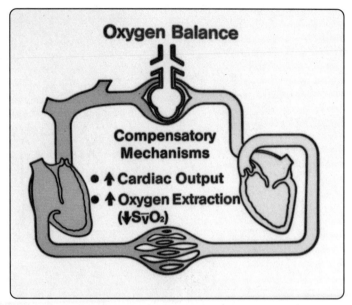

FIGURE 9-18 The body utilizes two fundamental compensatory mechanisms in response to inadequate O_2 supply. The first one is to increase the cardiac output. The second is to increase the amount of oxygen extracted from the blood. (Courtesy of Baxter Healthcare Corp., Edwards Critical-Care Division, Santa Ana, Calif.)

Simultaneously to implementing interventions designed to achieve optimal tissue oxygen delivery, efforts should be made to decrease tissue oxygen demand, thereby balancing supply to demand. Factors that increase oxygen demand are those which increase the metabolic rate, such as fever, agitation, activity, pain, and seizures.

INCREASED $S\bar{v}O_2$

An *increased* $S\bar{v}O_2$, >80%, generally indicates an increased O_2 supply, a decreased demand for O_2 at the tissue level, or inability of the tissues to utilize O_2. Increased O_2 supply can occur with an increase in SaO_2, PaO_2, CO, or hemoglobin. Decreased tissue demand for O_2 occurs with conditions that decrease the metabolic rate, such as hypothermia, anesthesia, heavy sedation, barbiturate coma, and sleep. The more common, and potentially clinically ominous, cause of an increased $S\bar{v}O_2$ is tissue inability to utilize O_2.

Decreased O_2 utilization occurs when there is an increased affinity of hemoglobin for oxygen (left shift of the oxyhemoglobin dissociation curve) because the tissues are not being offered the O_2 that they need. Decreased O_2 utilization also occurs in vasodilated states (e.g., sepsis, distributive shock) that lead to a maldistribution of blood flow at the capillary level. Perfusion of O_2-rich blood is adequate in areas not needing it and inadequate in areas of need. Toxic effects at the tissue level (e.g., thiocyanate toxicity, endotoxemia in late septic syndrome) can also lead to decreased O_2 utilization and an increased $S\bar{v}O_2$. Calculation of $\dot{V}O_2$ and the oxygen utilization ratio (see Direct and Derived Variables of Tissue Oxygenation Obtained With the Pulmonary Artery Catheter, below) assists in differentiating the cause of a tissue oxygenation defect when it is not apparent with the $S\bar{v}O_2$ alone and the patient has a complex critical illness.

Dual Oximetry

The simultaneous use of pulse oximetry and continuous $S\bar{v}O_2$ monitoring is termed *dual oximetry*. The main advantage of dual oximetry is that when a change in $S\bar{v}O_2$ occurs, the contribution of the pulmonary system to that change can be immediately, objectively evaluated and not speculated on or delayed while an arterial blood gas is obtained.

Dual oximetry can also be utilized to calculate the oxygen extraction index (O_2EI) and the intrapulmonary shunt. The O_2EI appears to be valid at an SpO_2 reading of 90% or greater. It is calculated as follows:

$$O_2EI = \frac{SpO_2 - S\bar{v}O_2}{SpO_2}$$

The reader is referred to the following section for interpretation of the oxygen extraction variable.

Calculation of the intrapulmonary shunt by dual oximetry may allow for continuous evaluation of pulmonary function during the titration of PEEP in a most cost-effective manner because multiple blood gas analyses may be eliminated. When the trend for intrapulmonary shunt is plotted by dual oximetry, the value is referred to as the ventilation-perfusion index ($\dot{V}\dot{Q}I$). It is calculated as follows:

$$\dot{V}\dot{Q}I = \frac{1 - SpO_2}{1 - SvO_2}$$

Even without performing calculations, dual oximetry provides immediately useful data regarding whether changes in $S\bar{v}O_2$ are due to changes in cardiac performance or lung function. When the $S\bar{v}O_2$ decreases, a concurrent decrease in the SpO_2 indicates a defect in the pulmonary component of oxygen transport, whereas a stable SpO_2 indicates increased oxygen extraction, probably because of a decrease in cardiac peformance.

DIRECT AND DERIVED VARIABLES OF TISSUE OXYGENATION OBTAINED WITH THE PULMONARY ARTERY CATHETER

Respiration has both external and internal components. External respiration is the movement of gases into and out of the lung and includes the exchange of gases at the alveolar-capillary membrane. Internal respiration is the exchange of gases between the capillaries and the cells of the body, the ultimate respiratory units. Internal respiration, also known as tissue oxygenation, is the focus of this section.

The primary goal of internal respiration is to maintain aerobic metabolism because the oxidative metabolic pathways are the most efficient method of energy production. At the cellular level within the mitochondria (the energy factories of the cell), oxygen is consumed to produce energy in the form of adenosine triphosphate (ATP). The production of ATP occurs in the citric acid (Krebs) cycle. Aerobic oxidation will cease, however, if the amount of oxygen transported to the cells falls to a critical level.

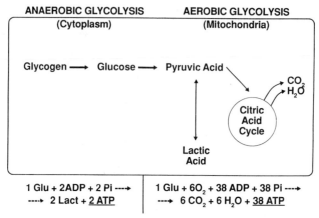

ANAEROBIC GLYCOLYSIS   AEROBIC GLYCOLYSIS
(Cytoplasm)   (Mitochondria)

1 Glu + 2ADP + 2 Pi ---→   1 Glu + 6O$_2$ + 38 ADP + 38 Pi ---→
---→ 2 Lact + <u>2 ATP</u>   ---→ 6 CO$_2$ + 6 H$_2$O + <u>38 ATP</u>

Figure 9–19 Glucose metabolism in the presence, or relative absence, of oxygen. Anaerobic glycolysis is much less efficient than aerobic glycolysis, creating significantly fewer high-energy phosphate bonds and lactic acid as a metabolic by-product. (From Mizock, BA, and Falk, JL: Lactic acidosis in critical illness. *Crit Care Med* 1992; 20(2):80–93.)

Hypoxia is a state of inadequate oxygen at the tissue level. When hypoxia is present, energy production continues because anaerobic glycolysis takes over; however, energy production then becomes much less efficient (Fig. 9–19). The by-product of anaerobic metabolism, lactic acid, begins to rise, creating a base deficit or metabolic acidosis. Therefore the patient's serum lactate level and pH are among the assessment parameters that may be utilized as indicators of the adequacy of tissue oxygenation (see Serum Lactate section, below).

Hypermetabolic and Hyperdynamic Response to Critical Illness

Recovery from critical illness requires a complex series of hemodynamic, metabolic, and immunologic adjustments. These adjustments provide the substrates needed to meet the body's high energy requirements for general maintenance of bodily functions, healing, immune system function, and so forth. During times of increased demand, large supplies of oxygen and substrates must be delivered to the cells for production of ATP via the oxidative pathways.

The body's response to the provoking stimuli of critical illness—such as surgery, trauma, fear, pain, inflammatory responses, wound healing, and infection—are mediated through the autonomic nervous system. Sympathetic nervous system stimulation results in an outpouring of catecholamines that increase ventilation, the amount of O$_2$ available in the blood, and the CO. These actions will increase the delivery of available O$_2$ and thus the transport of oxygen to the tissues. Many hormonal processes are also called into play to increase blood volume through the conservation of water and sodium, and to stimulate the release of substrates, such as glucose, needed for growth and energy production. The goal of the body in activating all of its compensatory mechanisms is to maintain adequate tissue oxygenation. Soon after injury, the tissues have large O_2 demands because of the stress imposed by critical illness, a hypermetabolic state ensues, and the body develops a hyperdynamic response to meet the high O_2 demands.

The clinical goal for the practitioner is to support the process going on in the body, and to augment it as needed when the patient's cardiopulmonary function limits the ability to mount a response sufficient to support the tissues. Recent evidence has shown that for sufficient O_2 transport to occur the patient's hemodynamics may have to reach supranormal states. The logic is that "normal" CO and oxygen delivery (DO_2) may be fine for a "normal" patient but will not meet tissue O_2 needs in a critically ill patient with huge O_2 demands. A prerequisite to appropriate patient intervention is an understanding of oxygen transport in the body and the ability to interpret tissue oxygenation variables.

Principle of Oxygen Supply and Demand

Formulating an understanding of oxygenation in terms of the principle of supply and demand provides a framework for the practitioner approaching the critically ill patient to determine the adequacy of tissue oxygenation. This framework also serves as a systematic way to determine which therapeutic measures should be taken to correct a state of inadequate tissue oxygenation.

COMPENSATORY RESPONSES TO INCREASED TISSUE OXYGEN DEMAND

A balance is ideally maintained between O_2 supply and O_2 demand in the body (Fig. 9–20). Both supply and demand can be monitored by objective measures of oxygen delivery (DO_2) and O_2 consumption ($\dot{V}O_2$), respectively. In response to increased oxygen demand by the tissues, the body activates

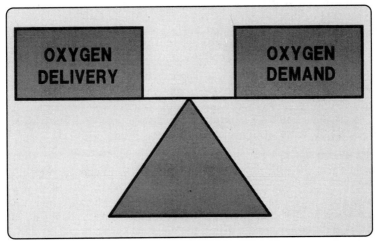

FIGURE 9–20 The primary function of the cardiopulmonary system is to provide an adequate supply of well-oxygenated blood to the tissues to meet tissue oxygen demand. The balance between O_2 delivery and O_2 demand can be monitored in the clinical setting with physiologic variables of oxygen transport and tissue O_2 utilization. (Courtesy of Baxter Healthcare Corporation, Edwards Critical-Care Division, Santa Ana, Calif.)

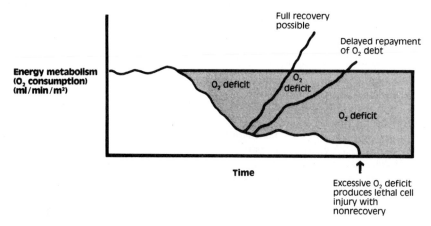

FIGURE 9-21 Oxygen debt (see text for discussion). (From Omert, L: Hemodynamic management. *Crit Care Report* 1990;1(3):376.)

compensatory responses mediated through the sympathetic nervous system. First, attempts to increase the O_2 supply, which include increasing the CO and increasing ventilation, are put into play. If attempts to increase the O_2 supply are unsatisfactory, the body then extracts a greater percentage of the available O_2 from the blood (Fig. 9–18). This results in less O_2 return to the heart in the venous blood, as evidenced by a decrease in $P\overline{v}O_2$ and $S\overline{v}O_2$ mixed venous blood gas values. These decreased values indicate diminished O_2 reserves.

When DO_2 is inadequate, variable amounts of tissue injury will occur, depending on the tissues' vulnerability to hypoxia. Tissue hypoxia translates into cellular dysfunction when aerobic sources of energy fall below the level required by the metabolic processes of those tissues. Tissues at greatest risk are the central nervous system and the myocardium, because these tissues utilize more O_2 than others in their resting state. When these vulnerable tissues must draw on reserve O_2, little is available. Conversely, some tissues tolerate hypoxia better than others. In general, it depends on the metabolic activity level of the cells. Each organ that suffers cell death from hypoxia will manifest its pathologic changes on the basis of the loss of the normal physiologic functions of that organ. Progressive damage, manifested by multiple organ dysfunction syndrome (MODS), is extremely significant to patient outcome.

OXYGEN DEBT

The fact that the body is utilizing its O_2 reserves in an effort to meet tissue O_2 demand is an excellent compensatory response. However, because oxygen cannot be stored by the body for times of increased need, when demand continues to exceed supply, anaerobic metabolism ensues, lactic acid accumulates and an actual O_2 debt accrues. The O_2 debt is the difference, with time, between the O_2 demand and the actual $\dot{V}O_2$ (Fig. 9–21). The debt will continue to grow if $\dot{V}O_2$ is limited by DO_2. If the O_2 supply is restored and the oxygen debt repaid before there is critical injury to tissue, then it is possible to preserve organ function. However, if the period of ischemia is prolonged, then irreversible damage will result.

OXYGEN DELIVERY (D_{O_2}): SUPPLY

The assessment of the patient begins with the question, Is adequate oxygen being delivered to the tissues? The amount of O_2 delivered to the tissues per minute is dependent on blood flow, CO or cardiac index, and the oxygen content of the arterial blood (CaO_2) (Fig. 9–22). Therefore:

$$O_2 \text{ Delivery } D_{O_2} = CO \times CaO_2 \times 10$$
$$\text{Normal } D_{O_2} = 1000 \text{ ml } O_2/\text{min}$$

CO is the major determinant of D_{O_2}. The CO occurs in response to metabolic demands, and individuals with an intact cardiovascular compensatory response to arterial desaturation or anemia will maintain D_{O_2}. If the patient cannot mount a sufficient response, because of new or preexisting myocardial dysfunction, then D_{O_2} falls. The clinician must then intervene to assist in augmenting the CO to maintain D_{O_2}.

A systematic examination of O_2 supply requires a CaO_2 assessment, which requires an understanding of the components of CaO_2. The O_2 content is the actual amount of O_2 in the blood. O_2 is carried in the arterial blood in two ways (Fig. 9–23): dissolved in the serum, which is assessed with the PaO_2 and in combination with hemoglobin (Hb), which is assessed with the SaO_2 (or the SpO_2 when measured with a pulse oximeter).

The O_2 dissolved in the serum accounts for only 2% to 3% of the total O_2 transported in the blood: 0.0031 ml of O_2 per 1 mm Hg per 100 ml blood. Clearly the PaO_2 provides information regarding only a very small part of the total CaO_2. If O_2 was carried in the blood only in this way, then the CO would have to be

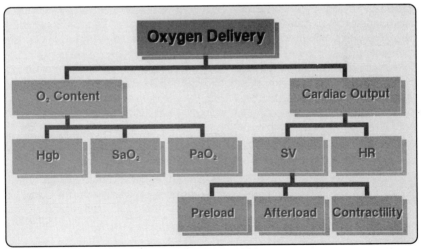

FIGURE 9–22 Oxygen delivery (D_{O_2}) is determined by the adequacy of blood flow and the oxygen content of the blood. When optimizing D_{O_2} in the clinical setting, a systematic assessment of the pulmonary (Hb, SaO_2, PaO_2) and cardiac (SV, HR) aspects of delivery will differentiate where therapeutic interventions will best be targeted. *Hb*, Hemoglobin; *SV*, stroke volume; *HR*, heart rate. (Courtesy of Baxter Healthcare Corporation, Edwards Critical-Care Division, Santa Ana, Calif.)

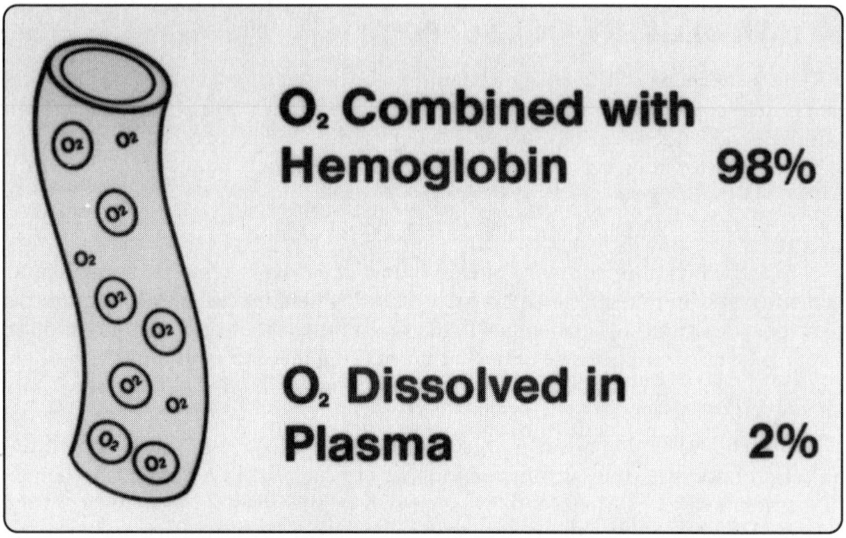

FIGURE 9–23 The majority of oxygen in the blood (98%) is carried in combination with hemoglobin and is assessed with the SaO_2. Only 2% to 3% is carried dissolved in the plasma. Dissolved O_2 is assessed with the PaO_2. (Courtesy of Baxter Healthcare Corporation, Edwards Critical-Care Division, Santa Ana, Calif.)

almost 160 L/min to deliver enough O_2 to the tissues to meet resting metabolic needs! The O_2 carried in combination with Hb accounts for 97% to 98% of transported O_2. A total of 1.34 ml of O_2 is carried in combination with Hb per 100 ml of blood. Hb is therefore an important assessment factor because it plays a major role in the O_2 carrying capacity of the blood. The relationship between Hb and O_2 is illustrated in the oxyhemoglobin dissociation curve (see Chapter 2).

Knowing how the blood carries O_2 and how to calculate the amount of O_2 carried by each method, one can calculate the CaO_2 as follows:

$$CaO_2 = (Hb \times 1.34 \times SaO_2) + (PaO_2 \times 0.0031)$$
$$\text{Normal } CaO_2 = 19\text{–}20 \text{ ml of } O_2 \text{ per deciliter of blood}$$

It should be evident from the previous discussion that Hb and SaO_2 are the primary determinants of CaO_2. If either of these components decreases, a compensatory increase in CO would be required if DO_2 were to remain adequate.

The O_2 content of the mixed venous blood, the $C\overline{v}O_2$, can also be calculated and then utilized in the computation of additional tissue oxygenation variables. For example, the difference between the O_2 contents of arterial and venous blood is used to determine *tissue utilization* of O_2. The $C\overline{v}O_2$ value is calculated as follows:

$$C\overline{v}O_2 = (Hb \times 1.34 \times S\overline{v}O_2) + (P\overline{v}O_2 \times 0.0031)$$
$$\text{Normal } C\overline{v}O_2 = 14\text{–}15 \text{ ml of } O_2 \text{ per deciliter of blood}$$

OXYGEN CONSUMPTION ($\dot{V}O_2$): DEMAND

The most meaningful overall measurement of cellular metabolism is $\dot{V}O_2$. The $\dot{V}O_2$, the amount of O_2 consumed by the body per minute, represents the total of all oxidative metabolism. The amount of O_2 needed is determined by the metabolic rate. $\dot{V}O_2$ is calculated as follows:

$$\dot{V}O_2 = CO \times (CaO_2 - C\overline{v}O_2) \times 10$$
$$\text{Normal } \dot{V}O_2 = 180\text{–}280 \text{ ml of } O_2 \text{ per minute}$$

Flow-dependent Oxygen Consumption

Under normal physiologic conditions, $\dot{V}O_2$ is independent of DO_2 (flow) and is maintained over wide variations in DO_2 because of the oxygen reserve in the blood. As delivery declines, $\dot{V}O_2$ is preserved through the activation of compensatory mechanisms, such as an increase in oxygen extraction. If delivery continues to fall, however, a point is reached where the ability to increase extraction further is exhausted. This point is termed the *critical delivery threshold* (Fig. 9–24). Below this threshold the ability of the tissues to consume oxygen is dependent on the flow of well-oxygenated blood. $\dot{V}O_2$ limited by DO_2 is known as flow-dependent, or supply-dependent, $\dot{V}O_2$; that is, the rate of O_2 consumed is limited by the rate of O_2 delivered to the tissues. In the supply-dependent region, as $\dot{V}O_2$ declines, anaerobic metabolism increases because $\dot{V}O_2$ no longer meets cellular energy requirements.

In the clinical setting, simultaneous increases in DO_2 and $\dot{V}O_2$ may indicate that a state of flow dependency is present and also provides useful information

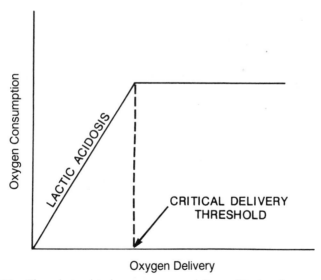

FIGURE 9–24   The relationship between oxygen delivery (DO_2) and oxygen consumption ($\dot{V}O_2$). The nonlinear response to decreases in O_2 supply is called oxygen regulation and is a normal physiologic phenomenon in man. The plateau portion of the curve represents the supply independent region where $\dot{V}O_2$ is maintained over a wide range of DO_2 as a result of vascular adaptations. Below the critical delivery threshold, $\dot{V}O_2$ becomes dependent on DO_2 (flow dependent oxygen consumption), the tissues must resort to anaerobic sources of energy production, and lactic acid ensues. See text for discussion. (From Mizock, BA, and Falk, JL: Lactic acidosis in critical illness. *Crit Care Med* 1992; 20(1):80–93.)

about the body's ability to further increase its $\dot{V}O_2$. Increases in DO_2 and $\dot{V}O_2$, but not in $S\bar{v}O_2$, indicate that tissue O_2 debt repayment is occurring. The $S\bar{v}O_2$ will not increase to normal values until the O_2 debt is repaid.

Causes of Abnormal $\dot{V}O_2$

Low $\dot{V}O_2$

Potential causes of low $\dot{V}O_2$ include the following:

1. Inadequate delivery of oxygen. A state of flow- or supply-dependent $\dot{V}O_2$ (see previous section) may be present, commonly due to a low CO state. Another example would be the early stage of hypovolemic or cardiogenic shock, in which sympathetic nervous system stimulation causes intense vasoconstriction in an effort to maintain blood pressure and venous return of blood to the heart. Capillary perfusion is restricted, limiting the delivery of oxygen to some tissue beds in need of oxygen.
2. Tissue inability to utilize O_2 because of a defect in normal cellular metabolism. This may occur with thiocyanate toxicity (which may develop when high doses of sodium nitroprusside have been used for a prolonged period) and sepsis-induced cytotoxic effects.
3. Maldistribution of capillary blood flow, primarily peripheral shunting of blood. In peripheral shunting of blood, the blood flows through capillary beds but no oxygen extraction occurs. For example, in sepsis, blood flow may be maldistributed to vasodilated areas and arteriovenous shunting occurs at the capillary level. It is also speculated that, in sepsis, oxygen extraction and consumption are reduced as a result of microcircuitry abnormalities caused by the presence of endotoxins or microemboli. Peripheral shunting also occurs with significant peripheral edema, which not only increases the diffusion distance for oxygen but may also impede capillary flow.
4. Increased metabolic demand, which may lead to a state in which $\dot{V}O_2$ is "normal" and yet inadequate to meet the higher demands imposed by critical illness.

High $\dot{V}O_2$

Potential causes of high $\dot{V}O_2$ include the following:

1. States that increase $\dot{V}O_2$ because they increase the metabolic rate. Examples include the presence of fever, shivering, seizures, hyperthyroidism, healing, increased work of breathing, and patient care activities such as turning, chest physiotherapy (CPT), bathing, and suctioning.
2. Repayment of O_2 debt.

Relation of $\dot{V}O_2$ to Survival

When $\dot{V}O_2$ is inadequate, an O_2 debt develops and various cells suffer ischemic damage depending on their vulnerability to hypoxia. Once the DO_2 improves, or the defect at the cellular level that is preventing O_2 extraction is corrected, $\dot{V}O_2$ exceeds the "baseline" demands for O_2 for a time. This excessive $\dot{V}O_2$ occurs to repay the O_2 debt and is a compensatory response with survival value. The increase in $\dot{V}O_2$ is a positive sign that the tissues are still able to utilize oxygen. Failure of the tissues to consume oxygen is an ominous sign that implies cellular defect and predicts a poor patient outcome. Unpaid O_2 debt may result in MODS. Patients who present with MODS or who die have been shown to have had greater, and more prolonged, reduced or inadequate $\dot{V}O_2$ and a greater calculated

O_2 debt than those who survive with or without organ failure. Therefore the maintenance of optimal $\dot{V}O_2$ should be a high-priority therapeutic goal in the clinical setting.

TISSUE OXYGENATION VARIABLES

A firm understanding of O_2 supply-and-demand dynamics prepares the clinician to analyze tissue oxygenation variables further. After an answer is found to the question of whether O_2 delivery is adequate to meet tissue O_2 demand, the next assessment question becomes, Is internal respiration adequate to maintain aerobic metabolism and prevent tissue hypoxia? Two variables, in addition to $\dot{V}O_2$ as previously described, will be analyzed in an attempt to answer this question: the arterial–mixed venous O_2 content difference ($AVDO_2$) and the O_2 extraction ratio (O_2ER).

Arterial–Mixed Venous O$_2$ Content Difference

The $AVDO_2$ measures the degree of oxygen extraction by the tissues. It identifies the extent to which O_2 transport matches tissue O_2 demands. $AVDO_2$ is calculated as follows:

$$AVDO_2 = CaO_2 - C\overline{v}O_2$$
$$\text{Normal } AVDO_2 = 4\text{–}6 \text{ ml/dl}$$

Because the CO is the primary determinant of oxygen delivery, the $AVDO_2$ has implications for flow and is often inversely proportional to the CO or cardiac index (CI). The following values, although not exact, are used for illustrative purposes:

AVDO$_2$	Cardiac Index
>6	<2
<3	>5

HIGH AVDO$_2$: >6 ML/DL

When the $AVDO_2$ is high, then the venous O_2 content is *decreased* because tissue O_2 extraction is increased. There is thus an inadequate supply of O_2 in relation to demand. Causes include the following:

1. Low flow states: decreased CO caused by problems with heart rate, preload, afterload, or contractility
2. Decreased arterial O_2 content caused by insufficient Hb or a defect in the pulmonary system resulting in a low PaO_2 or SaO_2
3. Increased O_2 demand because of fever, agitation, anxiety, pain, inflammatory processes, or healing; treatments such as weighing, bathing, or performing range-of-motion maneuvers; or interventions such as intubation, CPT, radiography, suctioning, or turning

LOW AVDO$_2$: <4 ML/DL

When the $AVDO_2$ is low, then the venous O_2 content is *increased* because tissue O_2 extraction is decreased. There is poor utilization of O_2. Potential causes include the following:

1. Tissues unable to utilize O_2 because of blockage of normal cellular metabolism, as may occur with thiocyanate toxicity or sepsis-induced cytotoxic effects.

2. Maldistribution of microcirculatory flow because of peripheral shunting of blood. In peripheral shunting of blood, the blood flows through capillary beds but oxygen extraction does not occur. An example is in the stage of sepsis in which blood flow is redistributed to vasodilated areas, causing arteriovenous shunting to occur at the capillary level. It is also speculated that, in sepsis, oxygen extraction and consumption is reduced as a result of microcirculatory abnormalities caused by the presence of endotoxins or microemboli. Peripheral shunting also occurs with significant peripheral edema, which increases the diffusion distance for oxygen and impedes capillary flow.
3. Increased affinity of Hb for O_2, that is, left shift of the oxyhemoglobin dissociation curve. This may occur with alkalosis, hypothermia, or administration of banked blood low in 2,3-DPG.
4. Error in mixed venous blood sampling. Aspirated blood is "arterialized" because the PA catheter is out too far or the sample was withdrawn too rapidly.
5. Oxygen delivery in excess of demand, such as when excessive supplemental oxygen is administered, hyperbaric oxygen therapy is given, or an induced high CO state is combined with a constant cellular demand.

Oxygen Extraction Ratio

The O_2ER is the percentage of oxygen delivered that is utilized by the tissues. This computation allows for the evaluation of the rate of $\dot{V}O_2$ normalized for the amount of oxygen transported. It is calculated as follows:

$$O_2ER = \frac{CaO_2 - C\bar{v}O_2}{CaO_2}$$

Normal range of O_2ER = 24–28%

Low O_2 Extraction, or Utilization

Low O_2 extraction, or utilization, is an ominous sign that, like low $\dot{V}O_2$, may affect patient survival. The underlying defect needs to be identified and corrective action taken before cell death occurs. Causes of low O_2 extraction include the following:

1. Impaired ability of the tissues to utilize O_2, blockage of normal cellular metabolism, as may occur with thiocyanate toxicity or microcirculatory abnormalities caused by sepsis.
2. Maldistribution of capillary blood flow. This may occur, for example, when doses of a vasopressor are used that result in intense vasoconstriction of some vascular beds. Because little or no blood flow is delivered to some areas, O_2 extraction cannot take place.
3. Increased affinity of Hb for O_2, indicated by a left shift of the oxyhemoglobin dissociation curve. This may occur with alkalosis, hypothermia, or administration of banked blood low in 2,3-DPG.

High O_2 Extraction, or Utilization

High O_2 extraction indicates that there is inadequate delivery in response to demand, and therefore the tissues are compensating by extracting more of the available oxygen in an attempt to maintain adequate consumption. Delivery needs to be improved so that tissues do not continue to utilize O_2 reserves.

Causes of high O_2ER may include the following:
1. Low hemoglobin concentration
2. Low PaO_2 or SaO_2 because of a pulmonary condition, such as adult respiratory distress syndrome (ARDS), pulmonary edema, an infiltrative-consolidative process, or pulmonary contusion; inappropriate ventilator settings; or technical problem with the patient-ventilator interface
3. Low CO because of a heart rate, preload, afterload, or contractility problem

Serum Lactate Concentration

A unifying factor in critically ill patients with inadequate tissue perfusion, whether it be due to hypovolemic, cardiogenic, or distributive shock, is lactic acidosis. Blood lactate levels increase with anaerobic metabolism and may represent the total O_2 debt or the magnitude of hypoperfusion. Lactate levels may also be increased in a variety of other conditions. Lactic acidosis is therefore classified as either type A (clinical evidence of tissue hypoxia) or type B (no clinical evidence of tissue hypoxia). Examples of causes of type B lactic acidosis include liver disease, malignancy, diabetes mellitus, drugs or toxins such as ethanol or salicylates, and inborn errors of metabolism. The focus of this section is on type A lactic acidosis, resulting from an imbalance of O_2 supply and demand.

Lactate is primarily metabolized by the liver. The normal amount of lactate produced under aerobic conditions is generally sufficiently managed by the liver. Therefore, under the conditions of aerobic metabolism and good liver function, there is no significant accumulation of lactate in the blood. Under anaerobic conditions, however, the amount of lactate produced will exceed the liver's ability to metabolize it, resulting in a metabolic acidosis. The patient's baseline liver function also affects the efficiency of lactate clearance and should be taken into consideration when lactate levels are interpreted.

Confirmation of a state of inadequate tissue perfusion may be assisted by obtaining a baseline lactate level drawn at the same time, or even before, the initial cardiopulmonary profile is obtained. The amount of lactate gives an indication of the severity of O_2 debt. Serial lactate levels monitored with time are then useful to determine the effectiveness of resuscitative therapies. Ideally, a steady decrease in the lactate level should be seen. If not, then the therapeutic plan should be systematically reevaluated for ways to further increase DO_2 and decrease O_2 demand. Serial evaluation of the patient's pH and base deficit may also serve as indicators of the adequacy of tissue perfusion.

TREATMENT OF TISSUE OXYGENATION IMBALANCES

Regardless of the type of shock a patient is experiencing, or the precipitating event, the common denominator is a disparity between the supply and demand of oxygen. This imbalance leads to inadequate oxygen consumption by the tissues. $\dot{V}O_2$ inadequate to meet tissue demand is related to decreased survival rates among patients with critical illness. Furthermore, persons who are critically ill often have increased O_2 needs because of a hypermetabolic state brought on by injury, inflammatory mediators, and the demands placed on the body for healing.

Optimize Do_2 and $\dot{V}o_2$

Recent evidence has shown that survivors of life-threatening critical illness demonstrate optimal oxygen transport and $\dot{V}o_2$ values that exceed those considered "normal." It has therefore been suggested that these supranormal values for physiologic variables should be used as therapeutic goals in the management of patients with perfusion deficit. These therapeutic criteria call for a CI 50% greater than normal (4.5 L/min/m²), Do_2 slightly greater than normal (600 ml/min/m²), $\dot{V}o_2$ about 30% greater than normal (170 ml/min/m²), and blood volume 500 ml in excess of the norm. Table 9–4 provides a quick reference of normal hemodynamic O_2 transport and O_2 utilization variables.

The goals of tissue resuscitation are to restore microcirculatory perfusion, stop the progression of O_2 debt, and repay any existing debt. The approach is to oxygenate, infuse, and perfuse. Sufficient FIO_2 should be used, possibly with mechanical ventilation, to ensure adequate oxygenation and ventilation and to maintain an SaO_2 of 92% or greater. The hemoglobin should be evaluated and packed red blood cells (PRBCs) administered as necessary to enhance O_2 transport.

The CI, and thus the Do_2, should be enhanced by first obtaining optimal preload. Fluid therapy titration should be based on improvements in O_2 transport (CI) and $\dot{V}o_2$, as well as physical assessment findings. Closely monitor the patient for signs of fluid overload, and if it seems that the optimal goals for volume resuscitation have been reached, and Do_2 and $\dot{V}o_2$ are still inadequate, then evaluate the need for pharmacologic support of the CI. The hemodynamic profile should be assessed to determine whether CI should be improved through agents that enhance preload, afterload, or contractility.

Contractility is enhanced with inotropic agents. An inotropic agent that increases CI without increasing systemic vascular resistance (SVR), such as dobutamine, is optimal because it increases $\dot{V}o_2$ not only by increasing Do_2 but

Table 9–4 O_2 Transport and O_2 Utilization Variables

Variable	Measurement or Calculation	Normal Value
Cardiac output (CO)	Direct measurement	4–8 L/min
Cardiac index (CI)	$\dfrac{CO}{\text{Body surface area}}$	2.5–4.0 L/min
Arterial O_2 content (CaO_2)	$CaO_2 = (Hb \times 1.34 \times SaO_2) +$ $(PaO_2 \times 0.0031)$	19–20 ml of O_2 per deciliter of blood
Venous O_2 content ($C\bar{v}O_2$)	$C\bar{v}O_2 = (Hb \times 1.34 \times S\bar{v}O_2) +$ $(P\bar{v}O_2 \times 0.0031)$	14–15 ml of O_2 per deciliter of blood
O_2 delivery (Do_2)	$Do_2 = CaO_2 \times CO \times 10$	1000 ml/min
O_2 delivery index	$Do_2 = CaO_2 \times CI \times 10$	520–720 ml/min/m²
O_2 consumption ($\dot{V}o_2$)	$\dot{V}o_2 = CO \times (CaO_2 - C\bar{v}O_2) \times 10$	180–280 ml/min
O_2 consumption index	$\dot{V}o_2 = CI \times (CaO_2 - C\bar{v}O_2) \times 10$	130–160 ml/min/m²
O_2 extraction ratio	$O_2ER = \dfrac{CaO_2 - C\bar{v}O_2}{CaO_2}$	24–28%
Arterial-venous oxygen content difference	$AVDO_2 = CaO_2 - C\bar{v}O_2$	4–6 ml/dl
Serum lactate		0.5–2.0 mEq/L

also by promoting more even distribution of peripheral blood flow. If the mean arterial pressure (MAP) and SVR are high, indicating that a high afterload may be impairing the ability to reach optimal CI, then a vasodilator may be needed. First ensure that other common causes of elevated SVR, such as pain, hypovolemia, hypothermia, anxiety, agitation, and excessive catecholamine administration, are treated. If treatment of other causes of elevated SVR are unsuccessful and shock is still refractory, use of a vasodilator is indicated. Vasodilators allow for an improvement in stroke volume by reducing afterload. The appropriate dose improves CI, Do_2, and $\dot{V}o_2$ without precipitating hypotension. An ultra-short-acting agent such as sodium nitroprusside will afford the clinician the greatest degree of control. Finally, if perfusion deficit continues, the use of a vasopressor may be indicated. A vasopressor is used to increase the MAP and is most often needed in neurogenic, anaphylactic, or septic shock or in support of a patient in arrest. Its use is contraindicated if volume status is inadequate, and caution must be used to prevent renal or splanchnic ischemia and arrhythmias.

Identify and Manage Underlying Pathologic Conditions

Patient management would be incomplete if the cardiopulmonary profile were the only focus. The underlying pathologic changes must be identified and the appropriate therapies initiated. The latter may include surgical drainage or debridement, antibiotic therapy, pulmonary toilet, and a myriad of other interventions. Adequate nutrition must also be ensured. Substrates are needed to produce ATP, for healing, to maintain immunologic function, and to ensure that visceral stores are not utilized for these processes. The goal of nutritional assessment and intervention is an anabolic state of healing. The critically ill patient must be fed early in the course of their illness, before a significant negative nitrogen balance develops.

Reduce Oxygen Demand

Reduction of O_2 demands should be made, where possible, concurrently with the achievement of optimal Do_2 and $\dot{V}o_2$ and is done by administering sedation if the patient is agitated or active. The use of neuromuscular blocking agents may also be needed, especially if the patient is difficult to ventilate and oxygenate. Febrile states should be treated because for every 1° C rise in temperature there is a 13% increase in metabolic rate and for every 1° F rise a 7% increase. Patient care activities should be organized to avoid excessive demands. The use of continuous $S\overline{v}o_2$ monitoring is particularly helpful in determining when activity, and thus O_2 demand, should be reduced.

Achieving maximal Do_2 in critically ill patients results in improved survival. Underlying O_2 deficits must be treated with the use of physiologic principles to ensure that adequate resuscitation has occurred at the cellular level, which is where the ultimate respiratory units lie.

APPLICATION OF TISSUE OXYGENATION VARIABLES: A CASE STUDY

A 52-year-old male pedestrian hit by a car was admitted to the trauma center. His injuries included a closed head injury; liver, renal vein, and superior mesenteric vein lacerations; an open fracture of the right femur; and multiple abrasions and lacerations. He was taken to the operating room, where an exploratory laparotomy was performed. Control of bleeding and repair of the liver, renal, and mesenteric lacerations was achieved. The right leg wound was irrigated and debrided, and a right tibial Steinman pin was placed for application of traction and fracture reduction.

When the patient was admitted to the ICU, his Hb and hematocrit values were 9.7 and 27.8, with a platelet count of 54,000. The patient was putting out moderate to large amounts of bloody drainage via an abdominal drain. Oozing from the femur wound and multiple abrasions was also evident. Hemodynamics after administration of dopamine, 2.5 μg/kg/min, dobutamine, 14.0 μg/kg/min, and epinephrine, 10 μg/min, were as follows:

- Sinus tachycardia rate = 110 beats/min
- Mean arterial pressure (MAP) = 65 mm Hg
- Central venous pressure (CVP) = 9
- Pulmonary capillary wedge pressure (PCWP) = 11
- CI = 5.4 L/min/m^2

An ABG sample was drawn on the following ventilator settings: assist/control (A/C) of 14, FIO_2 0.6, 5 cm H_2O PEEP, and VT 900. The following values were revealed:

pH	7.19	$Paco_2$	46		
Pao_2	144	HCO_3^-	18		
Sao_2	97.8%	Base excess (BE)	−9.9	Temperature	33.4° C

Therefore the pulmonary aspects of O_2 transport (Pao_2, Sao_2) were sufficient. The patient's ventilation ($Paco_2$) needed to be improved to correct that portion of the acidosis attributable to the respiratory system. The therapeutic goal was to increase preload and to assist in the weaning of the vasopressor (epinephrine), which because of its intense vasoconstrictive effect, would impair microcirculatory perfusion and $\dot{V}o_2$. The patient was given 1000 ml of 5% albumin and two units of PRBCs. Hypothermia was also noted to be a problem and warming measures were instituted. It was recognized that returning the body temperature to normal would result in dilation of vasoconstricted vascular beds and possibly in a drop in BP or CO.

After rewarming measures and volume administration, the epinephrine was reduced to 8.0 μg/min and the MAP increased to 72 mm Hg. A cardiopulmonary profile was then obtained (normal values in parentheses):

AVDO$_2$	2.4	(4–6)	CI	5.3
O$_2$Ext	21	(24–28%)	BP	104/50 (72)
$\dot{V}o_2$ (index)	124	(130–160)	PCWP	15
S$\bar{v}o_2$	79	(60–80)	Hb	8.0
Lactate	8.2	(<2.0)	Temperature	36.9° C

ABG: 7.32/168/31/HCO$_3^-$ 16/BE −8.2/Sao$_2$ 98% on A/C 14, FIO_2 0.6, 5 cm H_2O PEEP, and VT 1000

The following is the interpretation of the tabular material above: The AVDO$_2$ is low, indicating that C$\bar{v}o_2$ is increased, which is confirmed with an S$\bar{v}o_2$ of

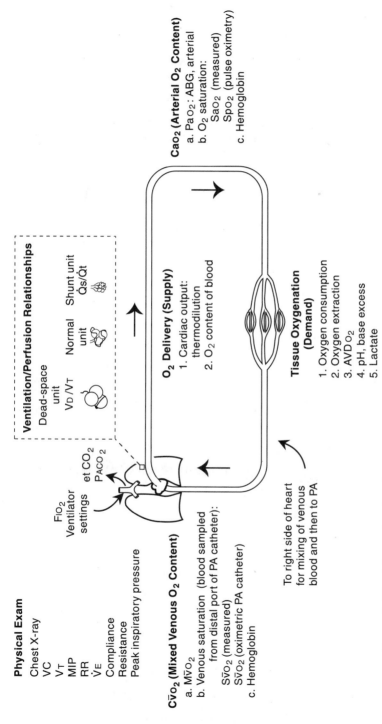

Physical Exam

Chest X-ray
VC
V_T
MIP
RR
$\dot{V}_E$
Compliance
Resistance
Peak inspiratory pressure

FIO_2
Ventilator
settings

et CO_2
$PACO_2$

Ventilation/Perfusion Relationships

Dead-space
unit
V_D/V_T

Normal
unit

Shunt unit
$\dot{Q}s/\dot{Q}t$

Ca_{O_2} (Arterial O_2 Content)

a. Pa_{O_2}: ABG, arterial
b. O_2 saturation:
   Sa_{O_2} (measured)
   Sp_{O_2} (pulse oximetry)
c. Hemoglobin

O_2 Delivery (Supply)

1. Cardiac output:
   thermodilution
2. O_2 content of blood

Tissue Oxygenation (Demand)

1. Oxygen consumption
2. Oxygen extraction
3. AVD_{O_2}
4. pH, base excess
5. Lactate

$C\bar{v}_{O_2}$ (Mixed Venous O_2 Content)

a. $M\bar{v}_{O_2}$
b. Venous saturation (blood sampled
   from distal port of PA catheter):
   $S\bar{v}_{O_2}$ (measured)
   $S\bar{v}_{O_2}$ (oximetric PA catheter)
c. Hemoglobin

To right side of heart
for mixing of venous
blood and then to PA

Figure 9–25 Advanced cardiopulmonary assessment data allow for the evaluation of external and internal respiration. Understanding which aspect of respiration each variable assesses is essential.

79%. The cause of the high $C\bar{v}O_2$ is revealed by the low O_2Ext. The $\dot{V}O_2$ is low because the tissues are not extracting quite enough O_2, probably because the O_2 supply is inadequate to meet the needs of this patient with huge O_2 demands. Regional O_2 supply is also being compromised peripherally because of the intense vasoconstriction caused by the epinephrine. Anaerobic metabolism is evident with the high lactate level.

Volume resuscitation continued, so that DO_2 could be increased further, with 250 ml additional 5% albumin, 2 more units of PRBCs, 4 units of fresh frozen plasma, and 6 platelet packs, until the CI continued to show no further improvement at 6.2 L/min/m^2. The epinephrine dosage was able to be reduced downward to 4 µg/min. This hemodynamic state was maintained and the trend of the progression was monitored with lactate levels. Within 7 hours the lactate concentration was 4.0. Four hours later it was down to a normal level of 2.2. Throughout this resuscitation, O_2 demand was minimized through the use of heavy sedation because the patient was very agitated. At one point the use of a neuromuscular blocking agent was also necessary.

SUMMARY

In the critical care setting a plethora of variables may be monitored by the critical care clinician for the purposes of completing an advanced pulmonary assessment, determining where deficiencies lie, and intervening appropriately. The use of sophisticated physiologic variables of O_2 transport and consumption provide the clinician with the insight necessary to manage the resuscitation, not of the vital signs, but of the tissues. Timely resuscitation of states of O_2 deficiency has been shown to reduce morbidity and mortality among critically ill persons.

It is imperative that the bedside practitioner understand how to interpret the data collected and what aspect of the cardiopulmonary system each variable assesses (Fig. 9–25). These variables, however, are useful only if collected with reliable equipment and interpreted in light of physical assessment of the patient.

RECOMMENDED READINGS

American College of Chest Physicians/Society of Critical Care Medicine Consensus Conference Committee (1992). American College of Chest Physicians/Society of Critical Care Medicine Consensus Conference: Definitions for sepsis and organ failure and guidelines for the use of innovative therapies in sepsis. *Crit Care Med* 20(6), 864–874.

Barone, J.E., and Snyder, A.B. (1991). Treatment strategies in shock: Use of oxygen transport measurements. *Heart Lung* 20(1), 81–86.

Bongard, F.S., and Leighton, T.A. (1992). Continuous dual oximetry in surgical critical care: Indications and limitations. *Ann Surg* 216(1), 60–68.

Cardiopulmonary Diagnostics Guidelines Committee (1992). AARC clinical practice guideline: Sampling for arterial blood gas analysis. *Respir Care* 37(8), 913–917.

Carlon, G.C., et al. (1988). Capnography in mechanically ventilated patients. *Crit Care Med* 16(5), 550–556.

Chulay, M., et al. (1992). Clinical comparison of two- and three-wavelength systems for continuous measurement of venous oxygen saturation. *Am J Crit Care* 1(1), 69–75.

Dracup, K., and Bryan-Brown, C.W. (Eds.) (1990). $S\bar{v}O_2$ monitoring: Research and clinical applications [Symposium proceedings]. *Heart Lung* 19(5); Pt 2 [suppl].

Graham, B., Paulus, D.A., and Caffee, H.H. (1986). Pulse oximetry for vascular monitoring in upper extremity replantation surgery. *J Hand Surg* 11A(5), 687–692.

Gutierrez, G., and Ronco, J.J. (1995). Tissue gas exchange. In R. Bone (Ed.). *Pulmonary and Critical Care Medicine* (pp. 1–18). St. Louis: Mosby–Year Book.

Hess, D. (1991). Noninvasive respiratory monitoring during ventilatory support. *Crit Care Clin North Am* 3(4), 565–574.

Lorenz, A. (1989). Lactic acidosis: A nursing challenge. *Crit Care Nurse* 9(4), 64–73.

Mackersie, R.C., and Karagianes, T.G. (1990). Use of end-tidal carbon dioxide tension for monitoring induced hypocapnia in head-injured patients. *Crit Care Med* 18(7), 764–765.

McGee, W.T., Veremakis, C., and Wilson, G.L. (1988). Clinical importance of tissue oxygenation and use of the mixed venous blood gas. *Res Medica* 4(2), 15–24.

Mizok, B.A., and Falk, J.L. (1992). Lactic acidosis in critical illness. *Crit Care Med* 20(1), 80–93.

Pierson, D.J., and Kacmarek, R.M. (1992). *Foundations of Respiratory Care*. New York: Churchill Livingstone.

Schnapp, L.M., and Cohen, N.H. (1990). Pulse oximetry: Uses and abuses. *Chest* 98(5), 1244–1250.

Shapiro, B.A., et al. (1989). Pulmonary artery oximetry. In B.A. Shapiro, et al. *Clinical Application of Blood Gases* (pp. 226–231). 4th ed. Chicago: Year Book Medical Publishers.

Shoemaker, W.C. (1987). Relation of oxygen transport patterns to the pathophysiology and therapy of shock states. *Intensive Care Med* 13, 230–243.

Shoemaker, W.C. (1992). Monitoring and management of acute circulatory problems: The expanded role of the physiologically oriented critical care nurse. *Am J Crit Care* 1(1), 38–53.

Shoemaker, W.C., Appel, P.L., and Kram, H.B. (1990). Measurement of tissue perfusion by oxygen transport patterns in experimental shock and in high-risk surgical patients. *Intensive Care Med* 16(suppl 2), S135–S144.

Shoemaker, W.C., Appel, P.L., and Kram, H.B. (1988). Tissue oxygen debt as a determinant of lethal and nonlethal postoperative organ failure. *Crit Care Med* 16(11), 1117–1120.

Shoemaker, W.C., Appel, P.L., and Kram, H.B. (1991). Oxygen transport measurements to evaluate tissue perfusion and titrate therapy: Dobutamine and dopamine effects. *Crit Care Med* (19)5, 672–688.

Shoemaker, W.C., et al. (1990). The efficacy of central venous and pulmonary artery catheters and therapy based upon them in reducing mortality and morbidity. *Arch Surg* 125, 1332–1338.

Sonnesso, G. (1991). Are you ready to use pulse oximetry? *Nursing*, 21(8), 60–64.

Sprung, C.L. (1993). *The pulmonary artery catheter: Methodology and clinical applications*. 2nd ed. Closter, N.J.: Critical Care Research Associates.

St. John, R.E. (1989). Exhaled gas analysis: Technical and clinical aspects of capnography and oxygen consumption. *Crit Care Nurs Clin North Am* 1(4), 669–679.

Swedlow, D.B. (1986). Capnometry and capnography: The anesthesia disaster early warning system. *Semin Anesth* 5(3), 194–205.

Szaflarski, N.L., and Cohen, N.H. (1991). Use of capnography in critically ill adults. *Heart Lung* 20(4), 363–372.

Tobin, M.J. (1988). Respiratory monitoring in the intensive care unit. *Am Rev Respir Dis* 138, 1625–1642.

Varon, A.J., Morrina, J., and Civetta, J.M. (1991). Clinical utility of a calorimetric end-tidal CO_2 detector in cardiopulmonary resuscitation and emergency intubation. *J Clin Monit* 7(4), 289–293.

Von Rueden, K.T. (1989). Cardiopulmonary assessment of the critically ill trauma patient. *Crit Care Nurs Clin North Am* 1(1), 33–44.

Welch, J.P., DeCesare, R., and Hess, D. (1990). Pulse oximetry: Instrumentation and clinical applications. *Respir Care* 35(6), 584–601.

◆ **10** ◆

──
──

Weaning From Mechanical Ventilation

Weaning from mechanical ventilation is the process of withdrawing the patient from mechanical ventilatory support in a staged manner. Patients who have required ventilatory support for only a short term and have no significant underlying pulmonary abnormality generally do not require an extensive weaning program. An example of this type of patient is one who requires postoperative ventilatory support after the administration of general anesthesia. Ventilatory support may simply be discontinued for this subgroup of patients once they are awake enough and have regained sufficient muscle strength to breathe on their own. True weaning is required in patients in whom the respiratory muscles are weakened and detrained. Repeated attempts at weaning may be unsuccessful and complicated by many factors such as malnutrition, stress, and immobility. The goal of a weaning program is to facilitate the strength and endurance of the respiratory muscles needed to sustain spontaneous ventilation. This goal may be achieved through good nutrition and the application of a planned, well-monitored program of exercise targeted at the respiratory muscles.

RESPIRATORY MUSCLE FUNCTION

The application of the principles of exercise physiology to the retraining of respiratory muscles requires an understanding of the types of muscle being retrained. The muscles of respiration are skeletal muscles and as such can be classified as slow (type I) or fast (type II) twitch fibers, terms that refer to the duration of muscular contraction. The respiratory muscles are mixed muscles; for example, the diaphragm contains about 50% type I and 50% type II fibers.

The duration of contraction of a skeletal muscle is, in general, adapted to the function of that muscle. Generally, slow muscles (type I fibers) are adapted for prolonged performance of work and are the most resistant to fatigue; they demonstrate greater endurance. Slow fibers are smaller, produce the lowest level of force when activated, and have a greater capillary supply and more mitochondria than fast fibers. They are the first to be recruited in motor efforts. They also contain myoglobin, a substance similar to hemoglobin in that it can combine with oxygen, storing it in the muscle cell until it is needed by the mitochondria. Therefore the slow fibers are ideal for a low-intensity, endurance activity such as quiet breathing, have a high oxidative capacity, and are specialized for aerobic energy yield. However, if subjected to sustained submaximal activity, slow fibers are also the first to exhaust their glycogen energy stores and to show fatigue.

Type II (fast) fibers have a more extensive sarcoplasmic reticulum; thus calcium can be rapidly released and taken up, allowing for rapid contraction. They reach peak tension in a very short time, and when higher-intensity respiratory activity such as vigorous coughing is required, the central nervous system recruits the fast-twitch fibers because they are adapted for strength. However, unlike slow fibers, they have low oxidative capacity and are very susceptible to fatigue when repeatedly activated.

EXERCISE PHYSIOLOGY APPLIED TO RESPIRATORY MUSCLE TRAINING

As we are all painfully aware, simply using our muscles does not constitute physical training, even if it does prevent disuse atrophy. To retrain respiratory muscles, a physical training program, with components of endurance and strength training, must be devised. A training effect can be achieved only if a sufficient load, in terms of intensity, duration, and frequency, is applied to the respiratory muscles. The duration of exercise periods is based on patient tolerance and the prevention of fatigue. The goal of a program designed to recondition the respiratory muscles is an improvement in muscle performance, as evidenced by the ability to sustain spontaneous respiration for increasingly longer periods.

Strength is the ability to develop force against resistance in a single contraction. Strength is developed when resistive or isometric exercise is applied. Strength conditioning is achieved by short bursts of intense activity or low repetitions of a high-intensity stimulus, such as sprints to the runner, heavy weights and limited repetitions to the weight lifter, or T-piece trials to the patient being weaned. This forceful type of muscular activity causes the muscle size to increase (hypertrophy). The individual muscle fibers (sarcomeres) increase in diameter, their nutrient stores increase, and they even gain in mitochondria. Both their motive power and their nutrient mechanisms for supporting increased motive power increase.

Strength conditioning of the respiratory muscles is achieved with high-pressure, low-volume work. High-pressure work calls for large airway and intrapleural pressure changes to accomplish minimal volume changes in the lung. It also requires high energy expenditure. When high-pressure work is applied to persons with normal lung function, they may be able to generate enough energy to achieve adequate volumes. However, persons with compliance or resistance abnormalities, or who are breathing through the increased resistance of a ventilator circuit, may become overwhelmed by the amount of energy required to sustain ventilation and experience fatigue. Under these conditions, it becomes necessary to limit the duration of the exercise periods or to implement strategies designed to decrease the work of breathing.

Endurance is the ability to exercise for prolonged periods before fatigue occurs. Endurance conditioning is achieved with numerous repetitions of a low-intensity activity, such as long-distance jogging by the runner, multiple repetitions with lower weights by the weight trainer, and the use of the pressure-support mode by the patient being weaned from a ventilator. This less intense muscular activity sustained for long periods promotes muscle endurance, not hypertrophy. It promotes mitochondrial enhancement and increases oxidative enzymes, myoglobin, and even the number of blood capillaries to support increased oxygen uptake and muscle metabolism.

Endurance is promoted through prolonged, mild exercise. Specific to the respiratory muscles, it is achieved with low-pressure, high-volume work. Endurance conditioning can be achieved with exercises that are both specific and nonspecific to the respiratory muscles. Nonspecific exercises involve general body conditioning.

The three basic principles of skeletal muscle training are overload, specificity, and reversibility. Overload means that the muscle must be challenged to the limits of its ability so that it will increase in size and functional ability. Specificity means that training needs to be applied specifically to the functional characteristic of that muscle, that is, endurance versus strength. Reversibility implies that if training ceases, the performance capabilities of the muscle will gradually decline.

VENTILATORY MUSCLE FATIGUE

During weaning, fatigue caused by excessive exertion should be avoided. Muscle fatigue is the inability of the muscle to continue to develop a force sufficient to perform a particular task. Fatigue results from muscle activity under a load (exertion) and is reversible by rest. Respiratory muscle fatigue therefore results in the inability of the respiratory muscles to continue to develop sufficient pressure changes to maintain adequate alveolar ventilation. Unlike fatigue of the biceps from carrying too heavy a load, fatigue of the respiratory muscles can be life-threatening. Much research is still needed in the areas of clinical diagnosis of respiratory muscle fatigue and the therapies that will assist in the recovery of fatigued muscles.

Fatigue is a function of the load placed on the ventilatory muscles and the muscle energy utilization capabilities. Prevention of muscle fatigue, therefore, requires maintenance of a balance between demand and supply factors affecting the ventilatory muscles. Demand factors include the work of breathing and the intensity of muscle contraction, whereas supply factors include provision and utilization of necessary substrates, such as flow of blood to the muscles, oxygen content in the blood, general nutritional status, glycogen reserves, and the muscles' ability to utilize energy (metabolic milieu).

Respiratory muscle fatigue may be manifested in the following conditions:

1. Decreased muscle strength due to factors affecting neuromuscular function. Causes may include defects in the contractile machinery as a consequence of atrophy (muscle cells become smaller), or as a consequence of loss of muscle mass, as in malnutrition. Neuromuscular diseases such as myasthenia gravis fall into this category of conditions that result in weak muscles, thereby contributing to the development of respiratory muscle fatigue.

2. An increase in the energy demand that exceeds the ability to produce work. Such imbalances occur with increases in airway resistance, decreases in pulmonary compliance, hypoxemia, and increases in abdominal volume or pressure.

3. An imbalance between energy supply and demand. A reduction in the energy supply to the muscles occurs during hypoxemia, anemia, low cardiac output states, hypophosphatemia, electrolyte imbalance (particularly sodium, potassium, and chloride), and starvation. Diaphragmatic blood flow

decreases in low cardiac output states and when diaphragmatic contraction is very intense. The increased energy demand in working muscle may also result in depletion of muscle energy stores, glycogen, and adenosine triphosphate (ATP). Such depletion has been established as being associated with muscle fatigue.

4. An accumulation of metabolic end products that inhibit or reduce muscle contraction. Accumulation of toxic by-products of muscle contraction, especially lactic acid, further contributes to fatigue. At a lower pH, a larger amount of calcium is needed to produce a given tension in muscle, and the increased amount of hydrogen ion exerts a direct negative effect on the contractile process.

Fatigue: Clinical Signs

Clinical manifestations of respiratory fatigue include a dysfunctional breathing pattern: increased respiratory rate (tachypnea) and shallow breathing, associated with a minute ventilation ($\dot{V}E$) in excess of 10 L/min. Despite the increased $\dot{V}E$, the alveolar ventilation is decreased because most of the increased inspiratory flow is through the anatomic dead space. Bedside pulmonary function tests show a reduction in vital capacity (VC) and maximum inspiratory pressure (MIP) (see Weaning Assessment Criteria, below). As the patient continues to breathe under fatiguing conditions, bradypnea and central apnea will ensue. It is unknown whether the reduction in central discharge is due to fatigue of the central nervous system or to an adaptive characteristic of the muscle that prevents its self-destruction by excessive activation.

Additional clinical signs that may indicate respiratory muscle fatigue include abnormalities of thoracoabdominal mechanics, such as respiratory alternans, which is an alteration between abdominal and rib cage breathing; asynchrony, or discoordinate breathing, which is characterized by a difference in the rate of motion of the chest and abdomen; and abdominal paradox, which is an inward movement of the abdomen during inspiration. Abdominal paradox, also seen with diaphragm paralysis, indicates that the diaphragm is not contracting properly. Reduction, or asynchronous activation of the chest wall and abdomen, reduces the efficiency of tidal volume distribution. This further increases the burden on the respiratory muscles, their use becomes even less efficient, and the problem of fatigue is compounded. The clinical observation of abnormal breathing mechanics has been shown to precede an increase in $PaCO_2$. Thus an increase in $PaCO_2$ is a late sign of respiratory muscle dysfunction.

The assumption that rib cage–abdominal motion abnormalities are reliable signs of fatigue and inevitably imply weaning failure is challenged by others (Tobin et al., 1987) who argue that abdominal paradox is due to an increase in load placed on the respiratory muscles rather than to fatigue. This conclusion was drawn after nonfatiguing exercise with significant inspiratory load resulted in rib cage–abdominal asynchrony within 1 minute of exercise initiation. Furthermore, the amount of abnormal motion did not progress as the exercise was continued. Abnormal motion of the ribcage and abdomen has been observed both in patients who are successfully weaned and in those whose weaning has been unsuccessful. Patients who fail weaning, however, may display more severe asynchrony and paradox than successfully weaned patients. Because there is considerable overlap between the two groups, abnormal rib cage–abdominal motion is probaby not discriminatory of fatigue or weaning failure.

Additional causes of rib cage–abdominal asynchrony include partial or complete upper airway obstruction, retained volatile anesthetic, which can selectively reduce rib cage activity, and residual neuromuscular blockade, even with full return of peripheral neuromuscular twitch.

When fatigue begins, bedside monitoring of respiratory rate (RR), $\dot{V}E$, tidal volume (VT), and breathing pattern signals changes that precede changes in pH and $PaCO_2$. All these parameters can be monitored by inspection at the bedside. Careful bedside monitoring may therefore preclude the need for repeated blood gas measures and may allow the clinician to determine when to return the patient to mechanical ventilatory support. If deemed necessary, blood gas analysis may be utilized to substantiate the diagnosis of fatigue.

When patients have respiratory muscle weakness, exercise training is useful. However, when respiratory muscle fatigue is the cause of the weakness, then rest is required, not training. Weakness is suggested by a chronic reduction in strength of the muscles, whereas fatigue is suggested by an acute decrease in strength, an abrupt increase in the $PaCO_2$ and possibly the development of abnormal rib cage–abdominal motion. It must be emphasized that fatigue occurs when there is an imbalance between energy supply and demand. It is reversible by ensuring adequate energy supply to the muscle, and by rest.

VENTILATORY MUSCLE REST

For successful, gradual reconditioning of the respiratory muscles, periods of exercise should be alternated with complete rest. The rationale for rest lies in an understanding of the previous discussion of how fatigue can lead to respiratory failure. Rest and nutrition are essential to replete necessary muscle glycogen and ATP. Adequate rest and prevention of fatigue are therefore key components in a respiratory muscle training program.

Returning the patient to ventilatory support or to a mode that assumes the work of breathing (WOB) will allow the respiratory muscles to rest. The metabolic cost of spontaneous, normal breathing is only 1% to 3% of total body oxygen consumption. Oxygen consumption necessary to support respiration increases with pulmonary disease and during weaning trials. $\dot{V}O_2$ may average as high as 25% of total oxygen consumption. Rest reduces the oxygen consumption of the respiratory muscles, thus improving availability of oxygen to other tissues. Whether an optimal ventilatory mode for providing rest to the inspiratory muscles exists still requires further investigation. Typical modes used for rest are assist/control (A/C) and high-level pressure support (PS_{max}). Sufficient rest time is needed to reverse the factors that led to fatigue. The recovery time necessary to return to normal resting conditions after exercise training is a function of the intensity and duration of the training program and the patient's work capacity. The amount of time devoted to rest should gradually decrease as the patient's muscle function improves.

WEANING ASSESSMENT CRITERIA

The purpose of weaning parameters is to identify the patient's readiness to be weaned in an effort to avoid premature weaning trials, which may stress the cardiorespiratory system, and to prevent prolonged ventilatory support and its associated complications. Weaning parameters are therefore theoretically utilized to predict whether a patient can be weaned successfully. However, the predictive power of weaning parameters is an area of much-needed research. Weaning parameters are also utilized to provide insight into the reasons for a patient's ventilator dependence and therefore provide a focus on which therapeutic interventions need to be implemented to prepare the patient for weaning. They may also assist in formulation of a weaning plan targeted toward the patient's specific needs. Serial measurements made after initiation of a weaning plan can be used to monitor the patient's progress. Throughout the literature, weaning parameters are also referred to as extubation criteria. Threshold values of adequacy are placed on the parameters, which implies that patients who meet these values may undergo successful extubation. The term *successful extubation* is generally considered to mean that the patient is able to remain free of ventilatory support for at least 24 hours. The predictive value of extubation criteria is also very limited.

It is imperative that weaning parameters be obtained in a standardized fashion so that useful, reproducible information is provided. Parameters that are dependent on patient cooperation and effort are the most susceptible to variability. These include vital capacity and maximum inspiratory pressure measures. Because studies have generally shown that the predictive power of standard weaning indices is poor, these measurements alone should not be used to determine a patient's readiness to be weaned, and the quest for more predictive indices must continue. Clinical judgment must play an important role in determining weaning readiness, especially if the patient lacks motivation or is unable to cooperate when weaning parameters are obtained. Weaning parameters facilitate assessment of component aspects of respiration and may be divided into the categories of oxygenation, ventilation, and respiratory muscle mechanics (Table 10–1).

Oxygenation

Patients are generally considered ready to be weaned when they can maintain a PaO_2 >70 mm Hg on an FIO_2 <0.5 and PEEP of 5 cm H_2O or less. Oxygenation is also assessed by evaluating the PaO_2 in relation to the FIO_2 by means of the simple-to-calculate PaO_2/FIO_2 ratio. A value of 200 indicates an intrapulmonary shunt of approximately 17.5%, oxygenation difficulties, and potential weaning problems. The PaO_2/FIO_2 ratio should therefore be greater than 200 as an indication of readiness to wean. If a pulmonary artery catheter is in place, the intrapulmonary shunt ($\dot{Q}s/\dot{Q}T$) fraction can be calculated. It should be <20% (see Chapter 2 for further information on the PaO_2/FIO_2 ratio and the $\dot{Q}s/\dot{Q}T$ fraction).

Ventilation

With blood gas analysis used as an assessment of ventilation and readiness for a weaning trial, the patient ideally should have a $PaCO_2$ value around normal (35 to 45 mm Hg), with a pH of 7.30 to 7.45. Chronic CO_2 retention should be considered in the determination of an acceptable baseline $PaCO_2$ for any given patient. The ratio of dead space to tidal volume (VD/VT) should be <0.6. Values greater than 0.6 signal an increased ventilatory demand, which may exceed ventilatory reserve when a weaning trial is attempted. Further information regarding the patient's ability to adequately ventilate is also provided by most of the measurements used to evaluate the mechanical function of the respiratory system.

Table 10-1 Standard Criteria Utilized to Determine Readiness to Wean From Mechanical Ventilation

Parameter	Threshold Value
Oxygenation	
PaO_2	>70 mm Hg on FIO_2 <0.5; PEEP of 5 cm H_2O or less
PaO_2/FIO_2	>200
$\dot{Q}s/\dot{Q}T$	<20%
Ventilation	
$PaCO_2$	35–45 mm Hg with pH 7.30 to 7.45, or baseline $PaCO_2$ for chronic CO_2 retainers
VD/VT	<0.6
Ventilatory Demand	
Minute ventilation ($\dot{V}E$)	>5 L/min but <10 L/min
Respiratory Mechanics	
Endurance measures	
Maximum voluntary ventilation (MVV)	Twice the $\dot{V}E$
Tidal volume (VT)	>300 cc, or ≥5 cc/kg
Strength measures	
Maximum inspiratory pressure (MIP)	<−20
Vital capacity (VC)	10–15 cc/kg
Respiratory Frequency and Pattern	
Respiratory rate	≤25 breaths/min
Ratio of frequency to tidal volume (f:VT)	<105 breaths/min/L

Respiratory Mechanics

Respiratory mechanics attempt to quantify respiratory muscle function in terms of strength and endurance.

MINUTE VENTILATION

The minute ventilation ($\dot{V}E$) is obtained by attaching a handheld spirometer to the patient's airway and instructing the patient to breathe normally for 1 minute (Fig. 10–1). Depending on ventilator model, the $\dot{V}E$ may also be obtained from the front panel display after the patient has been allowed to breathe spontaneously through the ventilator circuit for 1 minute. The $\dot{V}E$ value, along with the $PaCO_2$, gives a good indication of the demands being placed on the respiratory system. Normal $\dot{V}E$ is about 6 L/min. Values >5 L/min but <10 L/min are desirable when considering the patient for a weaning trial. Requirements for a high $\dot{V}E$, to maintain an acceptable $PaCO_2$, place an increased workload on the respiratory muscles. $\dot{V}E$ values >10 L/min, together with shallow, rapid respirations, have been associated with respiratory muscle fatigue.

MAXIMUM VOLUNTARY VENTILATION

Maximum voluntary ventilation (MVV) is obtained by attaching a spirometer to the airway and instructing the patient to breathe as hard and as fast as pos-

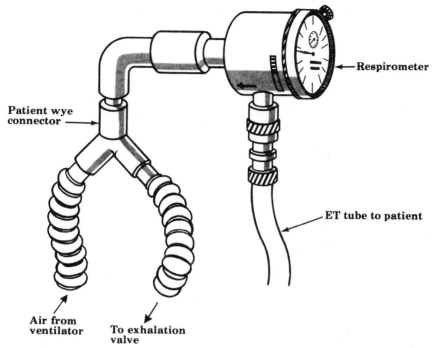

Respirometer

Patient wye connector

ET tube to patient

Air from ventilator

To exhalation valve

FIGURE 10-1 Handheld spirometer for measuring the volume parameters of tidal volume (VT) and minute ventilation ($\dot{V}E$). Exhaled volume is measured by attaching the respirometer directly to the endotracheal tube. Alternatively, the respirometer may be attached to the exhalation valve. Some spirometers are capable of measuring both inspiratory and expiratory flow. (From Pilbeam, SP: *Mechanical Ventilation: Physiological and Clinical Applications.* St. Louis: Mosby–Year Book, 1992.)

sible for 1 minute. The MVV assesses the patient's ability to sustain ventilation under stress. A normal MVV value is 50 to 250 L/min. The relation between the $\dot{V}E$ and the MVV provides a measure of ventilatory reserve and respiratory muscle endurance. The patient who is ready for a weaning trial should be capable, at least, of doubling the $\dot{V}E$ during the MVV maneuver. The patient must be cooperative and motivated to perform an MVV maneuver. In many intensive care settings the MVV is not measured because of the required level of patient cooperation.

TIDAL VOLUME

The average tidal volume (VT), measured in milliliters, is obtained by measuring the minute ventilation and dividing it by the respiratory rate (RR). The VT should generally be >300 ml before weaning is attempted. A VT <300 ml may indicate that the patient will have difficulty maintaining alveolar ventilation. More meaningful than a single value of adequacy for patients of all body sizes is an evaluation of the volume of gas that the patient moves in a tidal breath in relation to body weight. A normal spontaneous VT, the volume of gas inspired or exhaled in a single breath, is 5 to 8 ml/kg. Before a weaning trial the patient should be able to achieve a spontaneous $V_T \geq 5$ ml/kg. A decreased V_T indicates that the patient cannot generate sufficient muscular work to overcome the elastance and resistance of the lung. V_T is considered a measure of respiratory muscle endurance.

VITAL CAPACITY

Vital capacity (VC) is the maximum volume exhaled after a maximum inspiration. It is measured in milliliters per kilogram by a handheld spirometer that attaches to the endotracheal or tracheostomy tube. The patient is asked first to inhale to total lung capacity and then to exhale to residual volume. Obtaining a reliable VC measurement requires a considerable amount of patient cooperation.

The normal VC is usually between 65 and 75 ml/kg. A VC of >10 to 15 ml/kg is needed to sustain spontaneous respiration. The VC is a useful measurement of ventilatory reserve and strength. It reflects the patient's mechanical ability to take a deep breath, reverse atelectasis, and cough to mobilize secretions. A VC of <10 to 15 ml/kg suggests that the patient may become fatigued and have difficulty sighing, reversing atelectasis, and coughing. Measurements of VC have poor predictive value in terms of weaning outcome, probably because patient cooperation is required in obtaining the measurement.

MAXIMUM INSPIRATORY PRESSURE

The maximum inspiratory pressure (MIP) is measured in centimeters of H_2O by an inspiratory force meter, a gauge that is attached to the endotracheal or tracheostomy tube (Fig. 10–2). The patient is coached to exhale to residual volume and then to inspire with maximal attainable force against an occluded airway.

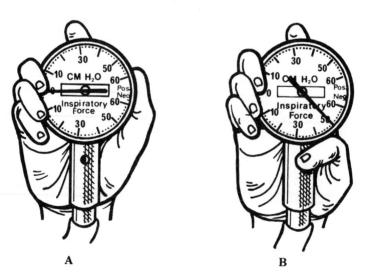

A   **B**

FIGURE 10–2 Inspiratory force meter. The meter is attached to the patient's airway. (A) Meter with gauge in zero position. (B) Maximum inspiratory force (MIP) is measured by instructing to the patient to exhale to residual volume and then to inspire with maximal attainable force while airflow is obstructed by occluding the open port on the front of the gauge. MIP = −50 cm H_2O pressure in this example. (From Pilbeam, SP: *Mechanical Ventilation: Physiological and Clinical Applications.* St. Louis: Mosby–Year Book, 1992.)

Mechanical performance is enhanced by beginning the effort from a low lung volume. Occlusion should be maintained for 5 to 10 seconds unless this degree of stress is contraindicated, deleterious side effects occur, or pressures are clearly observed to peak earlier. Repeated efforts are recommended because of considerable effort-to-effort variability, possibly because the patient becomes more proficient in the procedure. The maximal value observed during multiple trials should be recorded.

The literature contains many alternative terms for the MIP. These include negative inspiratory pressure (NIP), negative inspiratory force (NIF), maximum inspiratory force (MIF), peak negative pressure (PNP), and inspiratory force (IF).

In healthy men the MIP is normally around -115 cm H_2O. Values are approximately 25% lower in women. Patients capable of generating an MIP of < -20 are generally considered ready to be weaned. The MIP indicates ventilatory reserve and provides a global assessment of the respiratory muscle strength. It also assesses the patient's ability to take a deep breath and generate enough intrathoracic pressure to produce an effective cough.

RESPIRATORY FREQUENCY AND PATTERN

The respiratory frequency (f) or rate (RR) is obtained by counting the number of respirations in 1 minute. Respirations should be counted for a full minute, not some portion thereof, because the respiratory pattern may vary within 1 minute. Furthermore, for greatest accuracy, respirations should be counted by observation of the chest wall as opposed to being counted with a digital readout, even if the patient is connected to the ventilator and on the continuous positive airway pressure (CPAP) mode.

Normal RR is 12 to 20 breaths/min. A RR of <25 generally indicates ability to be weaned. A respiratory frequency in excess of 25 breaths/min may indicate that the patient has increased minute ventilation demands or has inadequate respiratory muscle strength to achieve an adequate tidal volume. Many factors, however, may cause an elevation of the RR. Common causes of tachypnea that need to be ruled out include fear, anxiety, pain, fever, hypoxemia, and hypercapnia. An elevated RR may indicate increased dead-space ventilation and decreased alveolar ventilation. It has generally been shown that RRs greater than 35 breaths/min cannot be sustained and signal respiratory muscle fatigue.

Possibly because the RR is such a simple measure to obtain, it is not always given the consideration it deserves, nor is it obtained with the necessary precision. However, the RR is a very sensitive measure of the ability to be weaned, even if it is not specific. In most weaning studies it is the single factor that correlates most highly with the ability to sustain spontaneous ventilation.

RATIO OF RESPIRATORY FREQUENCY TO TIDAL VOLUME

The ratio of respiratory frequency (f) to tidal volume (V_T) (f : V_T), a relatively new weaning parameter used to assess breathing pattern, is measured in breaths per min per liter. The f : V_T ratio measures the extent of rapid, shallow breathing, a common finding in patients whose weaning trial has failed. The normal f : V_T ratio is 40 to 60 breaths/min/L. Patients who have been successfully weaned have an f : V_T ratio <105 breaths/min/L. Most unsuccessful trials are associated with ratios exceeding this level, which indicates an inability to sustain ventilation. The f : V_T ratio has demonstrated a high predictive power and is easy to measure because it can be performed independently of patient effort or cooperation.

ADDITIONAL FACTORS AFFECTING READINESS TO BE WEANED

Evaluation of readiness to be weaned probably plays a greater role in successful weaning than does the mode of weaning chosen. As a complement to the objective weaning criteria discussed in the previous section, multiple physical assessment parameters must be evaluated to assess the patient's overall clinical status and readiness for weaning (Box 10–1).

Respiratory Factors

To form a clinical impression of the work of breathing, observe the patient's respiratory pattern during a trial of spontaneous breathing. Is the patient comfortable? Are any accessory muscles being used or any retractions or nasal flaring being demonstrated? Is the breathing pattern normal, or is there thoracic-abdominal asynchrony or abdominal paradox? Utilize this information in conjunction with measured indices of RR and f : VT ratio to form an impression of ventilatory work.

Before a weaning trial is initiated, it is imperative to achieve resolution of the underlying abnormality for which mechanical ventilation was initiated. Chronic

---

Box 10–1   Advanced Checklist of Factors to Consider When Determining and Maintaining Readiness to Wean From Mechanical Ventilation

Respiratory pattern
Resolution of underlying pathologic condition initially requiring ventilatory support
Static compliance of >25 ml/cm H_2O
Presence of auto-PEEP
Airway, size 7 mm (ID) or greater
Neurologically awake patient with intact drive to breathe
Intact gag and cough before extubation
Hemodynamic stability
Optimal oxygen delivery; optimal hemoglobin concentration and cardiac output
Balanced fluid status, adequate hydration
Electrolyte balance, particularly Na^+, K^+, Ca^+, Mg^+, and PO_4
Acid-base balance
Adequate nutrition with avoidance of overfeeding
Absence of fever, infection, or other hypermetabolic states
Adequate sleep
General body strength
Absence of elimination problems
Pain and anxiety in control
Psychologic readiness

ID = Inside diameter.

underlying disease processes should be under control. Assessment criteria include the chest x-ray examination, auscultation of the chest to detect the presence of wheezing or adventitious breath sounds, and assessment of the secretions, particularly to determine whether the volume of secretions is manageable. An underlying disease process may decrease lung compliance or increase airway resistance, both of which increase the work of breathing and energy demands on the muscle. Successful weaning is promoted by a respiratory system static compliance greater than 25 ml/cm H_2O. A compliance less than 25 ml/cm H_2O requires the patient to generate a significant amount of work just to expand the elastic lung tissues. It is unlikely that this level of ventilatory work could be sustained long enough to maintain adequate alveolar ventilation.

An assessment should also be made for the presence of overinflation of the lungs and dynamic hyperinflation (auto-PEEP). Inspiratory muscle contraction is optimal at low expiratory lung volumes, that is, volumes between functional residual capacity (FRC) and residual volume (RV). The pressure developed within the muscle and inspiratory endurance fall off sharply as lung volume is increased from FRC to total lung capacity (TLC). To minimize auto-PEEP formation in patients with chronic obstructive pulmonary disease, an airway size 7 mm internal diameter [ID] or greater should be in place, and bronchodilators may be administered as necessary before a weaning trial is initiated.

Weaning may be compromised by the amount of resistance to breathing created by the size of the artificial airway. In general, airways less than size 7 mm ID should be avoided. If the patient has an endotracheal tube, excess length should be eliminated by cutting the tube 2 inches from the teeth after ensuring correct placement with a chest x-ray film. Placement of a tracheostomy tube is another method of reducing airway resistance by reducing airway length.

Neurologic Factors

Neurologically the patient should be awake and should demonstrate an intact drive to breathe. The patient, however, does not have to be alert or completely oriented to be able to be weaned. Patients who have had a cerebrovascular accident or head injury may show impairments in their ability to concentrate, cooperate, and mentate; however, they may still undergo successful weaning. Before extubation, the patient must be able to cough and gag so that the airway can be protected.

Cardiovascular Factors

Before a weaning trial, hemodynamic stability must be ensured because oxygen demand is increased during weaning, therefore stress is placed on the cardiovascular system. Dysrhythmias should be controlled and the cardiac determinants of oxygen delivery—hemoglobin concentration and cardiac output—should be optimal to ensure that ample oxygen is being carried to the tissues. Furthermore, anemia may place stress on the cardiovascular system by requiring a higher cardiac output to ensure adequate tissue oxygen delivery.

Fluid balance should be monitored closely and achieved with the use of volume or diuretics as indicated. Electrolyte abnormalities must be corrected to promote optimal neural and muscular function. Of particular importance are sodium, potassium, and calcium and the minerals phosphate and magnesium.

Hypophosphatemia in particular is associated with respiratory muscle weakness and ventilatory failure. Acid-base disorders should be corrected and the patients who chronically retain CO_2 should be breathing at near their baseline Pa_{CO_2} with a compensated pH.

If a patient is requiring advanced methods of support, such as inotropic agents, vasopressors, or intra-aortic balloon pump therapy, to maintain hemodynamic stability, then weaning should generally be delayed. The initiation of exercise will add an additional stress to a cardiovascular system that already has limited reserves and may delay or prevent cardiac recovery. Exceptions include patients who seem to be ready for a weaning trial, and yet mild to moderate amounts of cardiovascular support are still necessary. In these patients the risks and potential complications of maintaining an artificial airway and mechanical support should be weighed against the benefits of progressing with weaning. Examples of such patients are (1) cardiac transplant candidates requiring cardiovascular support, while simultaneously all potential sources of infection such as an endotracheal tube must be eliminated, and (2) patients who have had cardiac surgery and who now have left ventricular dysfunction, requiring mild doses of inotropic support to ensure tissue oxygenation, yet whose lungs are clear and their fluid balance is manageable with diuretics.

Nutritional Status

Protein-calorie malnutrition, often a complicating factor in critical illness, impairs respiratory muscle structure and function. Specifically it creates a reduction in diaphragm muscle mass and contractility. With protein depletion, the patient may suffer significant impairments in endurance and strength, may demonstrate a decrease in the hypoxic ventilatory response, and is at greater risk of developing infection because of a decrease in both T- and B-cell immune function. Nutritional status plays a significant role in weaning success.

The goals of nutrition are to provide sufficient energy to sustain activity, prevent utilization of visceral protein stores, and promote the development of lean tissue. These goals may be achieved by providing protein and energy, as a balanced mixture of fat and carbohydrates, at rates slightly higher than the rate at which they will be used. Care must be taken not to overfeed the patient with carbohydrates and thus increase CO_2 production and ventilatory workload and possibly impair weaning progression. It is also important that the patient receive sufficient quantities of the minerals potassium, magnesium, phosphorus, and zinc to promote neural conduction, muscle contraction, and protein synthesis and thus lean tissue repletion.

Infection, Fever, or Other Hypermetabolic States

The presence of sepsis constitutes a contraindication to weaning because it increases the patient's metabolic requirements and CO_2 production, and therefore the ventilatory demand. Further increasing metabolic demand by initiating a period of exercise may place significant stress on the cardiovascular system, setting the patient up for weaning failure. An active pulmonary infection usually signals that the patient is not ready for weaning, especially if secretions are copious or thick and pulmonary compliance is reduced.

Sleep

Many factors in the ICU setting interfere with the patient's ability to complete sleep cycles, achieve adequate rest, and maintain patterns of sleep that are within the patient's norm. Inadequate sleep is associated with weakness, irritability, anxiety, inability to concentrate, and depression—all of which may limit the patient's capacity or willingness to participate in weaning. Uninterrupted sleep is essential to psychologic well-being. Measures to promote rest include consolidation of care in tolerable blocks that allow the patient rest periods between treatment periods, reduction of noise, administration of sedative-hypnotics at bedtime to promote sleep, and incorporation of the patient's usual sleep preparation routine as much as possible in evening care. Ensuring that the patient receives adequate rest may require considerable creativity and sensitivity on the part of the health care team.

General Body Strength and Endurance

In addition to respiratory muscle strength, the patient's general body strength in terms of peripheral muscle function and tolerance of exercise should be considered. Relative immobility and muscle disuse leads to weakness, atrophy, stiffness, and peripheral edema. If not contraindicated, general body strengthening should be promoted through progressive mobility. Assist and encourage the patient to perform exercises in bed, stand, sit out of bed in a chair, and eventually ambulate with assistance (while receiving ventilatory assistance with a manual resuscitation bag if necessary).

Elimination

Abdominal distention as a result of constipation, ileus, and gas impairs diaphragm function, reduces lung volumes, and may impede successful weaning. Management of gastrointestinal problems includes the evaluation of factors that decrease gut motility, such as narcotics, immobility, a diet low in fiber, and dehydration. Diarrhea caused by antibiotics, enteral feedings, or other factors leads to metabolic consequences that may interfere with normal respiratory function. When elimination problems are present, enteral feedings may not be tolerated and nutritional status may become inadequate, further compounding weaning problems.

Pain and Anxiety

When a patient is prepared for weaning, pain should be well controlled. Providing enough analgesia to provide pain relief without suppressing the respiratory drive is a balancing act that is more of an art than a science. The withholding of analgesia from a patient with pain may potentially cause weaning failure because of splinting of respirations and increased metabolic demands resulting from increased sympathetic nervous system outflow. Many options are now available for achieving pain control. In addition to traditional methods of analgesia administration, patient-controlled analgesia (PCA), epidural analgesia, nerve blocks, and transcutaneous electrical nerve stimulation (TENS) should be considered.

Psychologic Readiness

The patient's mental status and ability to cooperate are significant considerations in the approach to weaning. Impediments to weaning may be precipitated by medications, ICU psychosis, depression, and psychologic dependence on the ventilator. Psychologic readiness is promoted by providing clear explanations of the chosen weaning process to the patient. Each weaning trial should be accompanied by instructions. It should never be assumed that previous patient teaching sessions have provided all of the information considered essential by the patient or that the patient has remembered previously provided information.

Some patients may be fearful and anxious about the gradual withdrawal of ventilatory support, especially if they previously required reintubation or have had severe dyspnea associated with respiratory failure. It is important to be sensitive to the patient's fears and anxieties because they alone may cause shortness of breath. Pharmacologic intervention with anxiolytic medications may be necessary in selected cases.

Patients who demonstrate psychologic dependency on the ventilator require considerable reassurance that they will be monitored closely and that the staff will be ready to intervene if the patient requires ventilatory assistance. The clinician should ensure that a method of communication with the patient has been established, provide feedback to the patient about his or her progress, utilize distraction, and be encouraging and positive. Mental preparation must be valued as an essential component of a successful weaning program.

RESPIRATORY EXERCISES

Inspiratory Resistance Training

Strength of the inspiratory muscles is promoted through the repetition of a maximal inspiratory maneuver. Inspiratory resistance training is carried out through the use of a device that requires the patient to breathe through a narrowed orifice (Fig. 10–3). This increase in airway resistance causes the inspiratory muscles to contract in both an isometric and an isotonic manner. Thus the skeletal muscle training principle of specificity is applied. The principle of overload is also applied in that the muscles must work harder than normal to create a change in intrathoracic pressure that will result in a volume change in the

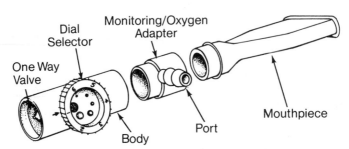

FIGURE 10–3 Inspiratory resistance training device (PFLEX). The device is designed to increase respiratory muscle strength and endurance. (Courtesy of Healthscan Products, Inc., Cedar Grove, N.J.)

lungs. Performance of these high-tension maneuvers increases muscle bulk and exercise tolerance. Focusing training on inspiratory muscles improves ventilatory efficiency because the inspiratory muscles play a greater role than expiratory muscles in both tidal and maximal breathing. The expiratory muscles are passive most of the time except in maximal expiratory maneuvers such as coughing, exercise, and pursed lip breathing. Inspiratory resistance training may be useful as an adjunctive measure in patients for whom standard weaning techniques have failed. Studies to date have shown conflicting results regarding whether inspiratory resistance training results in increased exercise capacity.

Resistance Training: Technique

Inspiratory resistance training devices have variable levels of resistance that can be applied. Generally the largest orifice (least resistance) is chosen first, and the patient inhales and exhales through the device for 10 to 15 minutes. Session duration is increased, every one or two treatments, by 5 to 10 minutes. Before progressing to the next level of resistance, the patient should be able to tolerate the chosen level of resistance for up to 30 minutes. When the patient demonstrates readiness to increase the level of resistance, the orifice size is decreased by 1 and the duration of training is decreased to 10 to 15 minutes. Training sessions are then gradually increased up to 30 minutes, and the sequence is repeated. Maximum training time for a 24-hour period is 30 minutes twice a day.

Failure to tolerate the resistance level and a need to stop the session is demonstrated by an increase in the RR to 40 breaths/min or more, or by other signs of distress. Subsequent treatment periods should be decreased in duration, or a larger orifice should be chosen. Supplemental oxygen may be administered during the procedure. Inspiratory resistance devices require carefully controlled patient training that can be labor intensive and time-consuming, and therefore expensive (even though the device itself is inexpensive). They are small and can be used in the home setting for ongoing pulmonary rehabilitation.

WEANING MODES

Numerous techniques are available for weaning and affect not only the quantity of work applied to the respiratory muscles but also the *quality*, that is, muscle-tension and volume-change characteristics of the load. Work quality affects patient comfort, the synchrony of patient-ventilator cycling, and whether the training period promotes strength versus endurance. Though the choice of weaning mode does affect comfort, synchrony, and workload application, it is uncertain how the various techniques affect weaning outcome. Furthermore, when each technique is used properly, none has shown superiority over the others. The technique chosen with a particular patient is probably not as important as the evaluation of readiness to be weaned and the employment of careful monitoring of patient tolerance after the trial has been initiated.

An optimal weaning program meets the patient's ventilatory demands and achieves optimal respiratory function, while ensuring that respiratory muscle fatigue is prevented. The kind of training program that can meet these goals is yet to be defined and can never be achieved without the skilled monitoring of a bedside practitioner. The amount of work required of the patient should remain at a tolerable level, and the ventilator should perform the balance of the work.

Finally, regardless of the weaning mode chosen, adequate periods of rest must also be ensured for the patient.

T-Piece or Blow-by Alternating With A/C

Until the early 1970s and the development of intermittent mandatory ventilation (IMV), the T-piece was the only method of weaning. With T-piece weaning the patient is disconnected from the ventilator to spontaneously breathe humidified oxygen for increasing periods. Between T-piece trials, the patient is reconnected to the ventilator and given full ventilatory support. Therefore periods of fully loaded spontaneous breathing are alternated with fully supported mechanical ventilation. The quality of work performed with T-piece weaning is high-pressure, low-volume work. This type of work promotes respiratory muscle strength. As trials increase in duration, respiratory muscle endurance is also enhanced. T-piece weaning is indicated for patients with a reliable respiratory drive. In comparison with IMV or CPAP weaning, the work of breathing (WOB) may be reduced because there is no demand valve to open or ventilator circuitry to breathe through.

Weaning from the T-piece begins by placing the patient on a T-piece setup at the same FIO_2, or 10% higher than on the ventilator. The first period of spontaneous breathing may be as short as 5 minutes. Periods of spontaneous breathing become progressively longer as the patient becomes capable of taking on more of the WOB. At the completion of the weaning period, the patient is returned to full ventilatory support, such as the A/C mode. The frequency of weaning trials may range from two to six per day, but it depends primarily on the duration of the trial and how much rest the patient requires before the next trial. As the duration increases, frequency decreases. Once the patient is capable of spontaneous ventilation for the entire day, then nighttime weaning may begin. The routine of alternating between T-piece and full ventilatory support continues until the patient has been disconnected from the ventilator for an entire day, at which time ventilatory support can be discontinued.

Continuous Positive Airway Pressure: CPAP Trials

The process of CPAP weaning is similar to T-piece weaning, but it is performed while the patient is still on the ventilator, so that CPAP can be applied. CPAP is used for patients at risk of having hypoxemia as a result of atelectasis, because CPAP improves alveolar stability, increases the functional residual capacity, and improves the distribution of ventilation to smaller airways. CPAP is indicated for patients whose oxygen saturation decreases during a period of spontaneous breathing and for patients whose ventilator parameters indicate readiness for weaning; however, PEEP is still required to maintain adequate oxygenation. The patient should not require PEEP greater than 5 to 8 cm H_2O.

The WOB may actually be increased during the administration of CPAP through some demand valve systems, which may interfere with weaning. Work may also be increased in comparison with T-piece weaning, because the patient is required to exhale against positive airway pressure.

The initial trial of spontaneous breathing with CPAP may be as short as 5 minutes. Periods of spontaneous breathing become progressively longer as the patient's respiratory mechanics improve and the patient becomes capable of taking on more of the WOB. At the completion of the weaning period, the patient is returned to full ventilatory support, such as PS_{max}, IMV at a rate that abolishes spontaneous respirations, or the A/C mode. The frequency of weaning trials may range from two to six per day but depends primarily on the duration of the trial and how much rest the patient requires between trials. As the duration increases, frequency decreases. Once the patient is capable of spontaneous ventilation for the entire day, then nighttime weaning may begin. Conversely, nighttime weaning may be eliminated because the amount of resistance work required by the patient to breathe unassisted through the ventilator circuitry may be too much to sustain for 24 hours. The routine of alternating between CPAP and full ventilatory support continues until patient assessment indicates the patient's capacity for sustained spontaneous ventilation. Ventilatory support may then be discontinued.

Intermittent Mandatory Ventilation

IMV was introduced in the 1970s, initially as a mode for weaning patients from mechanical ventilation. IMV provides a gradual transition from mechanical support to spontaneous ventilation, in comparison with T-piece or CPAP weaning. IMV may be more appropriate for patients who lack confidence in their ability to breathe without the ventilator.

With IMV the patient is allowed to breathe spontaneously between ventilator-delivered breaths. Weaning progresses by decreasing the number of ventilator breaths in stepwise reductions of 1 or 2 breaths per minute. Tolerance of the reduced level of support is assessed before the patient progresses to a new level of support. The rate of reduction depends on the patient's response and tolerance. Weaning below a rate of 2 to 4 breaths per minute may be unnecessary. Once the patient has reached an IMV rate of 2 to 4, a trial of spontaneous ventilation on CPAP or a T-piece may be initiated, or the patient may simply undergo extubation. Rest between weaning trials, and nocturnally, is accomplished with PS_{max}, A/C, or IMV set at a rate that abolishes spontaneous respirations.

With IMV weaning, the patient alternates between fully loaded spontaneous breaths and fully supported machine breaths over a few breathing cycles. The type of work applied to the respiratory muscles is high-pressure, low-volume work, which promotes respiratory muscle strength. Disadvantages of IMV weaning include patient discomfort and asynchrony with the ventilator as the patient attempts to alternate between the patterns associated with spontaneous and mandatory breaths. Another disadvantage is that high resistance in the inspiratory circuit can increase the WOB beyond the patient's capability. Circuit resistance varies with ventilator models, gas flow rates, and demand valves. The WOB to open a demand valve alone may be considerable, significantly contributing to the development of fatigue. A continuous-flow system, or flow-triggering (flow-by) system, should be considered to decrease the WOB associated with triggering the vent. When demand valve work is high, weak patients may tolerate T-piece weaning better than IMV. If neither is tolerated, then pressure support weaning should be considered.

Pressure Support

Pressure support (PS) was introduced in the 1980s as a mode of ventilatory support and weaning. With PS, every spontaneous breath is augmented by pressure assistance; therefore the patient is not required to take any fully loaded spontaneous breaths. By providing inspiratory flow assistance, internal impedance loads are overcome and pressure work is decreased while tidal volumes are augmented. By decreasing pressure work, PS approximates diaphragm tension characteristics of normal breathing. The work performed is of high-volume, low-pressure quality, which promotes endurance conditioning of the respiratory muscles.

As the level of PS is gradually decreased, the workload required of the patient is increased. When the patient is weaned with PS, oxygen consumption is decreased in comparison with other weaning modalities. PS is therefore beneficial for the patient with limited cardiac reserve and limited capacity for increasing oxygen delivery. It is also indicated for the patient who lacks the respiratory muscle strength to take on the WOB required during use of the T-piece, CPAP, or IMV mode.

With PS there is improved patient comfort and tolerance because the patient has control over the respiratory rate, tidal volume, inspiratory flow, and inspiratory time. Patients may report less dyspnea with PS because of the greater control afforded them over the respiratory cycle. PS weaning should be used with caution in patients prone to bronchospasm or secretion collection because exhaled tidal volumes will decrease. Low-level PS, such as 5 to 7 cm H_2O, is useful in overcoming inspiratory resistance caused by the endotracheal tube and the ventilator circuit. PS may facilitate weaning by preventing respiratory muscle fatigue caused by the additional load that these factors place on the respiratory muscles.

There are two methods of weaning with PS: PS alone and PS with synchronized IMV (SIMV). During weaning with PS as a stand-alone ventilatory mode, begin with a level of PS that ensures V_{T}s of 5 cc/kg and a RR <25 breaths/min. Proceed with weaning by reducing the PS in increments of 2 to 5 cm H_2O while assessing the patient for tolerance of the reduced level of ventilatory assistance. As the amount of PS is decreased, the RR should not increase substantially if lung mechanics are improving, and V_T should remain at least 5 cc/kg (monitor exhaled V_T on the ventilator). Weaning progresses until the patient is down to 5 cm H_2O PS, an amount that overcomes inspiratory circuit resistance. PS trials should also increase in duration, duration being guided by patient tolerance. Once the patient can breathe all day on a low level of PS, nighttime weaning may commence. Complete rest between trials is provided with either PS_{max} (a level of PS that provides full ventilatory support V_{T}s of 10 to 12 cc/kg) or the A/C mode.

The second method of weaning with PS is to combine it with SIMV. PS is usually used in this manner to assist spontaneous breaths of inadequate V_T or to overcome spontaneous-breathing resistance work necessitated by the demand valve and endotracheal tube. Weaning is accomplished by decreasing the number of ventilator (SIMV) breaths, followed by a gradual reduction in the PS level.

SYSTEMATIC APPROACH TO WEANING

1. Determine readiness for weaning.
2. Develop a weaning plan in collaboration with the health care team. Include mode, duration of weaning trial, end points, and periods of rest.

3. Prepare patient psychologically, include the patient in the planning, provide formal instruction, and establish a formal mechanism of communication. Explain that weaning is an exercise training program for the respiratory muscles, that they will gradually be taking on more of the WOB, and that they should provide feedback about how they feel, physically and emotionally, throughout the weaning process. Reassure the patient that ventilatory support will be reinstituted before fatigue develops.

4. Plan to initiate weaning during the day, when the patient is rested. Weaning should take priority and not be done after the patient has already had a full schedule of energy-depleting activities such as bathing, chest physiotherapy, suctioning, and ambulating. Patients who need to concentrate on their breathing should not be interrupted. Weaning should be restricted to the waking hours until the patient has been weaned successfully for one full day. Nighttime weaning can then be attempted.

5. Position the patient in a semi-Fowler's position to promote full respiratory excursion and prevent limitation of diaphragm movement by the abdominal organs. If the patient is assisted to a chair, allow a short period of rest before initiating the trial. Suction the airway as necessary and allow enough time for the patient's vital signs to return to baseline after the suctioning procedure.

6. Initiate weaning. Perform a baseline assessment of cardiac, pulmonary, and neurologic function. Stay with the patient initially and communicate in a calm, reassuring manner. Explain the weaning procedure as often as necessary to reduce anxiety. To increase confidence, provide positive, supportive feedback about how well the patient is doing.

7. Perform ongoing assessment of patient tolerance. Assess for signs and symptoms that the WOB is too great and the patient is beginning to fatigue. The following signs and symptoms indicate that mechanical ventilation should be reinstituted:

   a. RR exceeding 30 to 35 breaths per minute; abnormal respiratory pattern; asynchronous rib cage–abdominal motion or use of accessory muscle groups; exhaled V_T <5 cc/kg; decreased SaO_2 or increased $etCO_2$. The $etCO_2$ value may decrease with severe hypoventilation.

   b. Hemodynamic changes such as a change in the heart rate of 20 beats/min or more, angina, new dysrhythmia such as rapid atrial fibrillation, ventricular ectopy of 6 premature ventricular contractions per minute or more or salvos, conduction disturbances, ST segment changes, a change in the blood pressure of 20 mm Hg or more, skin temperature changes, or diaphoresis.

   c. Neurologic changes such as anxiety, confusion, agitation, or somnolence indicative of hypoxemia or hypercapnia.

   d. It is important to evaluate the individual's interpretation of the experience and not rely solely on physiologic criteria. Allow for the reporting of subjective symptoms such as dyspnea, which can progress to anxiety and tachypnea. Use of a visual analog scale provides the most objective method of reporting such a subjective symptom. A scale that ranges from no difficulty in breathing to extreme difficulty allows patients to quantify their perception.

8. Good clinical assessment should be utilized to determine when the patient is beginning to fatigue and should be reconnected to the ventilator to rest.

Ensure complete rest of the respiratory muscles by adjusting the ventilator settings so that the patient has no spontaneous respirations. Do not allow the patient to become so worn out during the trial that muscle energy stores are depleted. Return the patient to the ventilator before the $PaCO_2$ rises, which would be an indication of respiratory failure.

9. Throughout the process, provide psychologic support to the patient. The loss of the ability to breathe on one's own must be traumatic. The patient must be approached with compassion, empathy, and patience.

EXTUBATION

See Chapter 3: Airway Maintenance.

TERMINAL WEANING

Terminal weaning is the process of withdrawing mechanical ventilatory support when the patient is not expected to survive. It may be indicated when it is the patient's informed request or the request of an appropriate patient surrogate, when further continued ventilatory assistance has been deemed medically futile, and when further intervention serves no benefit. Efforts are therefore focused on reduction of patient pain and suffering.

As progress is made in medical technology, life-sustaining therapies become more readily available. The ability to prolong life in the ICU is increasing, and therefore it is advisable that individuals make their wishes clear through either an advanced directive or a detailed discussion with their family or physician. When the patient's wishes are not clear, however, the benefits and burdens of therapies must be weighed and the health care provider must act in the patient's best interest.

Ethical Principles

Ethical principles that apply to terminal weaning include autonomy and beneficence. Autonomy refers to one's right to control what happens to him or her. It is the basis for informed consent, which states that we may perform procedures and intervene with patients as long as they provide their consent after being fully informed. When an *informed and competent* patient withdraws consent, the patient's rights are being violated if a therapy is continued. Therefore, according to the principle of autonomy, treatment must cease. Such treatment may include life-supporting mechanical ventilation.

Beneficence is the obligation to promote good or to do no harm. In a consideration of terminal weaning, this principle seems to contradict the principle of autonomy. A good treatment regimen in the biomedical sense seems incompatible with removal of life-sustaining therapy. However, withdrawal of mechanical ventilation must be viewed in light of what is perceived as "good" by the patient in terms of quality of life and what makes life worthwhile to the patient.

The thought of withdrawing mechanical ventilation is disturbing to some who perceive the action as killing versus letting the patient die. Killing implies the performance of acts with the primary intention of causing death. However, when death is anticipated because of the nature of the disease or illness, but is not intended, terminal weaning is perceived as letting death occur more naturally.

There are many philosophical arguments and ethical issues surrounding the withdrawal and withholding of medical therapy. One such argument is about the administration of sedation during the removal of ventilatory support. Some believe that sedation should be administered in response to actual patient discomfort and not just given in anticipation of discomfort, because the latter method of administration could be interpreted as an attempt at euthanasia. The question is, Does the administration of sedation and/or analgesia significantly contribute to the patient's demise? The health care provider must remember that the purpose of narcotics is to eliminate patient suffering, not to intentionally contribute to the patient's death. It is a moral obligation to administer sufficient analgesia to prevent unnecessary suffering. Respiratory depression may be an unavoidable side effect of the primary purpose of the analgesic, relief of suffering.

Suggested Procedural Guidelines

The members of the health care team should be in agreement with, or at the very least understand, the rationale behind the decision being made. Collaboration between the members of the health care team and consultation with the hospital chaplain and an ethicist should occur, as necessary, to formulate a consensus. Ongoing, open, and effective communication between members of the health care team and the family and/or patient must occur to promote understanding and avoid unnecessary conflict. Staff members who disagree with the decision, or are ambivalent, should feel the right to withdraw from the case without sanction.

In a case of medical futility, the family must be provided with clear explanations of the patient's condition. The family should not be placed in the position of having to decide what is medically appropriate or to determine medical futility. Recommendations should be offered to the family on the basis of professional judgment and the family members should be assisted in making decisions. So that the family and patient can be fully informed, they should be provided with the information that further therapy will not improve outcome, that withdrawal of support is recommended, and that death is probable if the course of action being recommended is undertaken.

To make the decision, the family members will often require an explanation of what will be done. They will likely be fearful that the patient will suffer. Reassurance that measures will be taken to ensure comfort must be offered. At this time the patient and family may express wishes about the procedure itself, such as a desired level of sedation or the presence of family members, a member of the clergy, or a primary nurse or other health care provider with whom they have developed a trusting relationship. In some cases the family may request a delay to allow out-of-town family members to arrive or to have time to rethink their decision. Every effort should be made to accommodate their wishes, including the timing of terminal weaning. The patient and family should also be made aware that, although death is the expected outcome, it may not necessarily be imminent.

The drug generally recommended for the promotion of patient comfort during terminal weaning is morphine sulfate. Administration by continuous intravenous (IV) infusion is the most efficient method, and it eliminates the process of actively having to perform IV push to administer potentially large doses of morphine. Giving large doses of morphine by IV push may arouse a feeling of uncertainty within some health care providers as to whether they are actively assisting the dying process. The family may also perceive this action as such. Use of a continuous infusion may reduce feelings of active participation in the dying process. It also frees the bedside practitioner to concentrate efforts on the patient's and family's needs.

Ventilator withdrawal is then initiated. It must be emphasized that there is no one right technique by which this process should occur. The FIO_2 and the level of PEEP may be reduced while administering analgesia. Conversely, or simultaneously, the frequency of ventilatory breaths may be gradually reduced. The weaning process may proceed until the patient is spontaneously breathing through a T-piece or, if the patient has a tracheostomy, through a high-humidity tracheostomy collar. The extubation decision may be made on the basis of the expressed wishes of the patient and/or family or after consideration of the need for the artificial airway to manage secretions.

Sedation is titrated to signs of discomfort or distress such as tachypnea, agonal respiratory efforts, restlessness, tachycardia, or, in the case of the awake patient, self-report. The practitioner should be prepared to support the family and answer potential questions about agonal respiratory efforts, cyanosis, or muscle contractions. An atmosphere should be created in which the family feels comfortable talking to or touching the dying patient.

The process of terminal weaning generally takes hours, with primary attention concentrated on patient comfort. The use of medications that support the cardiovascular system, renal function, or metabolism is unnecessary during this time. Needless treatments should be eliminated and hygienic and comfort measures allowed to take priority.

Even though the decision to terminally wean the patient has been reached in a systematic, objective manner, the actual performance of the weaning procedure may arouse many troubling emotions in the patient, family, and bedside practitioner carrying out the process. The health care practitioners must provide the necessary support to the family and patient. Team members must also support each other as they proceed with the sometimes difficult task of letting the patient die.

SUMMARY

Weaning is the application of a planned exercise program for the respiratory muscles. It is achieved by systematic manipulation of the breathing workload. Successful weaning from mechanical ventilation begins with a thorough assessment of the patient's readiness for weaning and the elimination of any factors that will hinder the patient's progress. After initiation of a weaning mode, it is paramount that the patient be monitored closely for tolerance and that fatigue is prevented. Terminal weaning, or withdrawal, of ventilator support may become necessary if further treatment appears more burdensome than beneficial to the patient. The approach to withdrawal must be systematic, objective, and humane.

RECOMMENDED READINGS

Aldrich, T.K. (1988). Respiratory muscle fatigue. *Clin Chest Med* 9(2), 225–236.

Aldrich, T.K., Karpel, J.P., Uhrlass, R.M., et al. (1989). Weaning from mechanical ventilation: Adjunctive use of inspiratory muscle resistive training. *Crit Care Med* 17(2), 143–147.

Boysen, P.G. (1991). Weaning from mechanical ventilation: Does technique make a difference? *Respir Care* 36(5), 407–416.

Braun, N. (1984). Respiratory muscle dysfunction. *Heart Lung* 13(4), 327–332.

Burns, S.M. et al. (1995). Weaning from long-term mechanical ventilation. *Am. J. Crit. Care* 4(1), 4–22.

Campbell, M.L., and Carlson, R.W. (1992). Terminal weaning from mechanical ventilation: Ethical and practical considerations for patient management. *Am J Crit Care* 1(3), 52–56.

Cohen, C.A., et al. (1982). Clinical manifestations of inspiratory muscle fatigue. *Am J Med* 73, 308–316.

Daly, B.J., et al. (1993). Withdrawal of mechanical ventilation: Ethical principles and guidelines for terminal weaning. *Am J Crit Care* 2(3), 217–223.

Higgins, T.L., and Stoller, J.K. (1993). Discontinuing ventilatory support. In D.J. Pierson and R.M. Kacmarek (Eds.). *Foundations of respiratory care* (pp. 1019–1036). New York: Churchill Livingstone.

Knebel, A.R. (1991). Weaning from mechanical ventilation: Current controversies. *Heart Lung* 20(4), 321–334.

Knebel, A.R. (1992). When weaning from mechanical ventilation fails. *Am J Crit Care* 1(3), 19–31.

MacIntyre, N.R. (1988). Weaning from mechanical ventilatory support: Volume-assisting intermittent breaths versus pressure-assisting every breath. *Respir Care* 33(2), 121–125.

Marini, J.J., Smith, T.C., and Lamb, V. (1986). Estimation of inspiratory muscle strength in mechanically ventilated patients: The measurement of maximal inspiratory pressure. *J Crit Care* 1(1), 32–38.

McMahon, M.M., Benotti, P.N., and Bistrian, B.R. (1990). A clinical application of exercise physiology and nutritional support for the mechanically ventilated patient. *J Parenter Enteral Nutr* 14(5), 538–542.

Morganroth, M.L., Morganroth, J.L., Nett, L.M., and Petty, T.L. (1984). Criteria for weaning from prolonged mechanical ventilation. *Arch Intern Med* 144, 1012–1016.

National Heart, Lung, and Blood Institute Workshop Summary (1990). Respiratory muscle fatigue: Report of the respiratory muscle fatigue workshop group. *Am Rev Respir Dis* 142, 474–480.

Norton, L.C., and Neureuter, A. (1989). Weaning the long-term ventilator-dependent patient: Common problems and management. *Crit Care Nurse* 9(1), 42–52.

Pardy, R.L., Reid, W.D., and Belman, M.J. (1988). Respiratory muscle training. *Clin Chest Med* 9(2), 287–296.

Sahn, S., and Lakshminarayan, S. (1973). Bedside criteria for discontinuation of mechanical ventilation. *Chest* 63, 1002–1005.

Schneiderman, L.J., and Spragg, R.G. (1988). Ethical decisions in discontinuing mechanical ventilation. *N Engl J Med* 318(15), 984–988.

Sporn, P.H.S., and Morganroth, M.L. (1988). Discontinuation of mechanical ventilation. *Clin Chest Med* 9(1), 113–126.

Tobin, M.J. (1990). Which respiratory parameters can predict successful weaning? *J Crit Illness* 5(8), 819–837.

Tobin, M.J., Perez, W., Guenther, S.M., et al. (1987). Does ribcage-abdominal paradox signify respiratory muscle fatigue? *J Appl Physiol* 63, 851–860.

Tobin, M.J., et al. (1987). Konno-Mead analysis of ribcage-abdominal motion during successful and unsuccessful trial of weaning from mechanical ventilation. *Am Rev Respir Dis* 135, 1320–1328.

Truog, R.D., and Fackler, J.C. (1993). Withdrawing mechanical ventilation. *Crit Care Med* 21(9, suppl.), S396–S397.

Weilitz, P.B. (1993). Weaning a patient from mechanical ventilation. *Crit Care Nurse* 13(4), 33–41.

Yang, K.L., and Tobin, M.J. (1991). A prospective study of indexes predicting the outcome of trials of weaning from mechanical ventilation. *N Engl J Med* 324(21), 1445–1450.

Nonconventional Modes and Alternative Methods of Mechanical Ventilation

The application of positive-pressure ventilation and positive end-expiratory pressure (PEEP) are the cornerstones of therapy for acute respiratory failure. The condition of some patients, however, does not improve despite the employment of these therapies. Indeed, the condition of some patients may actually deteriorate when high levels of PEEP are utilized in an attempt to improve oxygenation, and when large tidal volume (VT) delivery results in high peak inspiratory pressure (PIP). Because conventional ventilation and PEEP sometimes ineffectively support the failing respiratory system, it becomes necessary to study alternative modes of mechanical ventilation. Nonconventional modes that will be discussed in this chapter are high-frequency ventilation (HFV) and independent lung ventilation (ILV). The use of nonconventional modes typically requires caregivers to learn new terminology associated with the modes, as well as new physical configurations of the airway, and possibly the ventilator, used to apply the mode. Alternative methods of mechanical ventilation also reviewed in this chapter include mandatory minute ventilation (MMV), airway pressure release ventilation (APRV), pressure-regulated volume control (PRVC), volume support (VS), and permissive hypercapnia (PHC).

HIGH-FREQUENCY VENTILATION

Historically, assisted ventilation has attempted to reproduce the mechanics involved in normal spontaneous breathing. Therefore conventional ventilation traditionally utilizes near physiologic respiratory rates (RRs), and tidal volumes (VT) greater than anatomic dead space. During the past 25 years, however, researchers have shown that adequate arterial oxygenation and alveolar ventilation may be achieved with the use of a substantially smaller VT (1 to 5 cc/kg) and higher respiratory frequencies (60 to 3600 breaths/min) than conventional ventilators. This group of ventilatory techniques, which utilize high-rate, low-VT delivery and do not attempt to reproduce the mechanics involved in normal spontaneous breathing, are known collectively as high-frequency ventilation. The three types of HFV are as follows: high-frequency positive-pressure ventilation (HFPPV), high-frequency oscillatory ventilation (HFOV), and high-frequency jet ventilation (HFJV) (Table 11–1).

HFJV is the most widely utilized of the HFV modes. Discussion will follow on the known and theoretic physiologic principles surrounding, and indications for, this therapy. Technical aspects such as the physical configuration of the ventilator system, the jet cannula, and the airway humidification system are described, and the terminology specific to this ventilatory mode is defined. Sections are also dedicated to patient monitoring, adjustment of the ventilator settings to correct arterial blood gas (ABG) values, weaning, and special patient care issues.

HIGH-FREQUENCY JET VENTILATION

HFJV is differentiated from other HFV modes primarily by the mechanism by which the gas is delivered. HFJV is the delivery of a small VT, 3.5 to 4.5 ml/kg, at a high breath frequency of 60 to 150 breaths/min through a small endotracheal catheter or cannula placed in the airway. The volume is delivered under considerable driving pressure, 20 to 50 pounds per square inch, through a cannula 1 to 2 mm in diameter. The cannula, referred to as the jet injector, is about the size of a 16/14-gauge needle. The "jetting" of humidified gases into the airway results in the entrainment of additional fresh gases (Fig. 11–1). Thus the volume delivered is a combination of insufflated and entrained gases and is generally targeted at two or three times the minute ventilation ($\dot{V}E$) delivered with conventional ventilation. The delivery of a very small VT at a rapid rate results in constant-flow, low-pressure ventilation.

The theoretic advantages of HFJV are its ability to lower peak airway pressures and to improve the efficiency of ventilation. Lower peak airway pressures may result in diminished pulmonary barotrauma. Ventilation efficiency is

TABLE 11–1 High-Frequency Ventilation

	HFPPV	HFJV	HFOV
Rate	60–120	100–150	600–3600 cycles/min (1–60 Hz)
Tidal volume	3.0–5.0 ml/kg	3.5–4.5 ml/kg	2–5 ml/kg
Technical Application	Time-cycled, pressure-controlled ventilator; may be achieved with some conventional ventilators.	Requires adjustable pressure source that can operate at driving pressures up to 50 psi; jet injector cannula 1.5–2.0 mm in diameter.	Device that can produce oscillatory flows at required frequencies, such as a piston pump. No oscillatory device for clinical use in adult patients is presently available.
Exhalation	Passive	Passive	The return stroke of the ventilator may generate subatmospheric pressure making exhalation active.

HFPPV = High-frequency positive-pressure ventilation; HFJV = high-frequency jet ventilation; HFOV = high-frequency oscillatory ventilation; Hz = hertz, where 1 Hz = 60 cycles.

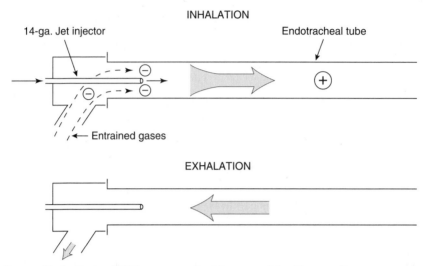

FIGURE 11-1 During HFJV, gases entrained because of the Venturi effect augment the alveolar ventilation provided by the pulsating jet. The Venturi principle states that as the velocity of flow of a gas increases, the pressure in the constricted part of the gas decreases, producing an area of negative pressure or a suction effect. During each HFJV inspiratory cycle, a pulsing jet of gas flows at an accelerated rate through the narrowed jet injector, developing an area of relative negative pressure at right angles to the jet injector. Previously humidified low-flow (20 L/min) gases are entrained into this area of relative negative pressure, continuously replacing those gases that have moved forward.

achieved in several ways. In the patient with airway disruption, such as tracheobronchial fistula, HFJV may prevent loss of a large portion of the VT through the disruption. HFJV may also improve the efficiency of ventilation because it is possible to increase the V̇E to two to four times the level accomplished with a standard ventilation mode, thereby enhancing CO_2 elimination.

Though not formally studied, HFJV has been reported to be better tolerated by patients, in terms of reduced requirements for sedation, than conventional ventilation. The increased tolerance of HFJV is attributed to the avoidance of the large changes in intrathoracic pressure that occur with each tidal breath during conventional ventilation. The loud sound of the high-frequency jet ventilator, however, has been difficult for some patients, families, and health care workers to tolerate.

History and Indications

The basis for HFJV evolved in 1967, when Sjöstrand and his colleagues were studying carotid sinus nerve impulses. They needed to develop a method of providing adequate ventilation while eliminating the circulatory artifact caused by artificial ventilation. They attempted different methods of ventilation, which eliminated blood pressure changes, but these caused CO_2 retention and therefore stimulated breathing. They observed that by increasing the RR to 60 to 80 breaths/min, combined with a small VT (3 to 5 ml/kg), adequate ventilation was provided, spontaneous breathing was eliminated, and airway pressures were low.

Current indications for HFJV include bronchoscopy and certain cases of bronchopleural or tracheoesophageal fistula to reduce gas loss through the airway defect. Theoretic clinical applications include ventilation during neurosurgical and cardiothoracic surgical procedures to produce a "quiet" surgical field, postoperative ventilatory management after pneumonectomy to reduce pressure on the site of surgical repair, ventilatory support in combined head injury and respiratory failure because reduced intrathoracic pressure can result in reduced intracranial pressure, primary and rescue treatment of respiratory distress syndrome, and upper airway surgery. Primarily, HFJV is used in infants. Its use in adults in the intensive care setting has been disappointing, having shown no distinct advantage over conventional modes.

Mechanisms of Gas Exchange

With HFJV, volumes less than anatomic dead space have been observed to result in adequate alveolar ventilation and oxygenation. The physiologic mechanisms of this achievement are not fully understood. Theories of gas exchange with HFJV involve two mechanisms: convection and enhanced diffusion. Convection is the process whereby flowing molecules carry other molecules along with them. Convective, or bulk, gas flow is the primary gas transport mechanism that results in alveolar ventilation under normal breathing conditions and is the principle of gas exchange behind conventional mechanical ventilation. During jet ventilation it appears that convection still plays a major part in gas exchange.

During HFJV, when gases are exiting from the distal port of the injector cannula, the pulsed gases acquire the characteristics of a jet stream. The kinetic energy of the jet stream transfers to the immobile gases present in the airway, which then begin to move in a convective manner in the same direction toward the distal airway. Another mechanism that plays a major role in gas exchange during HFJV is augmented, facilitated, or enhanced diffusion. Gas mixing and diffusion are augmented because the higher gas flows of HFJV result in increased turbulence and total movement of molecules.

Maintenance of oxygenation during HFJV is also achieved by the formation of auto-PEEP. High rates result in inadequate alveolar emptying and trapped volume in the lung. This trapped volume at end-expiration creates pressure in the lung known as auto-PEEP. Auto-PEEP results in an increased functional residual capacity (FRC), alveolar stability, and improved arterial oxygen tension. In either conventional ventilation or HFJV, it is the maintenance of an adequate FRC and mean airway pressure that determines the adequacy of oxygenation. Mean airway pressure during HFJV is similar to that during conventional ventilation, even though PIP and intrapleural pressure changes associated with the respiratory cycle are lower. The hemodynamic consequences of a higher mean airway pressure are therefore similar between the two modes.

The HFJV Therapeutic System

High-Frequency Jet Ventilator

Components of the HFJV system include a high-frequency jet ventilator, either a standard artificial airway fit with a jet adapter or an optional special jet artificial airway, a volume-controlled ventilator, and a humidification system (Fig. 11–2). The high-frequency jet ventilator serves as the high-pressure gas source (Fig. 11–3). The amount of pressure exerted on the gas is referred to as the drive pressure (DP) and is measured in pounds per square inch. DP is the primary determinant of V_T. The DP settings required to achieve an adequate V_T typically range from 14 to 40 psi. DP required to achieve adequate $\dot{V}_E$ depends on the compliance of the lungs. In conditions of noncompliant lung tissue, higher DPs may be needed.

The high-frequency jet ventilator contains a solenoid valve, or flow interrupter, and an electric timer. A solenoid valve is simply a valve that when open allows gas to flow and when closed prevents gas flow. A timer drives the flow interrupter, or solenoid valve, and allows selection of the RR and inspiratory time. After choosing the DP, RR, and inspiratory time, the jet ventilator delivers gas

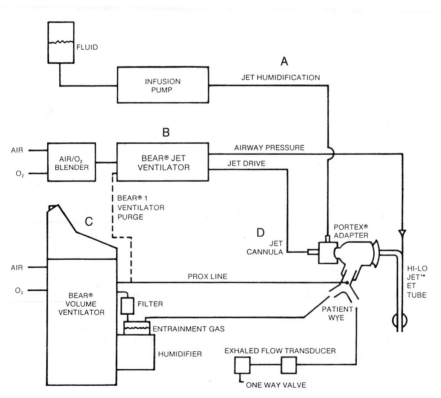

Figure 11–2 Example of configuration of HFJV therapeutic system. Primary components are (A) humidification system. (B) jet ventilator, (C) companion volume ventilator, and (D) jet injector cannula at site of airway. (From Bear Medical Systems, Inc., *Bear Jet Ventilator Instruction Manual*, Riverside, Calif., 1988.)

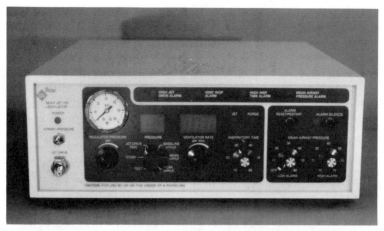

Figure 11-3   Bear jet ventilator, used to deliver high-frequency jet ventilation. (From Bear Medical Systems, Inc. *Bear Jet Ventilator Instruction Manual*, Riverside, Calif., 1988.)

in small, pulsating jets into the patient's airway. Therefore the gas control system of the jet ventilator is a conceptually simple device in which the high-pressure gas source is interrupted to produce delivered pulses, or small jets, of gas.

Artificial Airway

The next component of the system is the artificial airway, which may take on one of several configurations: a standard endotracheal tube (ETT) fitted with an adapter to which the jet cannula is applied, or a special HFJV ETT. Jet injectors differ in their diameter, their location in the airway, and their distance from the ventilator. All these factors affect performance and are a source of continued research. In general, the larger the injector diameter, the larger the volume of gas per jet pulse but the lower the peak gas velocity and therefore the entrainment capability. If the patient can tolerate reintubation, a Hi-Lo Jet tracheal tube may be placed (Fig. 11–4). The tube has a main lumen, as well as separate insufflation and monitoring-irrigation lumens. The main lumen serves as a channel for gas entrainment on inspiration and the elimination of expired gases. When the other lumens are capped, this lumen may function as a standard tracheal tube. The insufflation, or jet, lumen is a noncompliant tube embedded in the ETT wall. It permits the delivery of jet ventilation. This lumen can also be used for the administration of oxygen during suctioning or bronchoscopy. The monitoring, or irrigation, lumen may be used for monitoring of airway pressure, for irrigation to aid in the removal of secretions, for sampling of tracheal gases for end-tidal CO_2 (etCO$_2$) analysis, or for medication administration.

Companion Volume Ventilator

A volume-controlled ventilator is an essential component of the HFJV system, serving as the source of set-PEEP and entrained gases. The amount of set-PEEP initially used is generally the same that was set on conventional ventilation. Gases entrained because of the Venturi effect augment the alveolar ventilation provided by the pulsating jet. The Venturi principle states that as the velocity of gas flow increases, the pressure in the constricted part of the gas decreases, producing an area of negative pressure, or a suction effect. With

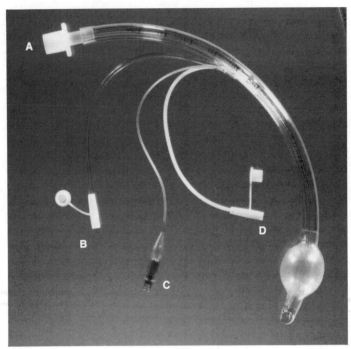

Figure 11-4 Hi-Lo Jet tracheal tube. (A) Main lumen for gas entrainment and exhalation. (B) Jet insufflation lumen. (C) Pilot balloon–valve for cuff inflation. (D) Monitoring–gas sampling lumen. (Courtesy of Mallinckrodt Medical, Inc., Mallinckrodt Anesthesiology Division, St. Louis, Mo.)

HFJV during each inspiratory cycle, a pulsing jet of gases flows at an accelerated rate through the narrowed jet cannula, developing an area of relative negative pressure at right angles to the cannula. From the companion volume ventilator, previously humidified low-flow (20 L/min) gases are entrained into this area of relative negative pressure, continuously replacing those gases that have moved forward (see Fig. 11–1). The companion volume ventilator also provides for monitoring of FIO_2, $\dot{V}E$, and exhaled VT. In the unforeseen and unusual event of jet ventilator failure, the companion volume vent may serve as a backup ventilator.

Humidification System

The final and essential component of the HFJV setup is a humidification system. Humidification of only the entrained gases is inadequate to protect the airway of patients receiving HFJV. Additional humidification is nebulized by the jet gas stream as normal saline solution is dripped through a channel exiting at the tip of the injector cannula (Fig. 11–5). The humidification solution is administered in a controlled fashion most easily with an intravenous-fluid infusion pump. The initial fluid rate is usually 20 to 30 ml/hr. The rate of infusion is empirically modified by assessing the consistency of the secretions. Inadequate humidification may result in severe necrotizing tracheobronchitis.

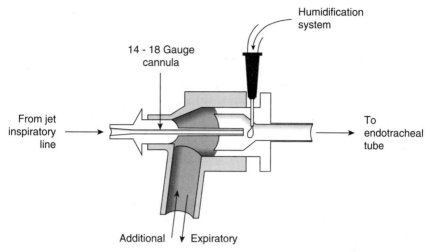

FIGURE 11–5   System for humidifying insufflated gases during high-frequency jet ventilation. (Reprinted with permission from Griffen, JP: Nursing care of patients on high frequency jet ventilation. *Crit Care Nurse* 1981;1:25.)

Effect of Changing Ventilator Settings on ABG Values

$PaCO_2$ is adjusted by manipulating the VT or RR. The VT may be increased by using a larger-bore injector cannula, increasing the DP, or increasing the inspiratory time. The PaO_2 is increased by adjusting the FIO_2 or the level of set-PEEP. PaO_2 may also be increased by manipulating factors that increase the mean airway pressure. Mean airway pressure is increased by increasing the DP as well as by decreasing the expiratory time, which leads to auto-PEEP formation. Caution should be used when the mean airway pressure is increased, because this increase may be associated with hemodynamic compromise.

RATE
Normally, rate is set at 100, and DP and inspiratory-to-expiratory (I:E) ratio are adjusted to affect alveolar ventilation. The effect of increasing and decreasing the rate is the same as with conventional ventilation. If rates are too high, expiratory time will be decreased, thus reducing CO_2 elimination.

DRIVE PRESSURE
Increasing the DP enhances CO_2 elimination by providing more gas exchange per cycle and by increasing the volume of entrained gas. Decreasing DP will decrease alveolar ventilation and thus increase $PaCO_2$. It may also decrease the mean airway pressure and therefore the PaO_2.

PEEP
With the addition of PEEP, the FRC is increased, mean airway pressure rises, and arterial oxygenation should improve. In this respect, PEEP with HFJV is no different from PEEP with conventional ventilation.

Ratio of Inspiratory to Expiratory Time

Increasing the percentage of inspiratory time provides a longer time for gas entrainment and exchange to occur; therefore it has the effect of increasing alveolar ventilation and thus decreasing $PaCO_2$. Lengthening the inspiratory time also reduces expiratory time, thereby creating auto-PEEP, which increases the FRC and decreases intrapulmonary shunt. If the inspiratory time is too long, it will occupy too much time, preventing passive expiration and thus increasing CO_2. Decreasing the inspiratory time has the effect of decreasing the alveolar ventilation and thus increasing $PaCO_2$.

Weaning from HFJV

Weaning may be achieved directly from HFJV or after transition to conventional ventilation. The process, as when any patient requires mechanical ventilatory support, begins with determining patient readiness for weaning, which includes resolution of the underlying pathologic condition and ability to oxygenate with an FIO_2 ≤0.5, and PEEP of 5 cm H_2O or less. Weaning from HFJV begins with decreasing the DP to decrease the $\dot{V}E$ delivered to the patient. Spontaneous ventilation will occur around the HFJV pulses, provided that arterial CO_2 tensions are not depressed. Stepwise decreases in DP and rate may be made as long as the patient is able to assume the balance of the work of breathing needed to maintain the desired level of ventilation. Weaning may also be achieved by alternating continuous positive airway pressure (CPAP) trials with periods of HFJV. As with any weaning plan, the patient should not be allowed to become fatigued, and adequate periods of rest should be ensured.

Patient Care Considerations for the Patient Undergoing HFJV

Patient-Ventilator System Monitoring

Because of the uniqueness of the method of providing respiratory support with HFJV, patient management principles also differ in some aspects from those applied during conventional ventilation. It is imperative that the practitioner be capable of adequately monitoring the patient-ventilator system by being thoroughly familiar with the display and control panels of both ventilators. The bedside practitioner must be capable of locating the following settings: DP, level of PEEP, set RR, inspiratory time, and FIO_2. The clinician should also be capable of rapidly assessing the following patient data: PIP, VT, and $\dot{V}E$.

Pulmonary Hygiene

Techniques of pulmonary hygiene distinctive to the patient receiving HFJV include maintenance of adequate humidification and special considerations during suctioning. Without adequate humidification, because of the high $\dot{V}E$ achieved with HFJV, there is a significant potential for airway desiccation. A continuous humidification system must be maintained, as previously discussed. Secretion consistency is observed to determine need for adjusting infusion rate.

A common question from nurses is whether the volume used to humidify the insufflated gases should be tallied into the patient's daily intake. The likely reason for this question is that the fluid is usually dripped into the airway by an infusion pump. The answer is that it is not necessary to include this volume in the intake. This approach is consistent with the fact that no other fluids used to humidify inspired gases are calculated as part of the daily intake.

Suctioning should be done as rapidly as possible, with the jet turned off. The jet is turned off to prevent aerosolization of patient secretions and therefore potential contamination of caregivers. It is also turned off to prevent blockage of the exhalation route for gases by the suction catheter, which could lead to overdistention and potentially to barotrauma. No special suction catheter is needed. When HFJV is first begun, secretion mobilization may be increased, necessitating frequent suctioning. The exact mechanism for this phenomenon is unknown but is believed to be due to the retrograde flow of gases through the airway, an additional benefit of HFJV that may reduce the incidence of aspiration during use of this mode.

Monitoring of breath sounds may be difficult as a result of the "jet" turbulence. The practitioner should be prepared to perform auscultation when the jet is on standby for suctioning, while an assistant provides manual ventilation for the patient.

PATIENT SAFETY

Patient safety is ensured by ventilator alarm systems. The most important alarm during HFJV is the high-pressure alarm. Immediate attention must be paid to all high-pressure alarms because of the significant potential for barotrauma if a large volume of gas is allowed to be delivered under the considerable pressures generated with HFJV.

PSYCHOLOGIC NEEDS

Finally, the psychologic aspects of using a nonconventional technique must be considered. As with any patient who is undergoing intubation, there is a potential for fear and frustration related to impaired communication. With HFJV there is also an alteration in the breathing pattern and the sensations associated with breathing. Differences in physical sensations associated with breathing should be explained to the patient. Breaths delivered by the HFJV are different because they are smaller in volume and more rapid in frequency. The ventilator sounds different from the conventional ventilator and may disrupt sleeping patterns and frighten the patient or family members. Respiration is not associated with the familiar rise and fall of the chest. Because the sensations are so unfamiliar, the patient may require sedation to promote adequate, healing rest. On the other hand, as previously stated, some researchers state that HFJV is actually better tolerated by patients, possibly because of reduced interference with the patient's own breathing patterns. The caregiver should be reassuring, should approach the patient calmly and with confidence, and should provide sedation and frequent explanations as necessary.

INDEPENDENT LUNG VENTILATION

The patient with pulmonary disease that is more predominant in one lung than the other illustrates a situation in which inadequate oxygenation may persist despite conventional methods of treatment. In fact, in patients with predominantly unilateral lung disease, the application of PEEP may be followed by a deterioration in blood gas values. The two lungs, in comparison with one another, have varying degrees of pathologic changes and thus are functioning very differently. One approach to the problem of unilateral, or asymmetric, lung disease is to insert a double-lumen endobronchial tube, which allows for independent ventilation of each lung. In this way, therapy directed to each lung can be tailored toward the mechanics that it, alone, demonstrates. This method of ventilation is known as differential lung ventilation, or independent lung ventilation (ILV). *Simultaneous independent lung ventilation* (SILV) is the term utilized when the timing of inspiration is synchronized between the two lungs, as opposed to *asynchronous independent lung ventilation* (AILV), in which no concern is given to the timing of inspiration and expiration between the two lungs.

History and Indications

In 1949 Eric Carlens described a double-lumen endobronchial tube that he had developed for use with differential bronchospirometry. In 1950 Björk and Carlens adapted this tube, called the Carlens catheter, for the administration of anesthesia during thoracic surgery. They stated that the catheter's use was indicated for prevention of the spread of secretions from one lung to

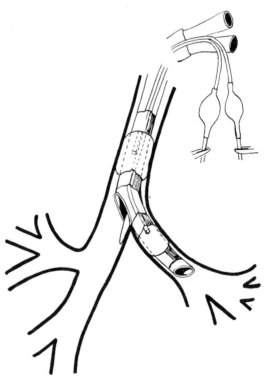

Figure 11-6 Diagram of original double-lumen endobronchial catheter developed by Carlens in 1949. The catheter, made of red rubber, featured a small hook that engaged the carina to promote tube stabilization. (From Björk, VO, and Carlens, E: The prevention of spread during pulmonary resection by the use of a double-lumen catheter. *J Thoracic Surg* 1950;20:151–157.)

the other during pulmonary resection. By 1962 the literature reported many cases in which the Carlens catheter had proved useful in all types of thoracic surgery.

The Carlens catheter (Fig. 11–6) was made of red rubber and had a small hook, which, when properly placed, engaged the carina and promoted tube stabilization. The distal lumen opened to aerate the left lung and the proximal lumen the right lung. The tube had two cuffs, the distal cuff lying in the left bronchus and the proximal in the trachea. Problems with the catheter precluded its use for long-term intubation in postoperative and intensive care settings. These problems included unreliable low-volume, high-pressure cuffs; increased resistance to gas flow because of smaller lumen sizes; difficulty in passing a suction catheter and in tube placement; dislodgment; and tracheal trauma caused by the carinal hook.

Advances in materials and techniques for the production of endobronchial tubes have led to the development of tubes whose use is more feasible for longer-term intubation. These new catheters have a more satisfactory lumen size, they have high-volume, low-pressure cuffs, and they come in a range of sizes. However, not all problems associated with endobronchial tubes have been obviated, and the clinician's role in monitoring for complications related to the artificial airway is a significant aspect of care of the patient undergoing ILV.

The development of a better catheter led to the evolution of many applications. It is generally agreed that ILV is indicated when conventional ventilatory support fails in the presence of asymmetric lung disease. It has proved useful in lobar pneumonia, unilateral contusion, refractory unilateral atelectasis, bronchopleural fistula or massive air leak, and nonuniform posttraumatic and septic adult respiratory distress syndrome (ARDS).

Pathophysiology of Asymmetric Lung Disease

Full appreciation of the indications for ILV is achieved through an understanding of the regional maldistribution of ventilation and perfusion in the lung, under the conditions of mechanical ventilation and asymmetric lung disease. When a patient is being mechanically ventilated, the volume of gas received by different regions of the lung is dependent on regional compliance and resistance differences. Areas of the lung with decreased compliance and increased resistance (longer time constants) are relatively underventilated in comparison with normal lung regions. The patient with unilateral, or asymmetric, lung disease presents a classic example of the situation in which ventilation is maldistributed because the two lungs demonstrate significantly different time constants.

In asymmetric lung disease, when parallel (conventional) ventilation is applied, the diseased lung receives a smaller portion of the VT because of its decreased compliance and increased resistance. The less diseased lung, because it is more compliant and has a lower airway resistance, receives a greater portion of the VT. The delivered VT is therefore unevenly distributed to the more normal lung, while the affected lung, because of its longer time constant, receives proportionately less volume. Maldistribution of the VT leads to overdistention of the more compliant lung. Hyperinflation causes the airway pressures to rise and results in an increased potential for barotrauma in the more compliant lung. The high pressure within the overinflated alveoli is transmitted to the alveolar capillary bed, compressing the alveoli so that blood flow through them is minimal to

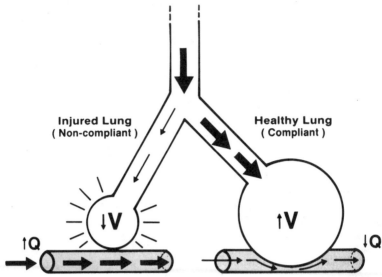

FIGURE 11-7 Maldistribution of ventilation and perfusion during conventional ventilation with asymmetric lung disease. Tidal volume is preferentially distributed to the more compliant lung, overdistending the alveoli *(right)*. Compression of adjacent pulmonary capillaries increases pulmonary vascular resistance and shifts pulmonary blood flow to the poorly ventilated, less compliant lung *(left)*. $\dot{V}/\dot{Q}$ mismatch is increased with overventilation of the compliant lung (increased dead space and therefore increased $PaCO_2$) and overperfusion of the noncompliant lung (increased shunt and therefore hypoxemia). (From Simon, B, and Borg, U: Independent lung ventilation. *Crit Care Report* 1990;1(3): 398–407.)

absent. These areas of high $\dot{V}/\dot{Q}$ or dead space, predominant in the more compliant lung, are clinically manifested by a rising $PaCO_2$.

The compression of the pulmonary capillary bed in the hyperinflated normal lung, together with the regional increase in the pulmonary vascular resistance, causes a diversion of blood to lower-resistance capillary beds in the pathologic lung. Blood flow, being shifted to the relatively underventilated diseased lung, creates low $\dot{V}/\dot{Q}$ or intrapulmonary shunt ($\dot{Q}s/\dot{Q}T$) areas, which are clinically manifested by failing oxygenation despite the delivered FIO_2 (Fig. 11–7). In an effort to improve oxygenation, the application of PEEP worsens the hyperinflation of the good lung and the diversion of blood to the bad lung. The therapeutic paradox in asymmetric lung disease, therefore, is that volume-controlled ventilation and PEEP are necessary to ventilate the less compliant lung; yet these same required volumes and level of PEEP increase pulmonary barotrauma in the more compliant lung and worsen overall $\dot{V}/\dot{Q}$ matching.

Criteria for Determining Asymmetric Lung Disease

The criteria for determining asymmetric lung disease and thus whether the patient may benefit from ILV can be divided into clinical findings and physiologic criteria. The chest x-ray film may provide anatomic evidence of the presence of asymmetric pathologic changes. However, physiologic asymmetry may not always be radiographically apparent. An asymmetric pattern will become apparent on occasion *after* PEEP is applied, when the nondiseased lung demonstrates hyperinflation and there is a shifting of the cardiac silhouette to the opposite hemithorax.

An asymmetric pattern of thoracic injury may create a high index of suspicion that the pulmonary pathologic changes are predominantly unilateral. Examples of such patterns are prevalent in the thoracic trauma population and include an injury such as flail chest and pulmonary contusion in one hemithorax.

Physiologically, asymmetric abnormality may be confirmed by measuring the compliance of each lung. This requires the placement of an endobronchial tube to isolate each lung and therefore is not practical as a means of deciding whether ILV is indicated. A maneuver that is more realistically performed in the clinical setting is the determination of oxygenation in each lateral decubitus position. If a disparity exists, the lung disease is likely asymmetric in nature. Patients with asymmetric lung disease will demonstrate their best oxygenation in the position where the better lung is dependent, because in this position there is the best matching of ventilation and perfusion. In the good-lung-down position, ventilation is greatest in the dependent lung because it has the best compliance. Perfusion, being affected by gravity, will also be best in this dependent lung. This optimal $\dot{V}/\dot{Q}$ matching in the good-lung-down position results in the best oxygenation. See Chapter 2 for further discussion on the effect of body position on $\dot{V}/\dot{Q}$ matching.

SILV Therapeutic System

ENDOBRONCHIAL TUBE

After determining that the patient's lung disease is asymmetric in nature and that conventional ventilatory support has failed to improve oxygenation, the practitioner can make the decision to use ILV to improve $\dot{V}/\dot{Q}$ matching. Necessary for the institution of SILV is intubation with a double-lumen endobronchial tube (Fig. 11–8). Double-lumen tubes are available in a variety of sizes measured in French (F) units, such as size 35F, 37F, 39F, and 41F tubes. They can be angled right or left for cannulation of the right or left main-stem bronchus and are available with or without the carinal hook. The use of the carinal hook, which aids in stabilization of the tube, should be limited to the operating room, where use of the tube will be short term. If the patient will be mobilized, as in the ICU, the carinal hook can be irritating and can lead to erosion of the carina. A left-angle tube is preferred, regardless of which lung demonstrates the greatest pathologic changes, because the right-angle tube is difficult to place without obstructing the right upper lobe segmental bronchus. This complication of use of the right-angled tube is addressed by a specially designed fenestrated bronchial lumen, which allows for ventilation of the right upper lobe (Fig. 11–8, *right*).

The endobronchial tube has two cuffs. The proximal cuff is situated in the usual tracheal position. The proximal lumen opens into the airway below the tracheal cuff and just above the carina. The distal balloon is on the bronchial extension of the tube. The distal airway lumen opens at the end of the bronchial extension. Inflation of the bronchial cuff allows for differential ventilation. The

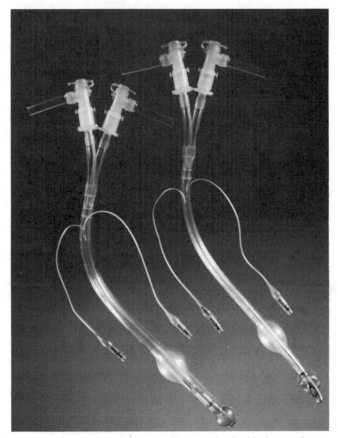

FIGURE 11–8 Broncho-Cath endobronchial tubes. The double-lumen design permits an airtight seal of the trachea and one bronchus. *Left:* Left-angled double-lumen endobronchial tube. *Right:* Right-angled endobronchial tube. The right-angled tube has a specially designed bronchial cuff and fenestrated bronchial lumen to allow ventilation of the right upper lobe. Both tubes come in a variety of sizes measured in French units. Color-coded cuffs, pilot balloons, and proximal lumens help identify bronchial and tracheal lumens. (Courtesy of Mallinckrodt Medical, Inc., Mallinckrodt Anesthesiology Division, St. Louis, Mo.)

cuffs, pilot balloons, and airway extensions are color coded for rapid differentiation between bronchial and tracheal lumens (Fig. 11–9).

TWO VENTILATORS

Each endobronchial-tube lumen is attached to a separate ventilator circuitry attached to its own ventilator. The two ventilators are most commonly synchronized for the start of inspiration. No significant differences in cardiac output have been shown between SILV and AILV. Servo ventilators (Servo 900C and 300, Siemens-Elema AB, Solna, Sweden) are synchronized by means of a cable that communicates between the two ventilators: one serving as the master, the other as the slave (Fig. 11–10). Individual ventilator settings will be dictated by the

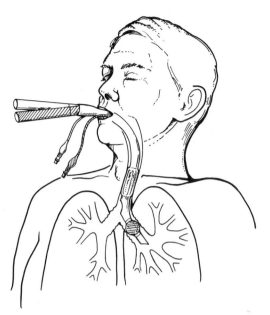

FIGURE 11-9 Left-angled endobronchial tube in proper position. For rapid differentiation, the bronchial cuff, pilot balloon, and proximal lumen are color coded blue, whereas the tracheal cuff, balloon, and lumen are clear. (From Traver, GA, and Flodquist-Priestley, G: Management problems in unilateral lung disease with emphasis on differential lung ventilation. *Crit Care Nurse* 1986;6:4.)

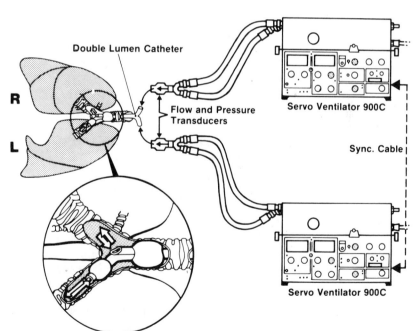

FIGURE 11-10 Therapeutic system for ILV includes the special dual-lumen endobronchial tube and two ventilators. The ventilators may be synchronized for the start of inspiration through the use of a cable. One ventilator serves as the master, the other as the slave. (From Siegel, JH, et al: Quantification of asymmetric lung pathophysiology as a guide to the use of simultaneous independent lung ventilation in posttraumatic and septic adult respiratory distress syndrome. *Ann Surg* 1985;202(4):425–439.)

particular lung mechanics demonstrated by each lung. It is feasible to have a variance between the two lungs in the delivery of VT, level of PEEP, I:E ratio, and even ventilatory mode.

Institution of ILV

The purpose of ILV is to provide therapy that will optimize $\dot{V}/\dot{Q}$ matching in each lung. Isolating each lung allows for the delivery of sufficient PEEP and VT to the affected lung to promote its reexpansion. Hyperinflation of the good lung and the resulting diversion of perfusion to the affected lung are also avoided.

Initially the total VT may be divided, with half being delivered to each lung. Airway pressures are then monitored for each lung and tidal volumes are adjusted to achieve acceptable airway pressures and alveolar ventilation. The ideal mechanism for guiding the selection of the appropriate VT and PEEP level for the right and left lungs is a compliance study on each lung. A compliance curve is developed, and VT and PEEP are adjusted until the inflation of each lung is at an optimal position on the pressure-volume curve.

The delivery of a relatively small VT to the noncompliant lung may result in relatively higher airway pressures. With time, the sick lung should begin to reexpand and demonstrate an improved compliance. The VT delivered to this lung should increase while airway pressures are decreasing. As air spaces in the less healthy lung reexpand, the percentage of shunt decreases, improving oxygenation and allowing the FIO_2 and the level of PEEP to be weaned.

Trend monitoring of static compliance is extremely useful for evaluating the effect of therapy on each lung. When the lung mechanics between the two lungs are nearly equal, the double-lumen tube may be replaced with a single-lumen tube. Deflation of the bronchial cuff and use of a Carlens (Y) adapter attached to the two lumens allows for a trial application of conventional ventilation before reintubation with a conventional ETT.

Advantages of ILV in Asymmetric Lung Disease

ILV is a physiologically directed therapy aimed at correcting $\dot{V}/\dot{Q}$ abnormalities caused by pathologic changes in the lung and exacerbated by conventional ventilation. The increase in VD/VT in the normal lung that was caused by hyperinflation and shunting of blood to the diseased lung is decreased through the delivery of a VT that places it in a more optimal position on the pressure-volume curve. The percentage of $\dot{Q}s/\dot{Q}T$ in the diseased lung is decreased by the recruitment of more air spaces through the selective application of PEEP. ILV can reverse persistent atelectatic changes associated with ARDS by applying a sufficient VT and level of PEEP to reexpand these atelectatic areas.

ILV generally produces a higher combined total compliance by achieving optimal compliance of each lung through a more appropriate distribution of ventilation. The healthier lung is no longer hyperinflated and pushed beyond its limits of elasticity. The diseased lung is ventilated with higher PEEP levels, which opens air spaces, gradually leading to an improvement in compliance.

With ILV there is a larger net VT delivery when the two lungs' tidal volumes are combined, in comparison with what can be delivered by conventional ventilation. This larger net VT delivery is achieved with lower airway pressures in the more compliant lung, which places it at a much lower risk of barotrauma.

Another definite benefit of ILV is that because the percentage of shunt is decreased, the FIO_2 required to maintain adequate oxygenation is often much less than was needed with conventional ventilation. High levels of oxygen are toxic to pulmonary tissue and can lead to fibrosis, especially if used for a prolonged period. Finally, tissue oxygen delivery is also improved because of a reduction in the pulmonary vascular resistance (PVR) and an increase in the cardiac output. Under the conditions of asymmetric lung disease and conventional ventilation, PVR is high because of hyperinflation of the compliant lung and transmission of high alveolar pressures to the pulmonary capillary bed. When PVR is reduced, cardiac output increases because the stroke volume of the right side of the heart improves.

Finally, with placement of an endobronchial tube, transbronchial contamination is reduced. The spillage of secretions and purulent drainage from the diseased lung to the healthier lung is diminished or prevented.

Patient Care Considerations for the Patient Undergoing ILV

Airway Clearance

Some aspects of bronchial hygiene are facilitated by the double-lumen tube, but new problems are also created. Because of the smaller lumen, a smaller suction catheter is required. A larger catheter is difficult to pass and can also lead to obstruction of airflow. A size 10F catheter is generally acceptable. A disadvantage of the smaller catheters is that retrieval of plugs and tenacious secretions may become more difficult. Suction catheter length is another consideration when an endobronchial tube is used. Standard adult suction catheters are 22 inches in length. Endobronchial tubes are usually packaged with four or five suction catheters 24 inches in length. These should be reserved for use in the longer bronchial lumen. Use of the longer catheters, however, is not required because, provided the suctioning procedure is not being performed through lengthy adapters and the full length of the catheter is inserted, standard catheters will reach beyond the tip of the bronchial lumen.

The actual depth of insertion of a suction catheter tip must be governed by clinical judgment. Adequate depth through either lumen is necessary to achieve secretion removal and prevent airway occlusion by accumulated mucus. Vigorous insertion of a suction catheter should be avoided, and when resistance is met, the catheter should be withdrawn. Suctioning through the proximal lumen generally results in slightly more resistance to catheter insertion, compared with suctioning through the bronchial lumen, possibly because of the location and shape of the side opening of the proximal lumen. Resistance, however, may indicate some obstruction of the proximal lumen by the tracheal wall, a potential complication.

Hyperoxygenation and Use of Manual Resuscitation Bag

Before each pass of the suction catheter, the patient must always be hyperoxygenated. It is also ideal to ensure the maintenance of PEEP during suctioning. The patient may be hyperoxygenated either through the ventilator or with a manual resuscitation bag (MRB). The maintenance of PEEP is also ensured by providing hyperoxygenation through the ventilator and by using a ventilator adapter with a sealed suction port. When a MRB is used for hyperoxygenation, it is possible to ventilate both lungs manually at the same time with the use of the Carlens Y-adapter that comes with the endobronchial tube. Suctioning is performed through ports provided by the Y-adapter. When not using the Carlens Y-adapter with the MRB, the clinician must keep in mind that only one lung is being ventilated and that volumes and pressures may need to be modified.

Maintenance of Ventilator Synchrony

When the ventilators are synchronized for inspiration with the use of a cable, disconnection of the master ventilator circuit from the patient's airway will result in erratic cycling of the slave ventilator. Therefore, when the master ventilator circuit is interrupted, manual ventilation with the Carlens Y-adapter is necessary to prevent complete interruption of ventilation by the slave ventilator.

Patient-Ventilator System Monitoring

The patient-ventilator system monitoring performed for the patient undergoing ILV is the same for the patient undergoing conventional ventilation except that twice the monitoring is required. Each ventilator's control panel must be checked for correctness of settings; and the display panel for the patient data on airway pressures and exhaled V_Ts. Before ILV is instituted, the risk of pulmonary barotrauma was greatest to the more healthy lung. However, after ILV initiation the lung with reduced compliance is at greater risk because of higher peak inspiratory pressures (PIPs) and required levels of PEEP. The exhaled V_T should be monitored to determine V_T in pressure modes and whether the set V_T is actually being delivered in volume-cycled modes. Exhaled V_T and PIP data are also useful in confirming tube placement (see below).

Endobronchial Tube Placement

The use of the endobronchial tube is associated with many unique patient care needs and potential problems. There is a great potential for bronchial injury related to excessive endobronchial tube cuff pressures or incorrect tube placement. Maintaining the correct position of the endobronchial tube is of prime importance. A tube that is too small may slip downward, whereas one that is too large has been associated with tube migration in an upward direction. The tube has to be positioned so that the proximal lumen is above the carina and the distal lumen is in the main-stem bronchus. When one is turning or tilting the patient, it is essential that the tube be held stationary and that the ventilator tubing not exert any traction on the airway. Tube placement at the teeth should be marked on the tube and noted in the medical record after chest x-ray confirmation.

Methods to assess tube placement include auscultation of the breath sounds. After inflation of both cuffs, one lung at a time is ventilated to ensure that breath sounds are audible on the side being ventilated and absent on the other. Auscultation of the breath sounds should also be performed when occlusion of the proximal lumen by the tracheal wall is suspected. When this complication occurs, the lung being ventilated with the proximal lumen, usually the right lung, will demonstrate decreased breath sounds, an elevated PIP caused by the increased resistance to gas flow, and potentially a decreased exhaled V_T.

Because the affected lung is going to have decreased breath sounds relative to the healthier lung, auscultation of breath sounds is not the only ongoing assessment that should be performed to assess tube placement. Inspired V_T and expired V_T should be frequently recorded for each lung. Tube misplacement may be accompanied by a sudden change in volumes. If the exhaled V_T of one lung acutely changes, assess the exhaled V_T of the other lung to see whether the volume is shifting to the other side. Volume lost from an endobronchial cuff leak will escape to the other lung. Volume lost from a tracheal cuff leak will likely vent to the atmosphere.

ENDOBRONCHIAL CUFF PRESSURES

The importance of measuring cuff pressures on both cuffs at least once every 4 hours cannot be overstressed. Excessive cuff pressure may result in tracheal or bronchial damage with granuloma formation on healing. Bronchial scarring may result in significant morbidity in that ventilation to the left lung may be persistently impaired. Interventions to the scarred bronchial segment, such as dilation, stent placement, or surgical repair, may eventually be required to correct the ventilation problem. Overinflation of cuffs may also result in cuff rupture, distortion, or herniation.

PSYCHOLOGIC NEEDS

The psychologic needs of the family and patient undergoing ILV must also be addressed. Direct patient care time is increased when a dual ventilator system is employed, and yet time must also be devoted to maintaining a caring and empathetic stance in this technologic environment. Frequently patients are sedated and medically paralyzed to prevent movement, to increase their tolerance to so many invasive apparatuses, to achieve optimal oxygenation and ventilation, and to reduce tissue oxygen demands. The clinician must remember, however, that despite heavy sedation and paralysis, it is still important to talk to the patient and explain what is being done when he or she is being touched, moved, and having procedures performed on him or her. If the patient is awake, ensure that a method of communication is developed.

Case Study: Application of ILV

A 24-year-old man was admitted to the trauma center after being injured on a construction site, where he was struck by a front loader. He suffered a crush injury to the left chest, hepatic fracture, fractured right humerus, and fractured left tibia. His pulmonary injuries consisted of fractured ribs and a severe left pulmonary contusion. In the field and during the acute resuscitation phase, he had significant blood loss and multiple hypotensive episodes, and he required massive volume resuscitation. Within days his chest x-ray film revealed ARDS. On day 7, HFJV was started in an effort to decrease high airway pressures and $PaCO_2$ levels and to improve the patient's oxygenation. HFJV provided satisfactory respiratory support for 3 days and then was deemed no longer necessary; the patient was therefore returned to conventional ventilation.

Four days later the patient demonstrated a $\dot{Q}s/\dot{Q}T$ of 28% and a deteriorating oxygenation status despite delivery of a high FiO_2 and increasing levels of PEEP. When he was turned on his side, with the more diseased lung in the dependent position, his oxygenation deteriorated relative to the period when the good lung had been dependent. The persistent severe asymmetry of his pathologic condition was also radiologically evident. The decision was made to reintubate with a double-lumen endobronchial tube and to initiate ILV.

Initially the total V_T of 1 L was divided in half, and each lung was ventilated with 500 cc. By using V_T values both above and below 500 cc, compliance curves were developed for each lung. These were examined to determine which V_T most ideally placed each lung on the pressure-volume curve (Fig. 11–11).

While the patient's hemodynamics and tissue oxygenation were monitored with a pulmonary artery catheter and oxygenation with a pulse oximeter, the V_T and PEEP were adjusted so that each lung's mechanical properties were optimal. Resulting ventilator settings were as follows:

	F_{IO_2}	Mode	Rate	V_T	PEEP	Static Compliance
Right lung	0.4	Assist/control	14	800	8	20 ml/cm H_2O
Left lung	0.4	Assist/control	14	200	15	5 ml/cm H_2O

ABG: pH 7.44/Pa_{O_2} 151/Pa_{CO_2} 42 $\dot{Q}s/\dot{Q}T$: 20%

Compliance studies provided the most specific and quantifiable manner by which the delivered V_T and PEEP level for each lung were determined. Additionally, the use of pulse oximetry as a noninvasive method of monitoring oxygenation meant that repeated drawing of ABG samples could be avoided while the ventilator settings were fine tuned.

After 90 hours of ILV, the patient had shown considerable improvement in the static compliance of the left lung (Fig. 11–12). Ventilator settings were altered as follows:

	F_{IO_2}	Mode	Rate	V_T	PEEP	Static Compliance
Right lung	0.3	Assist/control	13	600	8	20 ml/cm H_2O
Left lung	0.3	Assist/control	13	↑500	↓10	12 ml/cm H_2O

ABG: pH 7.42/Pa_{O_2} 150/Pa_{CO_2} 41 $\dot{Q}s/\dot{Q}T$: 10%

A trial of conventional ventilation was performed by attaching the Carlens Y-adapter to the endobronchial tube, letting down the bronchial cuff, and ventilating the patient's lungs with one ventilator. The patient demonstrated stability and therefore underwent reintubation with a standard endotracheal tube and continued to be supported with conventional mechanical ventilation.

MANDATORY MINUTE VENTILATION

Description

Mandatory minute ventilation (MMV) is a method of providing mechanical ventilation in which a constant minute ventilation ($\dot{V}_E$) is guaranteed. This is achieved by the ventilator as it monitors specific respiratory parameters and alters the level of support as necessary. If the patient's $\dot{V}_E$ falls below the prescribed level, the ventilator responds by delivering volume or pressure breaths at whatever level of support is necessary to maintain the preset $\dot{V}_E$. The degree of ventilator support is computer controlled through a closed-loop system. Therefore the amount of mechanical support decreases as the patient's $\dot{V}_E$ increases and vice versa.

MMV may presently be provided with either volume or pressure modes of ventilation. Sophisticated algorithms typically monitor a moving time-averaged

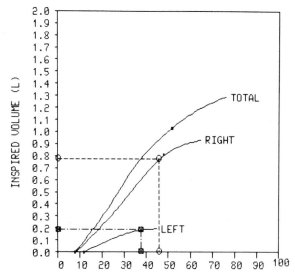

FIGURE 11–11 Comparison of static compliance curves in right and left lungs at onset of ILV. (From Siegel, JH, et al: Quantification of asymmetric lung pathophysiology as a guide to the use of simultaneous independent lung ventilation in posttraumatic and septic adult respiratory distress syndrome. *Ann Surg* 1985;202(4):425–439.)

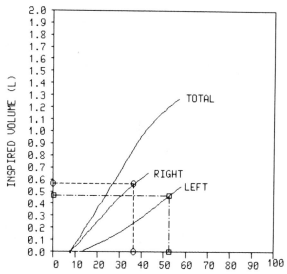

FIGURE 11–12 Comparison of static compliance curves in right and left lungs after 90 hours of ILV. (From Siegel, JH, et al: Quantification of asymmetric lung pathophysiology as a guide to the use of simultaneous independent lung ventilation in posttraumatic and septic adult respiratory distress syndrome. *Ann Surg* 1985;202(4):425–439.)

$\dot{V}E$ and vary the rate or level of inspiratory pressure as necessary. Manufacturers use a variety of terms to describe the modes available on their ventilators that provide MMV. These modes include minimum minute ventilation, augmented minute volume (AMV), and extended mandatory minute ventilation (EMMV). The patient may be breathing spontaneously or under controlled conditions, depending on the mode that is operating under the principles of MMV.

Indications

1. As a weaning tool, MMV may enhance the weaning process by promoting muscle strength while preventing fatigue.
2. MMV may be used to smooth transitions in the patient's ventilatory support needs, especially when there are fluctuations in ventilatory drive or effort.

Advantages and Disadvantages

The use of computers to maintain a constant $\dot{V}E$ may seem like science fiction. Because computers are capable of increasing the sophistication of clinical monitoring, it should be expected that their presence will become more commonplace. MMV certainly does not eliminate the need for the bedside practitioner to assimilate all the data and then to guide the ventilator's settings and monitor its function. However, the MMV system may prove advantageous in smoothing transitions from full to partial to no ventilator support, in that a stable $\dot{V}E$ and $PaCO_2$ may be achieved. Maintenance of a stable $\dot{V}E$ results in fewer arterial blood gas measurements and fewer manual ventilator adjustments and therefore may reduce the cost of ventilator weaning.

The main problem with most MMV systems is that they do not monitor the quality of the spontaneous breaths; thus the rapid, shallow breather, capable of generating the minimum $\dot{V}E$, defeats the basic premise of the system. Atelectasis may then develop. The incorporation of more sophisticated physiologic variables such as end-tidal CO_2 may eliminate an ineffective VT but also raises new questions regarding validity and reliability of the variable driving the system. Much research is still needed.

The second concern regarding MMV modes is that patient care may be adversely affected by the purported reduction in required patient assessment and intervention. The caregiver may be lulled into a false sense of security that the ventilator is "managing" the patient's ventilatory needs, and a less thorough assessment may ensue.

AIRWAY PRESSURE RELEASE VENTILATION

Definition and Description

During airway pressure release ventilation (APRV), the patient breathes spontaneously while receiving continuous positive airway pressure (CPAP). A valve opens intermittently during exhalation, releasing the pressure to either a lower set pressure level or ambient pressure. Therefore two levels of pressure—the CPAP level and the airway pressure release level—are applied (Fig. 11–13). After the airway pressure release, the CPAP level is restored. The ventilator settings are the CPAP level, the frequency of the airway pressure release, the level

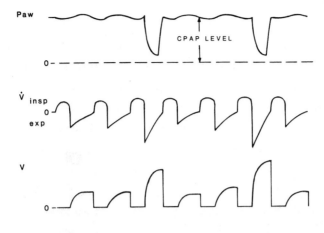

TIME

FIGURE 11–13 Mean airway pressure (Paw), flow $(\dot{V})$, and exhaled volume (V) tracings during airway pressure release ventilation (APRV). Patient breathes spontaneously at continuous positive airway pressure (CPAP) level. In this example, pressure releases occur every third breath, resulting in an exhaled volume that is larger than that of the CPAP breaths. Ventilation is promoted by titrating the frequency of pressure releases (i.e., the APRV rate). (From Sassoon, CSH: Positive pressure ventilation: Alternate modes. *Chest* 1991;100:1423.)

of pressure at the airway pressure release, and the duration of the airway pressure release.

During APRV the FRC is maintained with the CPAP level. During the cyclical pressure releases, the FRC decreases to a new level as gases are allowed to leave the lung passively. Passive lung deflation during airway pressure release augments alveolar ventilation and promotes CO_2 elimination. The pressure release is similar to an end-expiratory pause. An optimal release time would be considered to be equal to four time constants because approximately 98% of V_T is exhaled during this time. The duration of the pressure release is operator controlled and is usually 1.5 seconds. In patients with severe restrictive disease, this amount of time is inadequate for complete exhalation; thus this patient population represents a relative contraindication.

Indications

1. Acute lung injury, resulting in a decrease in the FRC and lung compliance but no impairment in respiratory muscle strength or in respiratory drive.
2. Mild postoperative pulmonary insufficiency.

Advantages and Disadvantages

Because of limited studies of human subjects, much is still unknown about APRV. It is purported to be advantageous over other modes of positive-pressure ventilation for the following reasons: it increases lung volume and lung compliance while preventing disuse atrophy of the respiratory muscles; it promotes CO_2 excretion by reducing lung volume rather than increasing it; the mean airway pressure never exceeds the CPAP level; and patients achieve ventilation at a lower PIP, thus reducing barotrauma and circulatory compromise.

APRV and PC share the common goals of reduction of the PIP in patients with noncompliant lungs, reduction of barotrauma, and stabilization of collapsed alveoli. The two modes of ventilation are similar in that both have set inspiratory and expiratory pressure levels. The essential difference between them is that APRV is a spontaneous breathing mode, whereas PC is not. APRV also does not require paralysis and sedation.

A disadvantage of APRV is that it is not available on commercial ventilators in the United States. It is generally achieved with a variety of valve configurations and homemade setups, resulting in considerable variability in system resistances. Study of a large number of patients is still needed to determine the applications of APRV, how it compares with other readily available modes, and its effect on patient outcome. One area of APRV research asks how synchronous and asynchronous airway pressure release and restoration of CPAP affect the work of breathing (WOB). Synchronous airway pressure release occurs during spontaneous expiration, whereas synchronous restoration of CPAP occurs during spontaneous inspiration.

PRESSURE-REGULATED VOLUME CONTROL

Description

Pressure-regulated volume control (PRVC) is a control mode of ventilation in which the patient receives a preset number of breaths of a preset VT that is given in the form of a pressure breath. Initial ventilator settings include respiratory rate, inspiratory time, and the target VT/V̇E. The ventilator strives to achieve the target VT using the lowest possible pressure.

Initially, and after any patient disconnection from the ventilator, the machine gives a sequence of four test breaths. The initial test breath is given at a pressure level of 5 cm H_2O above the PEEP setting, and the delivered volume at this pressure is measured. The ventilator then determines the pressure needed to achieve the target VT by performing a calculation involving the pressure used for the previous breath, the target VT, and the actual VT of the previous breath. The next breath in the test breath sequence is delivered at 75% of the calculated pressure needed to deliver the target VT. This process continues for the final two breaths of the test breath sequence. The inspiratory pressure with each subsequent breath can then change up to ±3 cm H_2O, being regulated to a value based on the volume/pressure calculation for the previous breath compared to the preset target VT/V̇E.

The ventilator will always go to the lowest pressure possible to achieve the desired VT. Thus, if the measured VT is too large, the pressure decreases in the same manner as stated above until the preset and measured volumes are equal. PRVC is therefore a control mode of ventilation with a guaranteed VT that is achieved by an adjusting pressure control level. The maximum pressure control level allowed is 5 cm H_2O below the set upper pressure limit. For patient safety, the upper pressure limit should be set as low as possible.

Indications

PRVC is suitable for patients who do not have a reliable respiratory drive either because of underlying pathologic changes or because the respiratory drive is affected by sedation and/or paralytic agents. It is useful for patients who demonstrate noncompliant lungs due to disease processes that result in lung units with varying time constants. This mode of ventilation is currently available only on the Servo 300, and to date no clinical studies of its use have been published.

Advantages and Disadvantages

PRVC combines the advantages of pressure and volume-controlled ventilation: the patient can be ventilated with low pressure while the VT is guaranteed. A decelerating flow pattern is delivered, which promotes more even distribution of gas in nonuniform disease processes. The ventilator automatically regulates inspiratory pressure as compliance and resistance factors affect the volume/pressure relation. Under conditions where compliance can change rapidly and dramatically such as with a tension pneumothorax, the ventilator will react and attempt to maintain a steady alveolar ventilation until stabilizing interventions can be performed. A hazard of PRVC is that in the event of a large air leak the vent may continue to raise the pressure control level in a step-wise fashion, "chasing" the volume lost through the leak, and possibly aggravating air loss through the defect.

Focus Areas of Patient Monitoring

1. Monitor the patient's exhaled VT and V̇E to ensure the set parameters are being achieved.
2. Monitor the inspiratory pressure to determine the amount of pressure required to achieve the desired VT. Set the upper pressure limit 10 to 15 cm H_2O above the average required inspiratory pressure. When the peak inspiratory pressure reaches 5 cm H_2O below the upper pressure limit, inspiration will continue. If this occurs for three consecutive breaths, the upper pressure limit alarm sounds and the display reads "limited pressure." If the actual upper pressure limit is reached, inspiration is terminated.

VOLUME SUPPORT

Description

Volume support (VS) is a mode of ventilation that pressure supports every breath to a level that guarantees a preset VT. It is volume-targeted ventilation, identical to PRVC except that it is a spontaneous breathing mode—the patient triggers every breath. Initial ventilator settings include a value for the expected spontaneous RR and minimum VT/V̇E.

Initially, and after any patient disconnection from the ventilator, the machine gives a sequence of four test breaths. The initial test breath is given at a pressure level of 5 cm H_2O above the PEEP setting, and the delivered volume at this pressure is measured. The ventilator then determines the pressure needed to achieve the target VT by performing a calculation involving the pressure used for the previous breath, the target VT, and the actual VT of the previous breath. The next breath in the test breath sequence is delivered at 75% of the calculated pressure needed to deliver the target VT. This process continues for the final two breaths of the test breath sequence. The inspiratory pressure with each subsequent breath can then change up to ± 3 cm H_2O, being regulated to a value based on the volume/pressure calculation for the previous breath compared to the preset target VT/V̇E. If the patient breathes above the preset VT, the ventilator will lower the pressure support in a step-wise fashion until the target VT is achieved. Inspiration may be flow-cycled, when flow has decreased to 5% of peak flow, or time-cycled, after 80% of the set inspiratory cycle time.

The ventilator responds to a decrease in the patient's RR that is less than the expected spontaneous rate by calculating a new target VT based on the preset minimum V̇E and the measured RR. The ventilator uses the new calculated target VT as the reference to regulate inspiratory pressure. The new calculated target VT is compared to the preset VT, and if the new VT exceeds the preset VT by 50%, the increase in inspiratory pressure is stopped at the level required to achieve a volume that is 150% of the set VT. The patient is guaranteed the minimum minute volume up to 150% of the set VT. If the patient's RR drops below the apnea alarm threshold during VS, the ventilator automatically switches to PRVC and will remain in this mode until the alarm is reset by the clinician. The ventilator switches back to VS after the apnea alarm is reset.

Indications

VS is suitable for weaning and for patients who do not have sufficient respiratory muscle strength to consistently guarantee an adequate VT. This mode of ventilation is currently available only on the Servo 300. There are no scientific reports of its use in the literature.

Advantages and Disadvantages

VS may be viewed as refined pressure support (PS) and, therefore, has all of the advantages of PS ventilation (see Chapter 7). During PS ventilation, a maximum peak inspiratory pressure is assured, and VT is variable on a breath-to-breath basis. With VS, however, VT is guaranteed, and the pressure will vary depending on the compliance of the lungs and on ventilator circuit and airway resistance factors. Unlike MMV modes, the patient cannot achieve the set V̇E using a rapid, shallow breathing pattern. Patients may be more comfortable because they have control over RR and inspiratory time.

Focus Areas of Patient Monitoring

1. Monitor the exhaled tidal volume to ensure that the patient is receiving the target minimum VT/V̇E. Patients may receive tidal volumes as large as 150% of the target VT in the event their RR decreases.
2. Monitor the peak inspiratory pressure to determine the amount of pressure required to achieve the desired VT. Set the upper pressure limit 10 to 15 cm H_2O above the average required inspiratory pressure. When the peak inspiratory pressure reaches 5 cm H_2O below the upper pressure limit, inspiration will continue. If this occurs for three consecutive breaths, the upper pressure limit alarm sounds, and the display reads "limited pressure." If the actual upper pressure limit is reached, inspiration is terminated.

3. Ensure all parameters used in PRVC are preset for apnea ventilation.
4. Monitor the patient's RR. If the patient's RR increases to >25 breaths/ min and the $\dot{V}E$ demands are increasing, assess the patient's ability to continue to manage the WOB associated with a spontaneous breathing mode. The patient's $\dot{V}E$ may exceed the set value because the set value indicates minimum acceptable $\dot{V}E$. Be sure to set the upper and lower volume alarm limits.

PERMISSIVE HYPERCAPNIA

Permissive hypercapnia (PHC) is a ventilatory strategy designed to reduce barotrauma caused by high inspiratory airway pressures. Airway pressures are reduced by utilization of tidal volumes smaller than the 10 to 15 cc/kg traditionally used with mechanical ventilatory support. The decreased VT results in lower peak and mean airway pressures, reducing the incidence of alveolar overdistention and attendant acute lung injury. Smaller volumes are permitted because ventilatory requirements are reduced by allowing the $PaCO_2$ to rise gradually to 50 to 100 mm Hg. Staged, deliberate limitation of ventilatory support results in a gradual increase in $PaCO_2$ that is generally tolerable because intracellular pH levels change minimally, as partial to complete metabolic compensation occurs. Hypercapnia is contraindicated, however, in the presence of increased intracranial pressure and may be poorly tolerated by patients with a preexisting metabolic acidosis.

Rationale for Use

High ventilatory pressures are associated with alveolar overdistention and pulmonary barotrauma. The incidence of injury increases when VT is maldistributed, as occurs in nonhomogeneous disease processes. Therefore, when conventional ventilatory strategies are applied to patients with heterogeneous disease processes, and result in areas of alveolar overdistention, ventilatory support may become a contributing factor in the progression of lung injury. In animal studies it has been clearly shown that when airway pressures are high, creating either localized or generalized alveolar overdistention, acute lung injury occurs that is very similar to the pathologic changes seen in ARDS.

In retrospective human studies, permissive hypercapnia has been shown to reduce the mortality rate among patients with ARDS and acute, severe asthma. In ARDS, compliant and noncompliant alveoli are interspersed throughout the lung. Tidal volumes of 10 to 15 cc/kg are more favorably distributed to the more compliant lung areas, leading to overdistention and barotrauma. In acute, severe asthma, bronchospasm and increased secretions result in some areas of the lung that are overdistended by air trapping and auto-PEEP formation and other areas that are consolidated. Localized lung injury occurs in the hyperinflated areas. Factors that affect the degree of hyperinflation include VT, respiratory rate, and the I:E ratio.

Implementation

The primary goal of PHC is to limit pressure-related barotrauma. It remains unclear, however, which pressure—the peak dynamic pressure, static, mean, or transpulmonary pressure—is the most important indicator of the risk of barotrauma. The pressure that may be the best to target and monitor at the bedside, when PHC is instituted, is the end-inspiratory static pressure, because it reflects alveolar pressure. This pressure is also known as the plateau pressure.

It is recommended that plateau, or static, pressure should not exceed 30 to 35 cm H$_2$O. Damage may occur to the lungs after prolonged exposure to pressures above this level and may subject those alveoli that have retained a normal compliance to undue stress. Because the peak inspiratory pressure (PIP) is more easily monitored clinically, it may be chosen as the trend variable and should be kept under 35 to 40 cm H$_2$O pressure to reduce pressure-induced lung injury. The PIP, however, is not ideal as the trend variable because it is affected by changes in airway resistance, which can vary significantly in the clinical setting. If PIP is used, then controllable factors affecting resistance, such as the inspiratory flow rate and pattern, must be kept constant. Furthermore, the relationship between PIP and plateau pressure must be intermittently measured and reevaluated with changes in the V$_T$.

As the airway pressure is reduced during PHC initiation, the mean airway pressure may decrease, resulting in a decrease in oxygenation. Strategies to improve a deteriorating oxygenation status include the addition of PEEP or an extension of the inspiratory time.

To achieve the target airway pressure, a V$_T$ as small as 5 to 7 cc/kg may be needed. The PaCO$_2$ should be allowed to increase gradually as determined by tolerance of respiratory acidosis. No lower pH limits have been recommended, and the acceptable pH should be determined on a case-by-case basis. Potentially adverse effects of increased PaCO$_2$, which should be monitored for, include cardiac depression, neurologic depression, and increased pulmonary vascular resistance. The PaCO$_2$ is gradually increased to avoid an acute, intolerable reduction in the pH and to make the infusion of bicarbonate solutions unnecessary. During the escalation phase an increase in the ventilatory drive, in response to an increased PaCO$_2$, accompanied by an unacceptable increase in the work of breathing, may be blunted with the use of heavy sedation and paralysis.

As the underlying disease process resolves and the patient's clinical status improves, the PaCO$_2$ should gradually be brought back to the patient's baseline. Rapid reversal of PHC should be avoided because it will result in metabolic alkalosis, the magnitude of which is dependent upon the degree of metabolic compensation that has occurred during the therapy.

Though PHC is, at this stage, an experimental therapy, its use warrants serious consideration in patients with ARDS, for whom the mortality rate remains high despite today's sophisticated ventilators and multiple available modes of ventilation. Much research still needs to be performed. However, on the basis of present evidence, the theory that ventilator-induced lung injury may be reduced by aggressive management of airway pressures is logical. PHC challenges the premise that ventilatory support should ventilate the patient's lungs until normocapnia is reached.

CONCLUSION

Throughout history, common and accepted clinical practices have given way to new methods of patient management. The future of ventilatory support in the intensive care setting will likely challenge many of today's practices as academic discussions question present thought and dedicated researchers reveal new knowledge.

RECOMMENDED READINGS

Carlon, G.C., et al. (1978). Acute life-threatening ventilation-perfusion inequality: An indication for independent lung ventilation. *Crit Care Med* 6(6), 380–383.

Carlon, G.C., Howland, W.S., Ray, C., et al. (1983). High-frequency jet ventilation: A prospective randomized evaluation. *Chest* 84(5), 551–559.

Downs, J.B., and Stock, M.C. (1987). Airway pressure release ventilation: A new concept in ventilatory support. *Crit Care Med* 15(5), 459–461.

Geiger, K. (1983). Differential lung ventilation. *Int Anesthesiol Clin* 21, 83–98.

Griffin, J.P. (1981). Nursing care of patients on high frequency jet ventilation. *Crit Care Nurse* 1(7), 25–28.

Hickling, K.G., Walsh, J., Henderson, S., and Jackson, R. (1994). Low mortality rate in adult respiratory distress syndrome using low-volume, pressure-limited ventilation with permissive hypercapnia: A prospective study. *Crit Care Med* 2(10), 1568–1578.

Kacmarek, R.M., and Hickling, K.G. (1993). Permissive hypercapnia. *Respir Care* 38(4), 373–387.

Kopec, I.C., VanDervort, A.L., and Carlon, G.C. (1988). High-frequency jet ventilation. In R.M. Kacmarek and J.K. Stoller (Eds.). *Current Respiratory Care* (pp. 153–157). Toronto: B.C. Decker.

Kvetan, V., Carlon, G.C., and Howland, W.S. (1982). Acute pulmonary failure in asymmetric lung disease: Approach to management. *Crit Care Med* 10(2), 114–118.

Marini, J.J. (1994). Mechanical ventilation and newer ventilatory techniques. In R.C. Bone (Ed.). *Pulmonary and Critical Care Medicine* (vol. II, Part R, pp. 1–26). St. Louis: C.V. Mosby.

Quan, S.F., Parides, G.C., and Knoper, S.R. (1990). Mandatory minute volume (MMV) ventilation: An overview. *Resp Care* 35(9), 898–905.

Räsänen, J., et al. (1991). Airway pressure release ventilation during acute lung injury: A prospective multicenter trial. *Crit Care Med* 19(10), 1234–1241.

Siegel, J.H., et al. (1985). Quantification of asymmetric lung pathophysiology as a guide to the use of simultaneous independent lung ventilation in posttraumatic and septic adult respiratory distress syndrome. *Ann Surg* 202(4), 425–439.

Siemens-Elema AB. (1993). *Servo Ventilator 300—Operating Manual*. Art. No.: 60 26 608 E313E. Solna, Sweden: Siemens-Elema AB, Life Support Systems Division, Marketing Communications.

Simon, B., and Borg, U. (1990). Independent lung ventilation. *Critical Care Report* 1(3), 398–407.

Sjöstrand, U. (1980). High-frequency positive-pressure ventilation (HFPPV): A review. *Crit Care Med* 8(3), 345–364.

Standiford, T.J., and Morganroth, M.L. (1989). High-frequency ventilation. *Chest* 96(6), 1380–1389.

Stock, M.C., and Downs, J.B. (1987). Airway pressure release ventilation: A new approach to ventilatory support during acute lung injury. *Resp Care* 32(7), 517–524.

Traver, G.A., and Flodquist-Priestley, G. (1986). Management problems in unilateral lung disease with emphasis on differential lung ventilation. *Crit Care Nurse* 6(4), 40–50.

Tuxen, D.V. (1994). Permissive hypercapnia. In M.J. Tobin (Ed.). *Principles and Practice of Mechanical Ventilation* (pp. 371–392). New York: McGraw-Hill.

Villar, J., Winston, B., and Slutsky, A.S. (1990). Non-conventional techniques of ventilatory support. *Crit Care Clin* 6(3), 579–603.

APPENDIX
I

Pulmonary Symbols and Abbreviations

SYMBOLS

Primary Symbols

C	Content of a gas in blood phase
F	Fractional concentration (or percentage) of a gas
P	Partial pressure of a gas
Q	Blood volume
$\dot{Q}$	Blood volume per unit of time
S	Saturation of hemoglobin with oxygen
V	Gas volume
$\dot{V}$	Gas volume per unit of time

Secondary or Qualifying Symbols

GAS PHASE

A	Alveolar
B	Barometric
D	Dead space gas
E	Expired
I	Inspired
T	Tidal gas

BLOOD PHASE

a	Arterial
v	Venous
$\bar{v}$	Mixed venous
c	Capillary

EXAMPLES

Ca_{O_2}	Content of oxygen in arterial blood
$C\bar{v}_{O_2}$	Content of oxygen in mixed venous blood
$F_{I_{O_2}}$	Fraction of oxygen in inspired gas
Pa_{O_2}	Partial pressure of oxygen in arterial blood
Pa_{CO_2}	Partial pressure of carbon dioxide in arterial blood

P_{AO_2}	Partial pressure of oxygen in alveolar gas
P_B	Barometric pressure
P_{IO_2}	Partial pressure of oxygen in inspired gas
S_{aO_2}	Saturation of hemoglobin with oxygen in arterial blood
$S\bar{v}O_2$	Saturation of hemoglobin with oxygen in mixed venous blood
$\dot{V}_A$	Volume of alveolar gas per unit of time (alveolar ventilation)
$\dot{V}_E$	Volume of expired gas per unit of time (minute ventilation)
V_D	Dead space volume
V_T	Tidal volume

ABBREVIATIONS

Lung Volumes

V_T	Tidal volume
IRV	Inspiratory reserve volume
ERV	Expiratory reserve volume
RV	Residual volume

Lung Capacities

(When two or more volumes are added together, they are known as a capacity.)

IC	Inspiratory capacity (IRV + V_T)
VC	Vital capacity (IRV + V_T + ERV)
FRC	Functional residual capacity (ERV + RV)
TLC	Total lung capacity (IC + FRC)

Pulmonary Mechanics

C_{ST}	Static compliance
C_{DYN}	Dynamic compliance
C_{TL}	Total compliance (chest wall + lung)
Raw	Airway resistance
WOB	Work of breathing
$\dot{V}_E$	Volume of expired gas per unit of time (minute ventilation)
MVV	Maximum voluntary ventilation
V_T	Tidal volume
VC	Vital capacity
MIP	Maximum inspiratory pressure
f	Respiratory frequency
RR	Respiratory rate
$f : V_T$	Ratio of respiratory frequency to tidal volume

Perfusion

$\dot{Q}$	Blood flow
QT	Cardiac output; also abbreviated CO
PVR	Pulmonary vascular resistance
SVR	Systemic vascular resistance

$\dot{V}_{O_2}$ Volume of oxygen consumed per unit of time (oxygen consumption per minute)

$\dot{V}_{CO_2}$ Volume of carbon dioxide produced per minute

Ventilation/Perfusion Relationships

$\dot{V}/\dot{Q}$ Ratio of ventilation to perfusion

$\dot{Q}_S/\dot{Q}_T$ Ratio of shunted blood flow to total blood flow (physiologic shunt)

V_D/V_T Ratio of dead space to tidal volume ventilation (physiologic dead space)

APPENDIX

II

Drugs Used in Intensive Respiratory Care

PAMELA GUILLAUME, RN, MS, CCRN

ROUTE OF ADMINISTRATION

Drug therapy is often used as treatment for a variety of respiratory disease states. Respiratory drugs may be used on an emergent basis for life-threatening disorders or prophylactically for patient comfort and prevention.

The route of drug delivery chosen for a particular patient is often determined by the drug's onset of action, duration, and availability. The three main routes of delivery are parenteral, oral, and inhalation. The oral route usually provides a longer onset of action and gradual release, but with potential gastrointestinal side effects. The parenteral route offers a quicker onset but more systemic effects (e.g., tachycardia). The inhalation route allows rapid local delivery to the lung tissue with minimal toxic effects.

BRONCHODILATORS

Bronchodilators play a major role in managing airflow obstruction because of their ability to relax bronchial smooth muscle. This category of drugs achieves bronchodilation by exerting their action on either the sympathetic or parasympathetic nervous system (Fig. II–1).

In the sympathetic nervous system (SNS), bronchodilation can be achieved by either of two different mechanisms. The first mechanism involves stimulating adrenergic receptors of the SNS. Table II–1 provides a review of the adrenergic receptors of the sympathetic nervous system and the effect they exert when stimulated. Specifically, stimulation of beta-2 receptors will initiate a series of transactions that lead to the production of cyclic adenosine monophosphate (cAMP). Increased production of cAMP facilitates enzyme reactions resulting in bronchodilation. The second mechanism of enhancing bronchodilation is by inhibiting phosphodiesterase production. Normally phosphodiesterase would convert cAMP into an inactive form, but by inhibiting the production of phosphodiesterase, cAMP remains active and facilitates bronchodilation.

In the parasympathetic nervous system (PNS), a series of transactions that results in bronchoconstriction begins with stimulation of the cholinergic

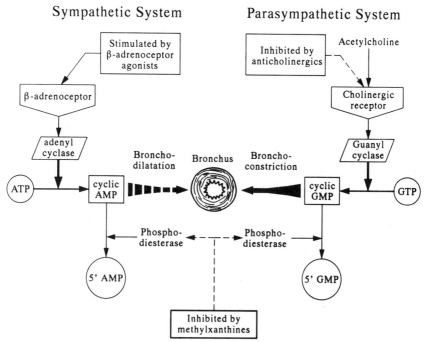

FIGURE II-1 Action of adrenergic and cholinergic bronchodilating drugs. (From Shenfield, GM: Combination bronchodilator therapy. *Drugs* 1982; 24:414–439.)

TABLE II-1 Adrenergic Receptors of the Sympathetic Nervous System

Receptor	Site	Effect
Beta-1	Heart	Increased heart rate Increased contractility Increased conduction
Beta-2	Blood vessels Bronchioles	Dilation
Alpha	Blood vessels	Constriction

TABLE II-2 Three Main Categories of Bronchodilators

	Beta-adrenergic Agonists		
Action	Smooth muscle relaxation via stimulation of beta-2 adrenergic receptors of the SNS Beta-2 receptor stimulation increases cAMP and causes bronchodilation		
Agents	*Selective* Albuterol Terbutaline	*Less specific* Isoetharine Metaproterenol	*Nonselective* Epinephrine Isoproterenol
Side effects	CNS: nervousness, headache, shakiness, tremor, insomnia, agitation CV: tachycardia, palpitations, HTN, arrhythmias		
Clinical implications	Inhalation route preferred because of rapid onset and ability to use smaller doses. Most potent group of bronchodilators. The ideal agent, to avoid cardiac side effects, is selective for beta-2 receptors. Preferentially act on distal airways and are therefore indicated for acute or chronic asthma and prophylactically for airway hyperresponsiveness. Secondary effect is stimulation of mucociliary clearance. Tolerance can develop with continuous treatment.		

SNS = Sympathetic nervous system; PNS = parasympathetic nervous system; cAMP = cyclic adenosine monophosphate; cGMP = cyclic guanosine monophosphate; CNS = central nervous system; CV = cardiovascular system; HTN = hypertension; GI = gastrointestinal tract; COPD = chronic obstructive pulmonary disease.

Methylxanthines	Anticholinergic Agents
Smooth muscle relaxation via the following possible mechanisms: Adenosine antagonism Phosphodiesterase inhibition Alterations in intracellular calcium transport Catecholamine release	Smooth muscle relaxation via blocking of cholinergic response of the PNS Cholinergic receptor inhibition decreases cGMP and causes bronchodilation
Theophylline Aminophylline (All drugs are theophylline derivatives.)	Atropine sulfate Ipratropium bromide Glycopyrrolate
CNS: restlessness, insomnia, seizures CV: flushing, arrhythmias, palpitations, tachycardia GI: nausea, vomiting, diarrhea	Atropine side effects: tachycardia, dry mouth, pupil dilation, drying of secretions Inhalation ipratropium bromide: very negligible side effects
Administer orally or intravenously. Indicated for acute asthmatic attacks or acute exacerbation of COPD. Low toxic/therapeutic ratio; therapeutic range 10–20 g/ml. Check levels intermittently because drug can be affected by many variables: liver disease, age, drug interactions. Metabolized by the liver. Secondary effects: Stimulate breathing Enhance ciliary function Inhibit histamine release Vasodilate pulmonary vessels Improve diaphragmatic contractility Mild diuretic, mild inotrope, slight central respiratory stimulant. Administer continuous drip on infusion pump.	Generally given via aerosol to reduce blocking of the muscarinic receptors in other parts of the body (heart, GI tract). Onset of therapeutic effect is more gradual than with beta agonists. Therapeutic effect with anticholinergics is 30–90 min. Preferentially act on proximal airways; therefore indicated for bronchitis and bronchospasm. Less effective than beta agonist for prophylactic use. May provide synergistic effect with beta agonist and methylxanthines. Give anticholinergic agent first when administering ipratropium with beta agonist.

receptors. These receptors facilitate the increased production of cyclic guanosine monophosphate (cGMP), which leads to bronchial constriction. Bronchodilators work on the PNS to inhibit this process and decrease the production of cGMP effectively blocking its bronchial constricting effects and resulting in relaxation of bronchial smooth muscle.

The three main categories of bronchodilators are the beta-adrenergic agonists, methylxanthines, and anticholinergic agents (Table II–2). All these agents are indicated for bronchial smooth muscle relaxation in either acute or chronic airflow obstruction and/or for prophylactic use when airway hyperresponsiveness can be predicted.

CORTICOSTEROIDS

Corticosteroids help alleviate airway obstruction through their anti-inflammatory action. Their ability to prevent histamine release, diminish hypersensitivity reactions, decrease edema, and reduce excessive production of mucus all contribute to decreasing airway obstruction. In addition, these drugs enhance the responsiveness of beta-2 receptors to sympathomimetic agents and methylxanthines, thereby promoting their bronchodilatory effects.

Corticosteroids are often used in combination with other bronchodilators for the management of acute and chronic asthma. They have been found to be beneficial in the acute management of chronic obstructive lung disease, although less success is associated with usage in the chronic stage of this disease. There are many questionable indications for using corticosteroids, in combination with other drugs, in the management of many forms of obstructive disease, such as aspiration pneumonia, acute respiratory distress syndrome, and pulmonary sarcoidosis. Corticosteroids are categorized according to their plasma half-life (Box II–1). The following clinical implications should be considered whenever any corticosteroid is given:

1. A corticosteroid can be given systemically (e.g., orally or intravenously) or by aerosol.
2. Give aerosolized form 10 to 15 minutes after administration of beta-adrenergic agent.
3. Aerosol form can cause fungal infection in oropharynx or larynx. Diminish possibility of side effects by having patient rinse mouth after treatment and/or add a spacer to the delivery system.
4. Systemic side effects include the following:
   - Acute adrenal insufficiency and/or recurrence of symptoms may occur with sudden withdrawal.
   - Prolonged use may lead to fat redistribution, increased appetite and weight gain, fluid retention, increased potassium excretion, osteoporosis, hyperglycemia, gastrointestinal distress (nausea, cramping, diarrhea), artificial sense of well-being, steroid psychosis.
5. Use of a corticosteroid may alter metabolism of theophylline, necessitating the monitoring of theophylline levels.

MAST CELL STABILIZERS

Mast cell stabilizers are used to prevent bronchospasm. They stabilize the mast cells and prevent the initiation of an allergic response and histamine release. The

---

Box II-1 Categories of Corticosteroids

Short Acting
Plasma half-life less than 2 hr
    Hydrocortisone
    Cortisone

Intermediate Acting
Plasma half-life 1–4 hr
    Prednisone
    Prednisolone
    Methylprednisolone
    Triamcinolone

Long Acting
Plasma half-life greater than 3 hr
    Dexamethasone
    Paramethasone

---

generic agent used as a mast cell stabilizer is cromolyn sodium. This agent is indicated for the prophylactic management of bronchial hyperactivity. Specifically it is beneficial in preventing both bronchospasm from exposure to allergens and exercise-induced bronchospasm. The following clinical implications are related to using cromolyn sodium:

1. Teach patient that drug is not a bronchodilator and cannot be used for treatment during an asthma attack.
2. Optimal drug effect is achieved if drug is given 1 week before allergen exposure or 15 minutes before exercise.
3. Agent is only available for inhalation.
4. Side effects are minimal, reversible, and stop when the drug is withdrawn. Immediately after inhalation, patient may have throat irritation, hoarseness, dryness of mouth, acute cough, sensation of chest tightness, or bronchospasm.
5. Side effects can be diminished by gargling with water after inhalation and/or by giving one or two puffs of aerosolized beta-adrenergic agent just before cromolyn sodium inhalation therapy.

MUCOKINETIC AGENTS

Mucokinetic agents promote the clearance of respiratory secretions. This is accomplished either by giving agents that help break up mucus into smaller particles or by increasing the amount of fluid in the respiratory tract (Table II–3). This may be necessary in the patient with thick, tenacious secretions. These agents will assist the patient in mobilizing their secretions so that they can be coughed up or suctioned out. The following clinical implications are related to using mucokinetic drug therapy:

1. Monitor systemic fluid status carefully. A patient with inadequate intake may become dehydrated, which may result in thick secretions. Excess in-

TABLE II-3   Categories of Mucokinetic Agents

Category	Action	Agents
Diluting/hydrating	Modify character of secretions	Saline solution Propylene glycol Oral expectorants, such as potassium iodide
Wetting	Lower surface tension of respiratory tract	Detergents, such as sodium bicarbonate Ethyl alcohol
Mucolytic agents	Disrupt mucoproteins responsible for high viscosity	N-Acetylcysteine
Proteolytic agents	Lyse protein material found in purulent sputum	Trypsin Deoxyribonuclease

travascular fluid may increase the hydrostatic pressure in the blood vessels and contribute to pulmonary edema.

2. Patient should have an effective cough so that the loosened secretions can be mobilized.
3. Implement pulmonary toilet to assist patient in mobilizing secretions. Consider postural drainage, percussion, and chest physical therapy.

ANTITUSSIVE AGENTS

Antitussive agents are used to help eliminate an ineffective cough that is not allowing a patient to rest or is preventing the use of the patient's energy on an effective cough. These agents act either centrally or peripherally (Table II–4). Centrally acting agents raise the threshold necessary to stimulate the cough center. Peripherally acting agents suppress coughing by reducing local irritation in the airways.

TABLE II-4   Categories of Antitussive Agents

Agents	Clinical Implications
Centrally Acting	

Narcotics
    Codeine
    Hydrocodone
	Narcotic dosage is less than that used to manage pain relief.
	Side effects of narcotics include constipation, dry mouth, impaired mucociliary clearance, and bronchospasm from histamine release.

Nonnarcotics
    Dextromethorphan
    Benzonatate
	Side effects of nonnarcotics include nausea, dizziness, and slight drowsiness.

Peripherally Acting	
Topical anesthetics Demulcents Expectorants	Topical anesthetics work well in preventing cough during bronchoscopy or endotracheal intubation.

DECONGESTANTS AND ANTIHISTAMINES

Decongestants and antihistamines are used to treat upper airway congestion. Decongestants work by their ability to constrict local blood vessels. This action decreases edema by reducing blood flow, which lowers hydrostatic pressure and prevents fluid exudation into the tissues. A typical decongestant is pseudoephedrine (Sudafed; Actifed). Decongestants are recommended for use on a short-term basis (3 to 7 days), because prolonged use can result in rebound congestion when the drug is discontinued.

Antihistamines help control cold or allergy symptoms such as sneezing, rhinitis, and itchy, watery eyes. A concern with antihistamines is their association with drowsiness, although the newer agents (e.g., terfenadine and astemizole) do not have this side effect.

RESPIRATORY STIMULANTS

Respiratory stimulants are used to increase the urge to breathe. This outcome may be effective in managing respiratory depression in patients with chronic obstructive pulmonary disease (COPD) or in patients who are awakening from anesthesia. They work by either a central or a peripheral mechanism. Centrally this class of drugs stimulates the respiratory centers in the brain stem. Drugs that work centrally include progesterone, protriptyline, naloxone, and acetazolamide. The peripheral mechanism of action is initiated by affecting the carotid and/or aortic chemoreceptors. Almitrine is an example of a peripherally acting respiratory stimulant. Some drugs, such as doxapram and theophylline, initiate both a central and a peripheral action. The patient must have an intact respiratory system for any of these drugs to be effective. Otherwise the increased respiratory drive would lead to worsening respiratory distress.

TREATMENT OF INFECTIONS

Infectious processes in the lungs are managed according to the nature of the organism (Table II–5). Some organisms, such as that found in tuberculosis, require multiple agents to combat the infectious process.

PARALYTIC AGENTS

Paralytic agents are indicated for either short-term or long-term paralysis. Short-term paralysis is often needed for intubation, either preoperative or emergent. Long-term paralysis is used in intensive care units to achieve optimal mechanical ventilation.

Selection of a paralytic agent is based on the agent's duration of action and potential side effects. Paralytics are classified as either depolarizing or nondepolarizing and act at the neuromuscular junction of the skeletal muscle. A depolarizing agent such as succinylcholine mimics acetylcholine and initiates muscle contraction. Its duration of action is extremely short. Nondepolarizing agents occupy the postsynaptic cleft but do not initiate muscle contraction. Their duration of action may be long acting, intermediate acting, or short acting (Table II–6). Long-acting agents can have a maximal duration of 120 to 165 minutes. Intermediate-acting agents have a maximal duration of 35 to

TABLE II–5 Categories of Drugs Used to Treat Infectious Lung Processes

Group	Description	Examples
Antibiotic	Binds to bacteria cell wall and inhibits growth or kills bacteria	Penicillins Cephalosporins Aminoglycosides Tetracyclines
Antiprotozoal	Interferes with DNA/RNA synthesis in protozoa	Pentamidine
Antituberculosis	Decreases tubercle bacilli replication	Isoniazide Rifampin Pyrazinamide
Antiviral	Interferes with DNA/RNA synthesis in viruses	Acyclovir Ribavirin Zidovudine
Antifungal	Interferes with fungal cell replication	Griseofulvin Nystatin Amphotericin B

45 minutes, and short-acting agents have a maximal duration of 15 to 30 minutes. Before giving a paralytic agent, consider the pathway of drug elimination, potential for vagolytic effects, or histamine release. Patients with underlying liver or kidney disease may have difficulty in metabolizing some agents. Vagolytic effects cause tachycardia and increase oxygen consumption. Histamine release from the mast cells causes vasodilation, leading to hypotension,

TABLE II–6 Categories of Nondepolarizing Paralytic Agents

Agent	Duration	Clinical Implications
Tubocurarine	Long	Renal and biliary excretion
Metocurine	Long	Primarily renal excretion Minimal biliary excretion
Gallamine	Long	Renal excretion Vagolytic action Histamine release
Pancuronium	Long	Renal excretion Some biliary excretion Vagolytic effects
Pipecuronium	Long	Renal excretion Steroid based
Doxacurium	Long	Renal excretion Most potent nondepolarizer
Vecuronium	Intermediate	Renal excretion Some biliary excretion
Atracurium	Intermediate	Eliminated via Hoffman degradation Histamine release
Mivacurium	Short	Hydrolyzed by plasma cholinesterases Histamine release

TABLE II-7   Adjunct Agents Used With Paralytic Agents for Sedation and/or Analgesia

Group	Action	Examples
Narcotics	Sedative and analgesic	Morphine Fentanyl
Benzodiazepines	Sedative properties Produce amnesia Reduce anxiety Promote muscle relaxation Anticonvulsant effects No analgesic properties	Midazolam Diazepam Lorazepam
Barbiturates	Sedative/hypnotic No analgesic properties	Long acting: phenobarbital Intermediate acting: pentobarbital Short acting: secobarbital

tachycardia, and flushing of the skin. Paralytics do not provide sedative or analgesic effect. Therefore additional agents must be utilized to provide comfort to the patient (Table II–7).

RECOMMENDED READINGS

Bukowskyj, M. (1988). Methylxanthines. In R. Kacmarek and J. Stoller (Eds.). *Current Respiratory Care* (pp. 52–55). Toronto: B.C. Decker.

Davidson, J. (1991). Neuromuscular blockade. *Focus on Critical Care* 18(6), 512–520.

Dettenmeier, P. (1992). Medications. *Pulmonary Nursing Care* (pp. 361–384). St. Louis: Mosby–Year Book.

Halloran, T. (1991). Use of sedation and neuromuscular paralysis during mechanical ventilation. *Crit Care Nurs Clin North Am* 3(4), 651–657.

Marley, R.A. (1994). Postoperative administration of aerolized medications: Part 1—The basics. *J Post Anesth Nurs* 9(5), 285–295.

Peters, J., Peters, B. (1990). Pharmacology for respiratory care. In C. Scanlan, C. Spearman, and R. Sheldon (Eds.). *Egan's Fundamentals of Respiratory Care* (pp. 455–482). St. Louis: C.V. Mosby.

Pierson, D. (1992). Drugs used in respiratory care. In D. Pierson and R. Kacmarek (Eds.). *Foundations of Respiratory Care* (pp. 175–193). New York: Churchill Livingstone.

Rau, J. (1994). Major drug families. In T. Barnes (Ed.). *Core Textbook of Respiratory Care Practice* (pp. 671–676). St. Louis: C.V. Mosby.

Seligman, M. (1988). Mucolytics. In R. Kacmarek and J. Stoller (Eds.). *Current Respiratory Care* (pp. 41–46). Toronto: B.C. Decker.

Snider, S. (1993). Use of muscle relaxants in the ICU: Nursing implications. *Critical Care Nurse* 13(6), 55–60.

Susla, G. (1993). Neuromuscular blocking agents in critical care. *Crit Care Nurs Clin North Am* 5(2), 297–311.

Traver, G.A., Mitchell, J., Flodquist-Priestley, G. (1991). Pharmacotherapeutics. *Respiratory Care: A Clinical Approach* (pp. 224–230). Gaithersburg, Md.: Aspen Publication.

Van Sickel, A., Spadaccia, K. (1991). Muscle relaxants and reversal agents. *Crit Care Nurs Clin North Am* 3(1), 151–158.

Zimet, I. (1991). Drugs used in respiratory therapy. In G. Burton, J. Hodgkin, and J. Ward (Eds.). *Respiratory Care: A Guide to Clinical Practice* (pp. 411–448). Philadelphia: J.B. Lippincott.

APPENDIX
III

—

Chest Drainage Systems
PAMELA GUILLAUME, RN, MS, CCRN

Chest drainage systems provide a mechanism to reestablish normal physiology of the pleural space. The source of disruption in the pleural space may be due to air, fluid, or blood. When occupied with air, such as a pneumothorax, the chest drainage system works to pull the air out from the pleural space, thereby reexpanding the lung. Fluid, such as a pleural effusion, or blood from a hemothorax requires a chest tube drainage system to drain the collection of fluid and reexpand the lung. A combined process may be occurring with both air and fluid, such as a hemopneumothorax.

Mediastinal chest tubes drain fluid from the mediastinal space. This is indicated for the patient after heart surgery.

CHEST TUBE INSERTION
Insertion Materials

The following items are necessary for implementation of chest drainage systems:

1. Chest tube: for drainage of air, a No. 16F to 24F gauge; for drainage of fluid or blood, a No. 28F to 36F gauge
2. Drainage system, such as a Pleur-evac system
3. Local anesthetic, such as 1% lidocaine with epinephrine
4. Antiseptic, such as povidone-iodine (unless contraindicated by allergy)
5. Sterile gloves
6. Large hemostats
7. Suture material
8. Dressing material: bacteriostatic ointment, petrolatum-impregnated gauze, 4×4 gauze pads, tape

Site of Insertion

To drain air, a chest tube is placed in the second, third, or fourth intercostal space in the midclavicular line. This higher placement is indicated to promote the drainage of air, which rises. For fluid, a chest tube is placed in the fifth or sixth intercostal space in the midaxillary line. Fluid is heavier and warrants a lower tube to use the principle of gravity for drainage.

Insertion Process

Initiation of a chest tube drainage system begins with the insertion of the chest tube. The steps for insertion are as follows:

1. Clean site with antiseptic, such as providone-iodine.
2. Inject local anesthetic to anesthetize insertion site.
3. Incise skin between ribs and dissect to pleural space.
4. Insert chest tube into pleural space (between parietal and visceral pleura).
5. Clamp chest tube close to the chest wall until connected to drainage system.
6. Pull suture in place around tube.
7. Connect drainage system to chest tube.
8. Release clamp from chest tube.
9. Apply dressing around chest tube insertion site.
10. Secure all connections; assess system.
11. Obtain chest x-ray film for placement.

ASSESSMENT AND TROUBLESHOOTING

From the time of insertion until discontinuation, the patient and system must be assessed for effectiveness. All components of a chest tube drainage system are assessed to determine proper functioning: patient, chest tube site, tubing, and drainage system. A typical three-chamber chest tube drainage system is shown in Figure III–1. A variety of chest drainage systems are on the market. Depending

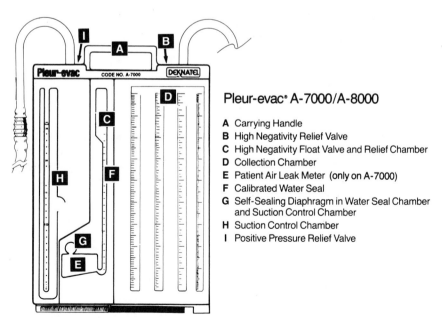

Pleur-evac® A-7000/A-8000

A Carrying Handle
B High Negativity Relief Valve
C High Negativity Float Valve and Relief Chamber
D Collection Chamber
E Patient Air Leak Meter (only on A-7000)
F Calibrated Water Seal
G Self-Sealing Diaphragm in Water Seal Chamber and Suction Control Chamber
H Suction Control Chamber
I Positive Pressure Relief Valve

FIGURE III–1   Three-chamber chest tube drainage system. Component parts are labeled. (Courtesy of Deknatel, Inc., Fall River, Mass.)

on the particular chest drainage system, it may have all or some of the features discussed in this section.

Patient

- Assess respiratory rate and breathing pattern.
- Auscultate lung sounds.
- Assess use of accessory muscles or abdominal breathing.
- Assess patient's comfort and anxiety level.

Site

- Assess dressing for drainage and change every 48 hours or more often as necessary.
- Palpate patient's skin around chest tube insertion site for subcutaneous emphysema. Subcutaneous emphysema indicates that air has escaped into the tissue under the skin. An increase in size of subcutaneous emphysema could indicate an air leak. Air may be escaping from the pleural space around the tube and into the tissue.

Tubing

The tubing should provide a straight passage down to the chest tube drainage system. There should be no kinks or dependent loops in the tubing. All tubing connections should be securely taped.

Assess tubing for the presence of drainage and/or clots. Passively empty any drainage in the tubing into the collection chamber. Clots can be dislodged by milking or stripping of the chest tube. Stripping is controversial and should not be done without a physician's order, because it is known to create transient high levels of negative pressure within the pleural space. Stripping of the chest tube requires anchoring the tubing with one hand while vigorously squeezing the length of the chest tube with the other hand. This process can create negative pressures in the pleural space up to -400 cm H_2O pressure and cause barotrauma to the lungs. Milking a chest tube is less stressful on the pleura. It is performed by gently squeezing the chest tube between your fingers and performing this process down the length of the tube.

Clamping of a chest tube is no longer recommended because it prevents the escape of a sudden increase in intrapleural pressure, as in a tension pneumothorax. A more commonly recommended practice is to place the patient on water seal when there is a need to discontinue suction, such as during transport or during weaning from a chest drainage system.

A sterile 4×4 pad with petrolatum-impregnated gauze should always be in the room in case a chest tube inadvertently comes out. Immediately placing the petrolatum gauze covered by a 4×4 pad over the insertion site will decrease the amount of air let into the pleural space.

Suction Control Chamber

The level of suction regulates the amount of negative pressure applied to the pleural space to facilitate lung expansion. Generally -20 cm H_2O pressure is used for the adult patient. There are two types of suction available, wet and dry.

With wet suction the amount of suction is regulated by the height of water in the suction control chamber. This level must be routinely assessed to verify that the water is filled to the appropriate level. When this chamber is assessed, it is necessary to pinch the suction line to stop movement in this column. This chamber should be refilled with sterile normal saline solution or distilled water. Water in the suction control chamber should gently bubble. More vigorous bubbling only contributes to noise and evaporation.

With dry suction, the amount of suction is regulated by a spring mechanism or screw valve mechanism attached to an external suction control dial. When the dial is turned, both mechanisms apply pull on a diaphragm in the drainage system, thereby controlling the level of negative pressure. There is visual confirmation of the level of suction on the front panel of the suction control chamber. The degree of pull will determine the level of suction. Although no water is used in these systems, they still require connection to a suction source in order to work. The level of suction must be routinely assessed to confirm the appropriate setting.

In either the wet or dry suction setup, there is a potential for increased positive-pressure buildup within the system if the suction tubing is inadvertently clamped, for example, by the rolling of a bed over the tubing. When positive pressure accumulates in the chest drainage system, a relief valve opens on the drainage system, allowing the positive pressure to be vented.

Water Seal Chamber

The water in the water seal chamber acts as a seal between the thoracic cavity and the environment. As air comes from the pleural space, it bubbles through the water in the water seal chamber and vents to the atmosphere. This prevents air from being pulled back into the pleural space from the chest drainage system every time the patient inhales. The water in this chamber is filled to the 2 cm line and must be assessed routinely for evaporation.

Tidaling is indicated by fluctuations in the water seal chamber that correlate with the respiratory cycle. This action reflects the changes in the pleural pressures that occur with respirations. Tidaling can be assessed only when the patient is not connected to suction. No tidaling will be observed if the patient's tubing is kinked or if the lung has fully expanded.

High negativity in the drainage system can result if the patient takes deep breaths before coughing or from stripping of the chest tube. This is indicated by a rising water level in the water seal chamber. Excess negative pressure can be relieved by depressing the high-negativity relief valve. This valve filters air into the system, relieving the pressure.

Air leaks are evidenced by bubbling in the water seal chamber. One reason that an air leak may occur is the natural escape of air from the pleural space as the lung reexpands. This is generally seen right after insertion of the tube. A second reason that an air leak may be present is that air may be leaking into the drainage system from a loose connection or a cracked drainage system. To locate the source of the air leak, clamp the chest tube close to the patient. If there is no bubbling in the water seal chamber, then the air is leaking either from around the dressing or internally from the pleural space. If the bubbling does not cease when the tube is clamped, then somewhere along the chest drainage system there is a leak. If the air leak persists after all tubing connections are checked, then consider replacing the chest drainage system.

Collection Chamber

Excess fluid in the pleural space drains into the collection chamber because of gravity. For gravity to work, the chest drainage system must be below the level of the patient's chest. After insertion of a chest tube, the volume of drainage should be assessed hourly, with levels marked minimally every 8 hours on the chest drainage system. The volume of drainage should gradually taper off and always be less than 100 cc/hr. However, trends should be monitored for each patient because sudden decreases or increases in drainage can also be significant.

Overall System

In the event that the entire chest drainage system tips over, reassess the fluid levels in each chamber. The unit does not need to be replaced unless it was cracked in the process.

If the chest drainage system does need to be replaced because it is broken or the collection chamber is full, follow this process:

1. Prepare new chest drainage system by appropriately filling the suction and water seal chamber.
2. Double-clamp the chest tube close to the patient.
3. Disconnect old chest drainage system and reconnect new system.
4. Release clamps.
5. Retape all connections and assess system for proper function.

DISCONTINUATION

Before the chest drainage system is discontinued, an assessment for patient readiness should be done. This assessment includes the following:

1. Auscultation of lung sounds
2. Assessment of patient's respiratory rate and breathing pattern
3. Absence of fluctuations in the water seal chamber
4. Absence of an air leak in the water seal chamber
5. Absence of or minimal drainage in the collection chamber
6. Confirmation of lung expansion by chest x-ray film

After assessment of the readiness of the patient, the chest tube may be removed as follows:

1. Medicate before procedure if needed.
2. Remove dressing around chest tube.
3. Cut anchoring suture.
4. Instruct patient to perform Valsalva maneuver by exhaling and bearing down while the tube is pulled. This will increase the intrathoracic pressure and decrease the potential for air to enter during the removal process.
5. Secure purse string suture.

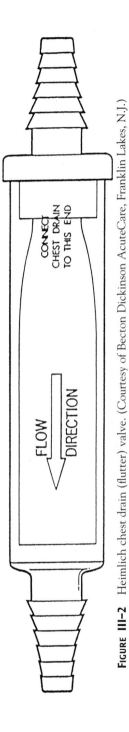

FIGURE III–2 Heimlich chest drain (flutter) valve. (Courtesy of Becton Dickinson AcuteCare, Franklin Lakes, N.J.)

6. Apply dressing with bacteriostatic ointment or petrolatum-impregnated gauze on chest tube site. Cover with 4×4 pads and elasticized tape.
7. Confirm lung expansion with chest x-ray film.

ALTERNATIVE SYSTEM: FLUTTER VALVE

The flutter valve is an optional chest drainage system indicated primarily for treating pneumothorax. The flutter valve consists of rubber leaflets encased in a transparent plastic chamber tapered at both ends (Fig. III–2). One end attaches to the chest tube, and the other end can be left alone or attached to a vented drainage bag. The flutter valve allows air or fluid to escape from the pleural space with normal respirations (Fig. III–3). On exhalation the rubber leaflets open and

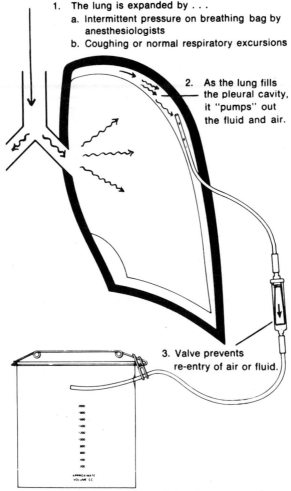

1. The lung is expanded by . . .
   a. Intermittent pressure on breathing bag by anesthesiologists
   b. Coughing or normal respiratory excursions

2. As the lung fills the pleural cavity, it "pumps" out the fluid and air.

3. Valve prevents re-entry of air or fluid.

Figure III–3 Flow of air and fluid with Heimlich valve connected to a vented drainage bag. Normal respiration promotes evacuation of the pleural space. (From Heimlich, HJ: Heimlich valve for chest drainage. *Medical Instrumentation* 1983; 17:1. [Association for the Advancement of Medical Instrumentation, Arlington, Va.])

allow air or fluid to escape, and on inhalation the leaflets close to prevent air from entering into the pleural space. This function mimics the water seal chamber in a traditional chest drainage system.

The advantages of the flutter valve are that it is less expensive than a three-chamber chest drainage system, and that it allows easy mobility by the patient. In some cases the patient may even be discharged with this tube in place. The disadvantages include the potential for occlusion caused by clots, the inability to detect an air leak, and the absence of suction.

In caring for a patient with a flutter valve, consider the following:

- Secure chest tube to dressing to prevent dislodgment.
- Ensure that drainage bag is vented to prevent pressure buildup within drainage compartment.
- Monitor valve for fluttering, which corresponds to closure of the valve before inhalation. The absence of fluttering could mean that the lung has fully expanded or that the valve has become obstructed by drainage.

RECOMMENDED READINGS

Carroll, P. (1991). What's new in chest-tube management. *RN* 54(5), 34–40.

Carroll, P. (1992). *Understanding Chest Drainage*. Fall River, Mass.: Deknatel.

Carroll, P.F. (1992). *Understanding Chest Tubes*. Fall River, Mass.: Deknatel.

Conner, P. (1987). When and how do you use a Heimlich flutter valve? *Am J Nurs* 87(3), 288–290.

Erickson, R. (1989). Mastering the ins and outs of chest drainage. Part 1. *Nursing* 19(5), 37–43.

Erickson, R. (1989). Mastering the ins and outs of chest drainage. Part 2. *Nursing* 19(6), 47–49.

Gordon, D., and Lorenz, B. (1991). A simple way to treat simple pneumothorax. *RN* 54(12), 50–52.

Heimlich, H. (1983). Heimlich valve for chest drainage. *Medical Instrumentation* 17(1), 29–31.

Kozier, B., Erb, G., and Olivieri, R. (1991). *Fundamentals of Nursing Concepts: Process and Practice*. Redwood City, Calif.: Addison-Wesley Nursing.

Merguert, S. (1994). S.T.O.P. and assess and chest tubes the easy way. *Nursing* 24(2), 52–53.

Miller, S., and Sahn, S. (1987). Chest tube indications, technique, management and complications. *Chest* 91(2), 258–263.

Swearingen, P. (1991). *Photo Atlas of Nursing Procedures*. Redwood City, Calif.: Addison-Wesley Nursing.

Index

Note: Page numbers in *italics* refer to illustrations; page numbers followed by t refer to tables.